HIV/AIDS AND DEMOCRATIZATION IN MEXICO

A Tale of a Globalized Struggle for Human Rights and Development

Antonio Torres-Ruiz

HIV/AIDS AND DEMOCRATIZATION IN MEXICO

A Tale of a Globalized Struggle for Human Rights and Development

Antonio Torres-Ruiz

COMMON GROUND RESEARCH NETWORKS 2018

First published in 2018
as part of the Interdisciplinary Social Sciences Book Imprint

Common Ground Research Networks
2001 S. 1ˢᵗ St., Suite 202
University of Illinois Research Park
Champaign, IL
61821

Library of Congress Cataloging-in-Publication Data

Names: Torres Ruiz, Antonio, author.
Title: HIV/AIDS and democratization in Mexico : a tale of a globalized
  struggle for human rights and development / Antonio Torres-Ruiz.
Description: Champaign, IL : Common Ground Publishing, 2018.
Identifiers: LCCN 2016024974 (print) | LCCN 2016033054 (ebook) | ISBN
  9781612298931 (pdf) | ISBN 9781612298917 (hbk : alk. paper) | ISBN
  9781612298924 (pbk : alk. paper)
Subjects: LCSH: HIV infections--Government policy--Mexico. | HIV
  infections--Social aspects--Mexico. | Sexual minorities--Mexico. |
  Democratization--Mexico.
Classification: LCC RA643.86.M6 (ebook) | LCC RA643.86.M6 T67 2018 (print) |
  DDC 362.19697/9200972--dc23
LC record available at https://lccn.loc.gov/2016024974

Cover Photo Credit: Dr. Antonio Marquet

Table of Contents

Abbreviations and Acronyms   ix

Acknowledgements   1

Introduction   5

Chapter 1   13
Mexico's Elusive Quest for Development in a Globalized Context

Chapter 2   49
Globalization, HIV/AIDS, and Human Rights

Chapter 3   93
Political Liberalization and Health Policies in Mexico

Chapter 4   141
HIV/AIDS and Sexual Minorities in Mexico

Chapter 5   187
General Conclusions

References   207

Appendices by Chapter   245

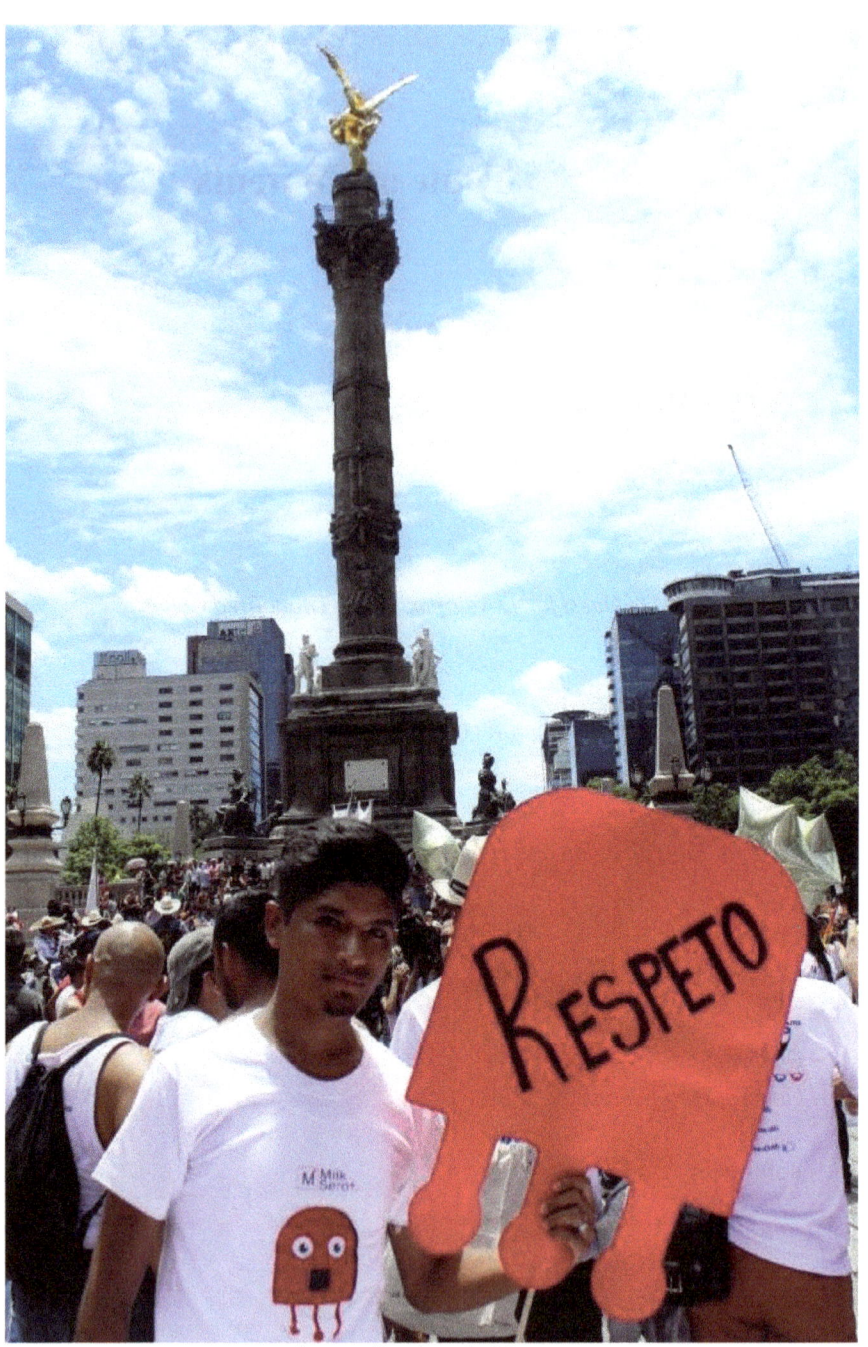

Source: Dr. Antonio Marquet

Abbreviations and Acronyms

AIDS/SIDA	Acquired Immune Deficiency Syndrome/ Síndrome de Inmuno Deficiencia Adquirida
ARVs	Anti-Retro Viral Drugs
CCE	Consejo Coordinador Empresarial/ Co-ordination Entrepreneurial Council.
CENSIDA	Centro Nacional de lucha contra el SIDA/ National Centre for the fight against AIDS, Mexico
CONASIDA	Consejo Nacional de lucha contra el SIDA/ National Council for the fight against AIDS, Mexico
CONAPRED	Consejo Nacional para Prevenir la Discriminación/ National Council for the Prevention of Discrimination
COPARMEX	Confederación Patronal Mexicana/ Mexican Association of Employers
CONEVAL	Consejo Nacional de Evaluación de la Política de Desarrollo Social/ National Council for the Evaluation of Social Development Policies.
FUNSALUD	Fundación Mexicana para la Salud/ Mexican Foundation for Health
GAPC	Global Aids Policy Coalition
GNP	Gross National Product
GPA	Global Program on AIDS
HICs	High Income Countries
HIV	Human Immunodeficiency Virus
IDB	Inter-American Development Bank
IFE	Instituto Federal Electoral/ Federal Electoral Institute
IGOs	International Governmental Organizations
ILO	International Labour Office
IMF	International Monetary Fund

IMSS	Instituto Mexicano del Seguro Social/ Mexican Institute of Social Security
INGOs	International Non-Governmental Organizations
INDESOL	Instituto de Desarrollo Social/ Institute for Social Development, Mexico
ISSSTE	Instituto de Seguridad y Servicios Sociales de los Trabajadores del Estado/ Institute of Security and Social Services for State Workers, Mexico
LGBT	Lesbian Gay, Bisexual, and Transgender/Transsexual
LMICs	Low-and-Middle Income Countries
MSF	Médecins sans Frontieres/ Doctors without Borders
MSM	Men who have Sex with Men
NAFTA	North American Free Trade Agreement
NGOs	Non-Governmental Organizations
OECD	Organization for Economic Co-operation and Development
PAHO	Pan-American Health Organization
PAN	Partido Acción Nacional/ National Action Party, Mexico
PEMEX	Petróleos Mexicanos/ National Oil Company, Mexico
PRD	Partido de la Revolución Democrática/ Party of the Democratic Revolution, Mexico
PRI	Partido Revolucionario Institucional/ Institutional Revolutionary Party, Mexico
PVEM	Partido Verde Ecologista de México/ Green Ecologist Party of Mexico
SAPs	Structural Adjustment Programs
SEDESOL	Secretaría de Desarrollo Social/ Secretariat of Social Development, Mexico
SHCP	Secretaría de Hacienda y Crédito Público/ Secretariat of Finance, Mexico
SPSS	Seguro Popular/ Insurance for the Poor
SSA	Secretaría de Salud/ Secretariat of Health, Mexico
STDs	Sexual Transmitted Diseases
TRIPS	Trade-Related Aspects of Intellectual Property Rights
UN	United Nations Organization
UNAIDS	Joint United Nations Program on HIV/AIDS
UNDP	United Nations Development Program

UNESCO	United Nations Educational, Scientific, and Cultural Organization
UNICEF	United Nations Children's Fund
UNPFA	United Nations Population Fund
USAID	United States Agency for International Development
WB	World Bank
WHO	World Health Organization
WTO	World Trade Organization

ACKNOWLEDGMENTS

I want to begin by emphasizing the importance of looking at HIV/AIDS from a social sciences perspective, especially so for those who have suffered the double discrimination of being infected by the virus or sick with the disease, and for being who they are, as gay men or other sexual minorities. In the struggle against the pandemic, the strong will, courage, and mobilization of gay men have had a major impact on the perceptions of people around the globe about HIV/AIDS, as well on the openings around sexuality politics and the public policies implemented. Their active public engagement has contributed to bringing about significant and positive changes. Thus, I want to especially thank, posthumously, Arturo Díaz Betancourt and Jorge Huerdo Siqueiros, who together with many other Mexican and Latin American activists, showed tremendous courage and great generosity towards others. And more personally, I want to thank them for helping others, including me, to understand the economic, social, and political significance of the issues at hand around the pandemic. It is important to give them the credit they deserve, since fighting for access to treatment and against discrimination literally became a matter of life and death for both.

On March 4, 2011, I was going about my daily academic life at York University, in Toronto, when sadly, I received the news from Mexico City about Arturo Díaz Betancourt's death. I met him in Mexico City, in November of 1996, while attending a workshop organized by the Autonomous Metropolitan University (UAM) on "Health in the Metropolis." Back then I was visiting Mexico, while in the middle of my master's in public policy at the University of Toronto. And I knew that I was interested in the political economy of health and the process of decentralization in Mexico, but I had no idea that that professional and personal encounter would clarify what a significant part of my future research would be about. Often, some people work on issues that might advance their academic careers, which might not be of much significance for real life or real people, but as a key figure in the struggle against HIV/AIDS, not just in Mexico but in all Latin America, Arturo was a good example of personal and professional commitment to a real cause. Throughout his life, he fought in favor of human rights, and was always very critical and combative in his approach to public policy and the governments' response to the pandemic. Among the many initiatives he led, he helped in the creation of a civil society association called Mexicans against AIDS (Mexicanos contra el SIDA) and was its first president. In that capacity, he contributed to the elaboration of what could be translated as the *Human Rights Passbook for People Living with HIV/AIDS* (Cartilla de los Derechos Humanos de las Personas que Viven con VIH/sida). Much earlier, in 1982, Arturo founded a university group at the National University (UNAM) called *Logos*, whose mission was to engage in the reflection and social communication around sexual identity and human rights. And in October 1994, together with journalists and activists Alejandro Brito, Carlos Bonfil, Manuel Figueroa, Arturo Vázquez, and well-known Mexican writer and intellectual Carlos Monsiváis, they created the special newspaper supplement on sexuality and HIV/AIDS titled *Letra S*, in *El Nacional*, which later migrated to *La Jornada*. Arturo also helped organized the *First National Encounter of Non-Governmental Organizations with work on HIV/AIDS* and participated in almost all of them until his untimely death. For many years, he was also part of the national body in charge of HIV/AIDS policies, CONASIDA, and together with Gilberto Rincón Gallardo was part of the creation of the *National Council to Prevent Discrimination* (CONAPRED[1]).

After that first encounter with Arturo, there were many more, and I ended up deciding to focus a significant part of my research and academic work on the political economy of HIV/AIDS. So, a few years later, in July of 2002, I was in Mexico City during a four-month fieldwork research stay and only a few days away from having an interview I had scheduled months before with Jorge Huerdo Siqueiros, when I learned about his death. Mr. Huerdo Siqueiros was also a committed activist in the fight against HIV/AIDS. He was a member of the *Commission for the Studies against Discrimination in Mexico*; the *Technical Secretary of the Committee for Citizen Observance and Vigilance of HIV/AIDS* (MEXSIDA); and, the director for Latin America of the *Global Network of People Living with HIV/A*IDS. Arturo had introduced me to Jorge the previous year, during the *Forum 2000* in Rio de Janeiro – the first biannual Conference for Latin America and the Caribbean on HIV/AIDS. Like Arturo, he was a key figure in the fight against the pandemic in Mexico and the rest of the Latin American region. And as will be shown in the book, their active participation in the process of policymaking, together with many other actors, has been central to the great progress made in HIV/AIDS and health-related policies in Mexico. To me, the news of their deaths – in Jorge's case from AIDS and in Arturo's due to the effects of cancer on his already compromised health due to HIV/AIDS - represented key moments in my research. At a very personal level, I was able to grasp the importance and emergency of HIV/AIDS and its political economy, and the need to pursue my research with even more motivation and a clear sense of purpose. The actions of individuals like Huerdo Siqueiros and Díaz Betancourt show a commitment that goes beyond the fight against HIV/AIDS. In their many roles, Jorge and Arturo, together with many other activists, public officials, and their supporters, demonstrated the need to address issues related to discrimination and marginalization that are commonly associated with the lack of sustainable human development. I am acutely aware of the fact that many names that should be part of the story I tried to tell are missing, but the hope is that by mentioning the organizations they collaborated with, and the successes they achieved, I will pay tribute to their lives and actions.[2] Furthermore, the serious consideration of an issue such as HIV/AIDS might contribute to making people in different fields and areas of activity to rethink many of the preconceived notions and believes that are often associated with human rights, development, and democratization.

---

[1] Consejo Nacional para Prevenir la Discriminación.
[2] For a complementary account and analysis of key actors involved in the struggle associated with the pandemic in Mexico see García Mucia et al. 2010.

There are many other people I would like to thank, such as family, friends, and colleagues, many of them falling into more than one category at once. And although I will not be able to list them all, I trust they know who they are. My immense gratitude for their love and/or support goes to Guillaume B., Judith T., Stephen C., Ana María B., David R., Joe W., Paul K., Antonio M., Francisco, C., Gabriel G.G., Nery S., Rafael D., Marina R.G., Antonio T.R., Aparna S., Michelle B., Laura T.R., Gabriela T.R., René T.R., Pedro T.R., Julián A.T., Mateo T.R., Anton K., Sofía T.R., Sebastián K., and a long and heartfelt etcetera. I also want to thank the team at Common Ground Research Networks, especially former editors Ian Holk and Dominique Moore, and current editor Phillip Kisubika, for their invaluable professional support throughout the editing and publishing process. Equally important and helpful were the critiques and feedback from the two anonymous peer reviewers. Lastly, I want to acknowledge and thank the following for their committed institutional and financial support: in Mexico, the National Council for Technology and Science (CONACYT[3]) and the Centre for the Research and Teaching of Economics (CIDE[4]); and in Canada, the International Council for Canadian Studies (ICCS), as well as the Department of Political Science and the Latin American Studies Program at the University of Toronto.

---

[3] Consejo Nacional de Ciencia y Tecnología.
[4] Centro de Investigación y Docencia Económicas, A.C.

Introduction

The Human Immunodeficiency Virus (HIV) and the Acquired Immune Deficiency Syndrome (AIDS) that sometimes follows the infection represent a public health issue with major global economic, social, and political implications. As of 2016, an estimated 36.7 million people were living with HIV, while another 1.8 million were infected and one million lost their lives to AIDS-related illnesses that same year (UNAIDS).[5] The numbers reported for 2016 were particularly staggering for Sub-Saharan Africa, where about 25.8 million of those people with HIV lived, and around 790,000 died due to HIV/AIDS-related causes. The region accounts for 66% of the world's new HIV infections every year, with at least five countries experiencing an adult HIV prevalence that exceeds 5 per cent (UNAIDS 2016). As such, the pandemic has had devastating effects on the development of some countries in the region and beyond, straining the few resources available for public health and highlighting the weaknesses of poorly structured health-care systems (See Yong Kim et al. 2000). And although the situation remains notoriously more severe in Sub-Saharan Africa, as a global health concern, the world epidemic (or pandemic) is also affecting economically and socially marginalized populations in the rest of the world, including Latin America, the Caribbean, and other Low-and-Middle-Income Countries (LMICs).[6]

Fortunately, the epidemic has not reached the same dramatic levels in Mexico; a country with a total population of about 120 million and an estimated 190,000 people living with HIV/AIDS. Yet as we will see below, it disproportionally affects some members of the sexual minorities population (or the Lesbian, Gay, Bisexual, and Transgendered/Transsexual [LGBTT] community).[7] Admittedly, we will not look at all groups within the LGBTT population, but the main focus will be on gay men and men who have sex with men (MSM), since they have been disproportionally affected by the epidemic and more actively engaged in opening up the policymaking process. Thus, the following analysis will provide sufficient evidence to assert that there have

---

[5] As we all know, the latest United Nations AIDS (UNAIDS) program's report offers figures for the previous year, but the agency updates its figures more regularly online: http://www.unaids.org/en/resources/fact-sheet.

[6] The terms low and middle, and high income countries (HICs) will be used, in opposition to the concepts of underdeveloped, Third World, developing, and other possible terms for very specific reasons. Considering the importance and the impact that language has on our own interpretations of reality, as well as how concepts change meaning throughout time and sometimes people tend to attach moral connotations to some of them, I rather use more neutral terms when referring to different groups of countries. Therefore, the following criteria will be used for the classification of countries: low-income countries: per capita income below $1,035 USD; middle-income countries: per capita income between $1,036USD and $12,615 USD; high-income countries: per capita income of $12,616 USD and above (See World Bank classifications for 2013: http://data.worldbank.org/news/new-country-classifications).

[7] For annually updated numbers and epidemiological analysis see: http://www.censida.salud.gob.mx; http://www.mexicovivo.org/30vih/30aniosdelvihsida.pdf

been important openings to greater civil society participation in the HIV/AIDS and health-related policymaking processes in Mexico. And based on that evidence, we will argue that these democratic openings are primarily explained by the formation of what will be defined as national and international HIV/AIDS policy networks. These networks represent the joining of forces of a variety of actors, such as national and international LGBTT and HIV/AIDS activists, governmental and inter-governmental institutions, and the scientific community, with a common goal; namely the control and future eradication of the pandemic and some of the conditions that make people vulnerable to it. Furthermore, it will be contended that these changes in HIV/AIDS and health-related policies ought to be seen as inextricably linked to the economic, social, and political transformations of the last few decades in Mexico, and to the international context defined by globalization.

If we had decided to simply look at the epidemiology or the statistics on HIV/AIDS in Mexico alone, we could conclude that it has not become a "real" public health or development crisis. Similarly, from an intellectual or an academic point of view, there might be some who question the significance of looking at the political economy of HIV/AIDS and sexual minorities in Mexico. However, for those affected by it, in terms of their health status and as a consequence of the stigma and discrimination associated with it, there has been some urgency associated to HIV/AIDS from the very beginning. Thus, apart from responding to a personal and academic interest in social justice for vulnerable minority groups and in the protection of human rights for all, the current analysis responds to a long-overdue need in the social sciences to look at the links between public health, HIV/AIDS, and sexual minorities. This neglect is especially true in the case of political economy and development studies focusing on Mexico. Furthermore, addressing this void will help us: a) to shed light on some of the opportunities and challenges faced by Mexico in its elusive quest for development and in the context of globalization; b) to understand how the HIV/AIDS pandemic accentuates the significance of the health sector, as a key component in the formulation of developmental policies and the protection of marginalized and vulnerable populations, and; c) in showing the ways in which the protection of public health increasingly relies on transnational linkages and co-ordination among governments, the private sector, and civil societies around the world. With these goals in mind, we will examine Mexico's response to the pandemic within an analytical framework that considers it part of a broader quest for democratization, human rights, and development.[8]

The HIV/AIDS pandemic represents a prime example of a truly global phenomenon, both in terms of its spread and the responses it elicited. For instance, it was the global sense of urgency associated with it, and the mobilization of civil society activists and other actors at the global level, that facilitated Mexican MSM and gay men's successful efforts at influencing the policymaking process at the national level. Additionally, the analysis of the national and international responses to

---

[8] All preceding concepts, such as globalization, democratization, human rights, and development will be defined and discussed in the following chapter.

the pandemic has broader implications for our understandings of democracy, development, human rights, and globalization, which go beyond the Mexican case and HIV/AIDS. And the analysis of social policies in general, and HIV/AIDS and health-related policies in particular, speaks loudly to issues related to state competence and inclusiveness in policymaking, to the linkages between state institutions and some civil society groups, and to patterns of marginalization and human rights violations.

In supporting the central argument, this book is divided into two main sections. The first half (chapters one and two) consists of a more academic or theoretical discussion, which focuses on the need to look at often ill-defined concepts such as development, democratization, human rights, globalization, NGOization (or civil society professionalization), and policy networks. The purpose is to clarify their meaning, examine their relevance, and consider their applicability to the current global reality, to come up with a more adequate conceptual framework for the analysis of HIV/AIDS and democratization from a social sciences perspective. The second part of the book (chapters three and four) looks at the specifics of the Mexican case, to identify the most important economic, social, and political transformations of the last few decades, and to provide a more detailed analysis of the political economy of the epidemic and the policymaking process in Mexico. The aim is to determine where the pressure for change in HIV/AIDS policies and the health sector has originated, the direction they have taken so far, and the role that national and international policy networks have played.

More concretely, chapter one will lay out the conceptual framework for Mexico's elusive quest for development. In it, we will draw from the well-known definition of sustainable human development and argue in favour of explicitly attaching a democratic dimension to it. The idea is to articulate and subscribe to a definition of development that promotes better living conditions through a process of democratization and the recognition, promotion, and protection of human rights for all, including sexual minorities. We will then provide and contrast the definitions of globalization and "globalism." The former will be defined as a multidimensional and long-term phenomenon, while the latter will refer to the ideas and policies behind the economic model that characterized the so-called 'Washington Consensus.' The aim is to emphasize the pros and cons of globalization and counter the monopolization of the term by those who subscribe to the neo-liberal ideology (i.e., globalism). A clear example of this attempt to monopolize the term took place on January 28, 2000, at the World Economic Forum (Davos, Switzerland). The then Mexican president Ernesto Zedillo Ponce de León (a convinced neo-liberal economist) made a memorable statement against those who participated in the 1999 Seattle protests during the World Trade Organization's ministerial meeting. Zedillo accused them of irrationally opposing globalization, calling them "globaliphobics." In his participation at the Forum, he referred to them as a "peculiar alliance" among the extreme right and the extreme left, as well as environmental activists and labour unions, all speaking in the name of civil society, "who had come together against globalization and around a common goal: to save people in developing countries .... from development." [9] According to Zedillo, what united protesters was their common "globaliphobia." Arguably, his words reflected most of the attendees' positions, both in favour of stronger economic integration and regarding their dismissal of critiques directed to the neo-liberal economic paradigm. Thus, the rationale for the emphasis on the distinction between these two concepts responds to a strong argument to be made in favour of a more complex and multidimensional understanding of the increasing interconnectedness associated with globalization. In turn, this distinction will facilitate a more balanced assessment of their impact at the international and national levels. It will also help us in defining the neo-liberal agenda for what it is; the current and predominant ideology driving the economic dimension of the broader world phenomenon known as globalization.

In fact, the multidimensional nature of globalization becomes particularly clear when one looks closely at civil society activists involved in the struggle against HIV/AIDS. Most of them are not phobic to globalization, on the contrary, they have embraced the advantages that come with their engagement at the regional and global levels. It is equally important to discuss development and democracy in the context of globalization, since they all represent inter-related phenomena that are central to our analysis. Furthermore, the clarification and discussion of the preceding concepts are meant to challenge the predominant labels and classifications of political regimes or developmental models, most of which tend to focus on procedural/electoral politics while prescribing economic and trade liberalization policies, respectively. Such models are generally developed in the Global North [10] and respond to analyses that show a bias against any non-liberal/non-globalist democratic political regimes, strategies, and set of public policies. These criticisms are part of a broader discussion that falls beyond the scope of this book, which entails an epistemological critique of the current and most dominant comparative development and democratic theory literatures (Torres-Ruiz and Ravecca 2014, Torres-Ruiz 2017; 2018). Among those criticisms, and one that we will address below, there is the need to avoid some of the generalizations made about political regime transformations that often characterize mainstream political science analyses in the Global North, especially when looking at the Global South. Instead, we propose to examine more closely concrete public policy issues, such as HIV/AIDS, in our examinations of democratization processes in Mexico and elsewhere, so that we can say more about the complexity and specifics of regime transformations.

Two other concepts that will be introduced and addressed in chapter one are NGOization and policy networks. On the one hand, we will refer to NGOization,

---

[9] See transcription of Zedillo's speech at http://zedillo.presidencia.gob.mx/pages/disc/ene00/28ene00n multiple forms.html.

[10] It is important to clarify here that the use of Global North and Global South is not a strictly geographical distinction, but rather an epistemologically rooted decision to distinguish between countries occupying very different positions in the global system, economically, politically, and historically speaking. These terms are also intentionally used *in lieu* of heavily loaded terms such as underdeveloped, Third World, or developing countries, which have been strongly contested in the social sciences' subfields of comparative political studies and development.

which is a neologism coined to refer to the process of increasing professionalization of civil society activism. And we will briefly discuss the implications and consequences of this phenomenon, since HIV/AIDS activists have increasingly formalized and structured their participation in public life. On the other hand, we will draw from the notion of policy networks, and adapt it to our description of the ways in which a variety of actors have come together in the formation of a complex network of formal and informal relationships with a common goal. This is part of another world phenomenon associated with globalization, defined by Manuel Castells (1996 and 2010) as the network society, which according to him represents a new social structure that could be seen as a reaction to the double global crisis of state legitimacy and economic instability. Furthermore, the concept of policy networks represents a helpful conceptual tool in the redefinition of one of the central features of the Mexican political system that will be discussed in chapter three; namely 'camarillas' (political cliques with very concrete characteristics).[11]

Based on the previous conceptual discussion, chapter two will focus on the global context. We will describe the growing links between external and domestic actors, and the centrality of the international human rights discourse and regime in the struggle for global justice and health for all (especially for those most vulnerable and disproportionately affected by the pandemic). Therefore, most of our attention will be directed to the formation of international HIV/AIDS policy networks, and their influence on the formulation and implementation of HIV/AIDS public policies, not just in Mexico but in other countries within the Latin American region and beyond. Additionally, the argument will be made that contrary to other international policy networks, such as those engaged in health-care financing, HIV/AIDS policy networks tend to be of a more inclusive nature. Among other actors, we will look at International Governmental Organizations, International Non-Governmental Organizations (INGOs), Trans-national Corporations (TNCs) in general and Pharmaceuticals in particular, Trade Agreements, and trans-national HIV/AIDS activism and civil society organizations. This will allow us to identify the members of some of the relevant international policy networks, and address questions such as; who benefits from globalization? and whose interests are represented by international actors?

Moving on to the second half of the book, we will examine the ways in which the globalization of public health policy intersects with national governmental functioning, and the extent to which HIV/AIDS policy is an example of concrete international policy influences on Mexico's democratization. Thus, chapter three will be devoted to an overview of the Mexican political system and its main features. For those readers who are not sufficiently familiar with the Mexican case, this brief revision will allow them to more fully understand the specific context, since it provides a general historical perspective of the economic, political, and social

---

[11] As will be discussed in chapter three, "camarillas" have played a key role in the formulation of public policy in Mexico. Hence, the special interest in understanding how increasingly internationalized policy environments are contributing to the transformation of some of the long-lived features of Mexico's political life.

circumstances within which Mexico's HIV/AIDS policies have evolved. And it will offer a general outline of the process of political liberalization with a special focus on the health sector, other related social policies, and the role of "camarillas." In chapter four, we will look at the roles of sexual minorities, conservative groups, private corporations, NGOs, and the Mexican government, as well as their participation in the establishment and functioning of the domestic HIV/AIDS policy network. This will allow us to elaborate on the central argument, and contend that although public health policies in general – including and especially HIV/AIDS-related policies - have been constrained by globalist economic policies, there have been significant openings in the process of decision making. In other words, although important limitations remain – imposed by some of the features of the Mexican political system, as well as a global and still influential neoliberal agenda – the formation of the domestic HIV/AIDS policy network has facilitated the inclusion of formerly marginalized groups in the process of decision-making and implementation of HIV/AIDS policies, with very concrete results. Among other successes, for instance, both the right to universal access to treatment and the existence of special public funds for prevention campaigns among Men who have Sex with Men (MSM) have been the result of the network's efforts. Our analysis will cover from the 1980s, when the first AIDS cases were registered, to the early months of 2013, when the new administration of Enrique Peña Nieto (the current Mexican President) took office. We focus on this period to explore the extent to which the policies adopted from the start of the pandemic to the transition period that runs from the late 1990s - the end of more than 70 years of uninterrupted Institutional Revolutionary Party's (PRI[12]) rule at the federal level - to the two presidential terms (2000-2006, 2006-2012) of the National Action Party (PAN[13]).

The last and fifth chapter will provide some general conclusions regarding the degree to which the current analysis, framed within the context of globalization, allows us to shed light on some aspects of Mexico's developmental efforts, especially when it comes to democratization and human rights, as they relate to public health and HIV/AIDS. And we will also consider the benefits of applying the policy networks analysis to our understanding of globalization, particularly the increasing interconnectedness that comes with it and its effects on people's wellbeing.

The following is a qualitative examination that draws from different bodies of academic literature and extensive fieldwork research. On the one hand, it engages with works dealing with the meaning and relevance of the key concepts mentioned above, such as development, democracy, human rights, and globalization, all of which are central for understanding of contemporary politics and Mexico's reality. It also draws from the most relevant works on Mexico's democratic transition of the past decades, as well as from the public policy literature about the establishment and consolidation of internationalized policy environments. From the latter, it adapts and applies the concept of policy networks - both domestic and international - in order to

---

[12] Partido Revolucionario Institucional.
[13] Partido Acción Nacional.

assess the extent to which these networks have contributed to the process of democratization. On the other hand, the data and the facts collected and accounted for in the course of the last fifteen years of research are the result of a series of fieldwork trips to Brazil, Cuba, and Mexico, as well as to some of the regional conferences on HIV/AIDS for Latin America and the Caribbean, and the World AIDS Conferences. Attendance to these meetings was essential for the establishment of contacts and the building of trust with interviewees.[14] And although some of the information shared by the latter is available through publicly accessible media, the personal encounters were essential to understanding the formal and informal links between members of the networks. Most of the 112 interviews were conducted in four locations (Havana, Mexico City, Rio de Janeiro, and Toronto). Among them, 70 consisted in open-ended conversations, which took place in Mexico and facilitated the identification and analysis of health political cliques ("camarillas") and the HIV/AIDS policy networks.[15] In Mexico, interviewees included public health officials, HIV/AIDS and sexual minorities activists (some of them members of NGOs), people living with HIV/AIDS, academics, and health-care providers. At the respective regional conferences in Havana, Rio de Janeiro, and Toronto, they were HIV/AIDS activists from across the region, as well as officials of some international organizations. Most of the interviews were confidential, while nineteen of the interviewees consented to the disclosure of their names. Some notes on the interviewing process and a detailed list (in alphabetical order) and a breakdown by category of all the interviewees are provided in Appendices 1.1 and 1.2. Additionally, several primary and secondary sources were consulted (Official governmental reports, relevant laws, minutes of national and international meetings related to health and HIV/AIDS, national journals and other periodicals, materials provided by the NGO community, etc.).

---

[14] For a brief discussion of the process of interviewing itself please refer to Appendix 1.1
[15] There are no previous works on the composition and role of these political cliques in the health sector.

CHAPTER 1

Mexico's Elusive Quest for Development in a Globalized Context

The end of the twentieth century and the first fifteen years of the new one represented a period of great transformations for Mexico. Domestic and international forces triggered a series of events that have redefined fundamental aspects of the Mexican reality. A series of social, economic and political processes led to a federal election, in July of 2000, which was regarded as a key moment in the transformation of Mexico's political life.

For some, the first years of the new millennium represented the culmination of a long process of democratization, for others these were only the first steps on a long road to democracy. In the context of such a complex reality and with the aim to contribute to the debate, the present analysis attempts to understand the meaning and evaluate the impact of some of these changes on Mexico's development and political transformations. It is in this context that it will be argued here that the establishment of what will be defined as national and international policy networks represents a catalyzing force. This is especially true for the case of domestic HIV/AIDS and sexual minorities activists, who have been engaged in the ongoing struggle for the protection of human rights and an increasing participation in the process of public policy-making.

It is also contended that through closely analyzing the formulation and implementation of HIV/AIDS and health-related policies we can uncover fundamental features of the broader process of Mexico's economic, political, and social transformations. Yet any serious attempt to understand the changing Mexican reality must begin by discussing the meaning of democracy within the larger analysis of development, human rights, and globalization. Therefore, the prevailing reality of a middle-income country like Mexico forces us to underline some of the differences between the Global North (mostly High Income Countries or HICs) and the Global South (mostly LMICs). These differences must not be overlooked, particularly if we consider the implications that trade agreements, extreme poverty, inequality, income polarization, and the lack of a strong welfare state in most LMICs have in limiting a country's capacity to respond to some of the new health challenges that accompany globalization. Furthermore, emphasis will be put on the varying effects that the reforms associated with the neo-liberal economic agenda have had on the capacity of the South to respond to the HIV/AIDS pandemic.

DEVELOPMENT AND DEMOCRACY

Is there one 'correct' way of conceptualizing development? How do democracy and development relate to each other? Is democracy a condition for development, or vice versa? How do we incorporate human rights into our analyses of health and development? These are central questions that will be addressed in the next sections, and which ought to be considered in analyzing HIV/AIDS and health-related policies. Although it is not the aim of the present analysis to come up with any definitive answers to these questions, an attempt will be made to provide a series of helpful reflections. More specifically, and given the history and characteristics of the pandemic, these are questions of major concern in studying the fight against HIV/AIDS. Similar to other diseases (e.g. cholera and tuberculosis, Ebola, etc.), HIV/AIDS has accentuated patterns of marginalization and lack of proper sanitary infrastructure, and it tends to thrive in poverty stricken regions and within vulnerable populations. Thus, an attempt to address the pandemic as a problem connected with development and democracy will allow us to define a solid conceptual framework for the analysis of HIV/AIDS and health-related policies in Mexico.

In an effort to understand the impact of the pandemic in Mexico and regardless of what definition of development one adopts, some kind of shorthand is needed to underscore the real differences in wealth and power between countries, particularly for the discussion of global inequality and its impact on health.[16] In 2015, and according to the World Bank about 87 percent of the world population lived in LMICs, enjoying less than one-fifth of the total world Gross National Product (GNP).[17] There are, of course, other major differences among countries besides income levels, to which we will refer below. At this point, however, it is important to stress the fact that in the context of major inequalities among nations, we need to acknowledge the diverse and complex realities of countries in the Global South (the world's majority), and the enormous gap between them and the Global North. In fact, most of the people in LMICs face major daily challenges that are quite different in nature from those present in HICs, such as large scale poverty and deprivation, as well as the lack of universal access to adequate health care facilities.

In spite of the differences between the Global North and South, formally at least, there are some values about which there is a high degree of 'declared consensus,' such as the centrality of basic human rights, the construction of more democratic regimes, and the universal responsibility to provide for the majority a human existence with dignity. In the public discourse, some of these individual rights have been extended to the equal rights of states to development and democracy, which were agreed upon at the 1993 Vienna Convention on Human Rights.[18] This recognition reflected Hoffman's (1981) and others' concerns regarding the need for states to have not just

---

[16] For the discussion of the relevance and validity of the concept of development itself, see the work of Swiss scholar Gilbert Rist (1996).

[17] World Bank Group: http://beta.data.worldbank.org/

[18] See the 1993 Vienna Declaration and Programme of Action: http://www.ohchr.org/EN/ProfessionalInterest/Pages/Vienna.aspx.

equal rights but also equal possibilities for development.[19] Yet when one looks at the world reality and considers the conditions under which people live globally, it is clear that the most apparent international injustice is the poverty of a great part of humankind; of hundreds of millions of people. For Mexico, a middle-income country (with a Gross National Income per capita of US$16,056.00 (2011 PPP), and 37.7 per cent of the national population surviving with less than US$2 dollars a day (UNDP Human Development Report 2015), any serious analysis of development must consider poverty not only as the lack of basic economic resources, including money and food, but as an indicator of vulnerability due to the lack of access to quality education and health care. Unfortunately, most quantitative measures of poverty cannot account for the double jeopardy experienced by some groups, such as sexual minorities, for whom poverty is often the result of, or exacerbated by, discrimination, overt or covert, with the resulting violation of their most basic human rights.

Additionally, although some scholars have argued that a state that is conducive to economic growth and "development" can be more or less democratic or authoritarian (See Robinson and White 1998), the argument will be made for the need to incorporate a democratic character to the state in order to achieve sustainable human development and guarantee human rights protections. A theoretical and principled defense is not the only justification for the importance of looking at democracy for the Mexican case. In fact, the processes of political liberalization and democratization that define the reality of Latin America in general, and of Mexico in particular, during the last few decades force us to consider it as a fundamental component of current developmental efforts.

Sustainable Human Development Defined

Ambitious attempts at defining development have resulted in the elaboration of meta-theories that have proven to be either flawed or too encompassing to be helpful in addressing the problems one identifies in the analysis of specific country cases. In the history of development theory, different schools have attempted to explain universal patterns with different degrees of success or acceptance. Modernization theorists, for example, came up with a linear and universal understanding of "phases" of development (See Hirschman 1958; Rostow 1971). For them, development represented a process through which 'backward' and traditional societies (mostly LMICs) could become 'modernized,' 'westernized,' or 'developed' (See Apter 1965; Pye 1966). As a reaction to this rather ethno-centrist interpretation of reality, dependency theory proposed a more systemic way of explaining the gap between wealthier and poorer countries. 'Dependentistas[20]' were of the opinion – to different degrees -that colonialism and imperialism were to be 'blamed' for the 'under-

---

[19] Stanley Hoffman (1981) has deeply analyzed these matters introducing issues like moral and ethical considerations. See also Amartya Sen (1997; 2009).

[20] As dependency theorists are known; the Spanish term reminds us of their focus on, and in some cases, background from Latin America.

development' of most, if not all, LMICs (See Amin 1974; Cardoso 1972; Frank 1967).

More recent versions of these two theories are still popular among some scholars. On the one hand, neo-classical economics approaches (to which we will refer below in our discussion of 'structural adjustment' and define later as the globalist agenda) have inherited the rationalistic and positivist stages-of-development approach put forward by modernization theorists. On the other hand, following the tradition of dependency theory, scholars have elaborated more complex versions of the systemic explanation for the lack of development (See for example Wallerstein's (1974, 1979) world-systems theory). Although a full revision of these theories falls beyond the scope of the present analysis, it is necessary to underline here that, without adopting a relativist position or dismissing the contribution of these theories to the study of LMICs, meta-theories are of little use in understanding the complexity of concrete countries' realities. Even more importantly, respect for cultural and historical diversity would prohibit broad generalizations.

This critical rejection for the adoption of all-encompassing theories in the analysis of the Mexican case should prevent us from coming up with a new theory that could be contrasted to others and exported to other places. On the contrary, it is important to emphasize the need to look at the reality of Mexico and think of development as a set of policies that respond to the specific context of a middle-income country. And even the official governmental subscription to the United Nations Development Program (UNDP) or other international agencies' developmental goals must be regarded critically, given the recent history of neo-liberal structural adjustment policies embraced by all federal administrations. Therefore, one of the central aims of the current analysis is to consider the Mexican reality as it is, rather than the propagation of theories that, more often than not, fail to explain such reality or distort it completely in an attempt to fit the theory. In fact, back in the 1990's, Schuurman (1993) spoke of the impasse that continues to characterize the field of development theory in the last decades, which has been the result of the realization that there is not just one single way to approach and define development. In turn, this has forced some scholars to focus more on the interaction of the economy, the state, and society, attending to specific geographic, cultural, historical and political circumstances. Several efforts have incorporated some of these concerns into less normative definitions of development. Martinussen (1997), for instance, defined it as "the societal reproduction and transformation processes of the developing [LMICs for the present analysis] countries, in conjunction with the international factors that influence these processes" (p.4). Similarly, Robert Bates (2001) explained that "students of development specialize in the study of the poorer countries," and defined development as "the growth of per capita incomes and the transformation of social and political systems" (p. 20). At the risk of stating the obvious, it is worth underlining that, as pointed out by Bates, a key feature of the notion of development is the temporal dimension of human societies: that is, the passage of time.

For the purposes of the present analysis, development is defined as sustainable human development, and it does not apply just to LMICs but to all countries, North and South. This definition allows us to underscore both the temporal and the human dimensions of the process. The temporal dimension is translated into the idea of sustainability, and is based on the definition put forward by the World Commission on the Environment and Development (Bruntland 1987), while the human element responds to the need to conceptualize development in terms of human security and vulnerability, and the respect for human rights and their enforcement. As such, sustainable development has been defined as 'development that meets the needs of the present without compromising the ability of future generations to meet their own needs' (Bruntland 1987, p. 43).[21] This definition has also been adopted by the UNDP as a central component of its stated mission. Yet it is important to acknowledge that the very same definition of sustainable development has been criticized for being a flag for many ships (See Adams 1993). However, and in spite of its limitations, the present analysis strongly supports the notion of sustainability, as a concept that allows us to incorporate a long-term view regarding the actual consequences of economic and political policies on people and their environment. Furthermore, for this study, sustainability is understood in a very concrete sense: as in Susuki and Dresel's (2002) analysis of hundreds of working solutions to a variety of very concrete problems. In their book, both authors provide a great number of examples of corporations, communities and individuals around the world, who spontaneously have come up with creative ways to survive 'sustainably'; in opposition to an endless set of economic and industrial demands for unlimited growth that lead to ongoing environmental degradation and climate change.

For its part, the human dimension of the definition of sustainable human development alludes to the notion of human security, which has also been defined before. In 1994, the United Nations (UN) document entitled *"New Dimensions of Human Security"* referred to this concept as symbolizing the "protection from the **threat of disease**, hunger, unemployment, crime, social conflict, political repression and environmental hazards" (p. 22). It further stated that "in the final analysis, human security is *a child who did not die, a disease that did not spread*, a job that was not cut, an ethnic tension that did not explode in violence, a dissident who was not silenced" (p. 22, in both cases, emphasis is the author's). Thus, as we can see, health is a central element of the notion of human security,[22] and it reinforces the purpose of emphasizing its centrality for sustainable human development. Additionally, as it will become clearer in our discussion of HIV/AIDS and health (chapter two), the notion of human security allows for the incorporation of vulnerability into our analysis; a particularly relevant concept given the positive co-relation between marginalization and poverty and the spread of the epidemic.

At this point, it must be acknowledged that some of these ideas are similar to and draw from some earlier alternative paradigms. For instance, in the 1970s the

---

[21] Of particular interest for the present analysis is the fact that the World Commission on Environment and Development was headed by Dr. Gro Harlem Bruntland, who later became the Director General of the World Health Organization (1998-2002).

[22] For a more detailed analysis of the links between health and human security see the piece edited by Chen, Leaning, and Narasimahn (2003).

International Labour Organization (ILO) advocated for a "basic needs" approach to development, and as indicated above the UNDP has promoted the idea of "human development" through its several reports. Regardless of the preferences for the adopted terminology, the important issue here is the incorporation of the human and temporal dimensions to the definition of development. This helps to underline the need to pay special attention to the control – or lack thereof - that the poor and marginalized are able to exert over aspects of their lives they consider to be important to them. This also allows one to keep in mind, at all times, the multidimensional nature of development (development will be used below in general to refer to sustainable human development in short), and to avoid falling into the facile economic analyses based mostly on efficiency and productivity.

The international consensus on development was manifested in the 1986 UN Declaration on the Right to Development (See Sengupta 2000, p. 559), and as indicated above, it was further agreed upon in the 1993 Vienna Declaration on Human Rights. Originally, Articles 55 and 56 of the UN Charter make explicit reference to the commitment to social progress and development, the need to address *health-related problems*, and the importance of international co-operation. This is further reinforced in the International Covenant on Economic, Social and Cultural Rights (Article 12 (1)), as the right of everyone to enjoy the highest attainable standard of physical and mental health. When considering the case of Mexico, a country that has subscribed to these international agreements, the recognition of the right to development forces the various social and political actors (especially the government) to accept it as a right that needs to be implemented by collective action.

Developmental Strategies: Whose Responsibility?

Instead of conceiving of 'A Developmental State' we should think of various possible types of developmental states, or rather, of a varied set of state policies conducive to development. Although there seems to be a widely spread inclination to come up with a typology of different developmental states, it is better to avoid the risk of reproducing the same habits of the previously mentioned theories that tried to come up with ideal types. Instead, the current analysis focuses on the specific policies adopted by concrete governments, and it argues that the democratic character of a political regime is a necessary component, although not a sufficient one, for the achievement of sustainable human development. Additionally, a central contention will consist of considering public policies conducive to development as integral and indispensable components of a truly democratic or democratizing regime.

The analysis of development and health forces us to look not only at the centrality of the state but, more importantly, at the interaction between the state and civil society, with the intention to identify where responsibilities lie within a continuum of state-civil society complementary roles. Thus, it is necessary to begin with a basic theoretical definition of both the state and civil society and outline the interactions between the two. With regards to the state, the present analysis adheres to Alfred Stepan's formulation, in which he asserts that the state must be considered as more than just the 'government' (In Evans et al. 1985). Following this formulation, Evans (1995; 1996) has defined the state as the continuous administrative, legal, bureaucratic and coercive system[23] that attempts not only to structure relationships between civil society and public authority in a polity but to structure many crucial relationships within civil society as well. A valuable component of this definition, and one which determines whether or not a state might be conducive to development is what Evans (1995) calls 'embedded autonomy': a combination of governmental corporate coherence and connectedness with society. By corporate coherence, Evans refers to a very selective meritocratic recruitment process and long-term career rewards for bureaucrats, which give the government a significant degree of autonomy from special vested interests in society. On the other hand, connectedness (or the 'embedded' part of the concept) refers to "a concrete set of social ties that binds the state to society and provides institutionalized channels for the continual negotiation and re-negotiation of goals and policies" (Evans 1995, p. 12).[24]

Although the idea of 'embedded autonomy' is a useful tool for the analysis of HIV/AIDS and health-related policies in Mexico, once again, one has to be careful and avoid a normative search for 'A Developmental State.' In fact, it is better to look at the actual characteristics of the Mexican state, and then identify the kind of relations that exist between the government and civil society, in order to determine whether these could be regarded as democratic and conducive to development. After all, it is well known that in Mexico, like in most Latin American countries, the state faces a series of circumstances that make it significantly weak. For example, in her analysis of Latin America, Teichman (1988) has identified two major reasons for the weakness of the state. On the one hand, often the lack of resources does not allow the state to carry out its legitimization function, while on the other, this same lack of resources makes it subject to manipulation from external actors and financial sources.[25] In addition to the ideas put forward above, and for the purposes of the present analysis, development is defined by the expansion of substantive freedoms and rights for the population, not only in terms of civil and political rights, but also social and economic rights, including the provision of health care. Therefore, although the state plays a central role, our analysis would be incomplete without considering the role that individuals and groups - as members of civil society - can play in the formulation of policies and strategies conducive to development.

For its part, as a conceptual tool, civil society has been defined as "[the] intermediate associational realm between state and family populated by organizations which are separate from the state, [which] enjoy autonomy in relations to the state,

---

[23] As we know, both Max Weber and Michel Foucault wrote extensively about the nature of the modern state, albeit from different perspectives and at very different historical moments. For a discussion of some of Foucault's ideas, especially in contrasting the notion of governance with governmentality, see Torres-Ruiz (2017).

[24] Classic cases of this type of state are South Korea and Japan (See Evans 1995; Johnson 1982; Robinson and White 1998).

[25] This point on external financial sources and actors is one we will be coming back to below, in order to explore the link between external agents and domestic politics, especially the case of International Financial Institutions, Transnational Corporations, and Trade Agreements.

and are formed by members of society to protect or extend their interests or values (Robinson and White 1998, p. 40). Obviously, in the context of the Mexican reality, this definition will simply serve as a point of reference in describing the actual characteristics of civil society in Mexico. In fact, in all instances, one must approach the analysis of civil society very carefully, given the "flabby thinking," that, as Standing (2000, p. 740) reminds us, is often behind the use of concepts such as participation and partnership. In other words, and echoing Standing's views, it is necessary to be wary of a good deal of well-intentioned nonsense that has been written in recent years on the allegedly positive relationship between civil society participation and development. This warning has the intention of helping us avoid a normative loading to the notion of civil society that could lead us to tautological conclusions. Although civil society's participation in public policymaking and in the pursuit of development can have a positive impact, this can also be detrimental to the wellbeing of some or all members of society.

Any domestic civil society is heterogeneous by nature, and as such it represents a set of varied groups whose actions can have positive or negative effects on a country's development. Internationally, global networks can produce nightmares (i.e. organized crime and terrorist groups) as well as miracles (i.e. human rights activists and humanitarian assistance groups). Domestically, small elite groups are usually able to exert far greater influence by means of their concentrated organizational and economic resources and power than rather large and disempowered groups. Thus, it is important to distinguish between clientelistic[26] (corrupt or otherwise) and institutional access (through parties and other organized and legal channels). Under some circumstances, however, the participation of civil society groups can have a positive effect, as part of what Brian Crisp (in Robinson and White 1998, p. 41) calls the 'consultative arena': a network of decision-making bodies linked to specific areas of policy which bring together state officials and representatives of key groups in civil society (a concept that is similar to what will be defined as policy networks – section 1.3 of this chapter). Another positive outcome that can result from the presence of strong civil society groups is to make government more accountable; but even in that case, as put by Landell-Mills (in Robinson and White 1998, p. 23), this does not necessarily guarantee a wiser or more successful government.

This emphasis on the interaction between the state and civil society leads us back to the discussion of the relationship between democracy and development. As stated before, although Robinson and White (1998) argue that a state that is conducive to "development" (which in their use should be referred to as economic growth) can be either democratic or authoritarian, the following section will further elaborate on the need to incorporate a democratic character to the state in order to achieve sustainable human development. Furthermore, the reality of Latin America during the last three decades forces us to consider democracy as a fundamental component of current developmental efforts. As we all know, several countries in the region, Mexico

---

[26] This is a concept to which we will come back and define in the next chapter, given its significance for the analysis of Mexican politics.

included, have undergone a major process of political transformation - termed by scholars as a 'transition' to democracy (See Karl 1990; O'Donnell 1991, 1992, 1994; Schmitter and Karl 1993). In the case of Mexico, and as part of this transition, various political and economic changes (local and international) are reshaping the structures of both the state and society, with its obvious consequences for development.

Democracy and Sustainable Human Development

Along with Nun's analysis of Latin America (2000), it is argued here that democracy can be conducive to development, given that it generally facilitates the emergence of a strong collection of civil society groups, with the potential of constituting and defining pluralist interests and generating zones of equality and solidarity (See also Przeworski et al. 2000). Yet as successfully discussed by White (in Robinson and White 1998), while it is still common to find "Western politicians and pundits talking about the hypothetically positive socio-economic consequences of democratization, there is by no means a consensus on the issue among development professionals and analysts" (p. 21). Admittedly, although multiple authors have argued that there is a positive correlation between liberal democracy and capitalist economic growth, it is not clear whether this kind of growth is conducive to long-term development for the majority. In fact, actual democracies can also be conducive to elite-dominated growth, which can be socially unequalizing and exclusionary, and politically disempowering (See Robinson and White 1998). Additionally, even in those countries where democracy has flourished and given way to the improvement of people's lives, its maintenance requires constant vigilance by society as a whole and especially by marginalized groups (See Friedman 1999).

In spite of some of its associated flaws and challenges, it is argued here, along with other scholars, that there are several reasons why democracy must be regarded as fundamental in the pursuit of sustainable human development. As pointed out by White (in Robinson and White 1998, p. 27), for example, democracy has gained ground because of its popular appeal among ordinary citizens as a means of protecting civil liberties and political rights. In historical terms, Amartya Sen (1999) sees the world-wide rise of democracy in the last decades as one of the great developments that occurred in the twentieth century. In his compelling discussion of the value of democracy, Sen argues that countries do not have to be fit for democracy; rather they can become fit through democracy. This has been a momentous change, Sen (1999) asserts, "extending the potential reach of democracy to cover billions of people, with their varying histories and cultures and disparate levels of affluence" (p. 4). As such, democracy can contribute to economic growth, social justice or to feed everyone within a country's borders.[27]

It is then necessary to define what we mean by democracy and identify the features that can, in fact, be helpful in the attainment of development. From a pluralist

---

[27] One of Amartya Sen's central arguments has been the fact that the presence of democratic regimes is associated with the absence of famines.

perspective, Robert Dahl (1971) argues that democracy is a regime through which citizens exercise some control over their leaders. Yet Dahl also emphasizes the importance of certain potential threats to democracy, such as the danger of the overwhelming power of the corporate sector, which forces us to think of the need to democratize all sorts of different spheres of public life and government functioning. Dahl (1971, 1989) proposes some criteria for identifying a country as democratic, these being; civil and political rights plus fair, competitive, and inclusive elections. The countries that meet these criteria are commonly referred to as 'liberal democracies.' Yet in reality there is a range of different regimes that do not necessarily fit this definition; countries somewhere in between democracy and authoritarianism are often referred to as "electoral democracies" (See Schedler 1998). Schedler's (1998, p. 93) analysis, for example, is based on a four-fold classification – authoritarianism, electoral democracy, liberal democracy, and advanced democracy. Electoral democracies face the challenge of the attainment of full democracy, or as Guillermo O'Donnell once put it, the accomplishment of a 'second transition' from a democratic government to a democratic regime (See O'Donnell 1991; 1992; 1994; See also Schmitter 1993). In fact, more substantive forms such as participative (See Rawls 1989) or deliberative (See Habermas 1994) models of democracy are crucial for the creation of the necessary conditions conducive to the introduction of institutional reforms that can help turn the possibility of democracy into an actuality (Hongju and Slye 1999, p. 157)[28].

As argued above for the case of development, one cannot fully discuss the implications of democracy for the lives of real people without referring to a time, a place, and a given set of circumstances. Accordingly, the transformation of a political regime into a democracy must be conceived as following different paths and responding to specific realities. As put by Sklars (in Robinson and White 1998, p. 32), "democracy comes to every country in fragments or parts." Under this logic, each fragment becomes an incentive for the addition of another one, and in a way this stresses the need for 'political invention and improved design' of democratic institutions in a specific context.[29] The various problems and obstacles faced by different countries in the struggle for democratization has increasingly become the focus of students of Latin America (See Schmitter and Karl 1993; Diamond and Linz 1989; Haggard and Kaufman 1994; Diamond, Hartlyn, Linz and Lipset (1999); Diamond and Morlino (2005); Hagopian and Mainwaring 2005). And as a consequence of the changing realities in most of the countries in this region, in some cases, issues related to democratic quality have gained the attention of scholars over issues associated with democratic survival. However, the degree of concentration of power in most of these "new" democracies and the manipulation of people's preferences by political campaigns and the media, raise concerns not only about their

---

[28] See also Robin Luckham's analysis of alternatives to liberal democracy in the context of the analysis of the developmental state, in Robinson and White (1998).

[29] For the case of contemporary Latin America, for example, Schedler (1998) points to two key fundamental issues that must be dealt with in order to transcend the electoral nature of democracy; these being 'state' and 'judicial reform.'

quality, but their stability as well (See Stokes 2001; O'Donnell 1991). Once again, the issue of electoral versus representative democracy comes to the fore, and is reflected in O'Donnell's call for a need to overcome the 'delegative' nature of Latin American electoral democracies in favour of representative democracy. The latter, involves multiple processes of accountability, beyond the isolated act of voting at the time of elections. This is reinforced by Stokes' (2001) analysis, in which she concludes that although democracy does not guarantee that politicians follow through on their campaign promises, it is important to be aware of the serious risks of corroding democratic legitimacy that mandate violations carry with them. She goes on to point out that although mandate violations may produce short or medium-term economic improvement, they will ultimately undermine Latin American democracies. Probably as a result of repeated cases of mandate violations, the perception of Latin Americans, in 2015, regarding democracy and its institutions shows that a meagre 57 per cent supported democracy, and only 37 per cent approved of the way in which the political institutions perform.[30]

It should be clear for all, as argued by Ralf Dahrendorf (1981; 1988; 1994; 1996), that the democratic illusion of a government of the people has always been an invitation to impostors and new power monopolies. In most cases, Nun (2000) argues, the Latin American bourgeoisie has not been an agent of democratization. As Nun further elaborates, the bourgeoisie has preserved its domination, while democratization is the result of pressures and demands that more often than not have been activated from below, by workers and their unions, as well as by other political organizations and social movements (Nun 2000, p. 84). In fact, often, social policies throughout Latin America have targeted the poorest sectors, not so much to level the inequalities, but to contain uprisings or as tools of political patronage (See Stahl 1996; Burt 1996). Although some of these targeting programs are based on the idea of participation, it is clear that participation per se is not sufficient for the consolidation of democracy; it all depends on who participates and under what circumstances. This is what Nun (2000) calls the paradox of Latin America; that is the challenge to consolidate representative democracy in the context of extreme poverty, inequality and polarization.

Although an in-depth discussion of the meaning of citizenship escapes the scope and purpose of the present analysis, it is necessary to acknowledge the need to define it in a way that allows individuals meaningful participation in the process of democratization. In fact, the notion of democratic citizenship can be helpful in understanding the limitations faced by most Latin Americans today. In principle, citizenship should guarantee not only civil and political rights but also economic, social, cultural and sexual rights for all. According to Marshall (1963), for example, there cannot be democratic citizenship without social rights. For Nun (2000, p. 64), the collective wellbeing is a precondition for the exercise of citizenship and a condition for the legitimacy of the state. As such, representative democracy does depend on the effective exercise of citizenship and a relatively equal allocation of

---

[30] See Latinobarómetro's report for 2015: http://www.latinobarometro.org/latOnline.jsp

resources and income distribution. This implies that the social basis and range of accountability of democratic politicians should go beyond a narrow group of elites, and embrace broader sections of society (Robinson and White 1998, p. 31; See also Brysk 2000). The question we are left with, of course, as Nun (2000, p. 91) points out, is how to determine what is the proportion of full citizens for a truly representative democracy to be called as such.

A useful way to investigate the extent to which democratization is taking place is to look at specific areas of public policy. Beyond electoral participation, the politics of economic and social policymaking can tell us much more about the non-electoral dimensions of democratization. In doing so, we will be better positioned to discern whether civil society and the government engage in a more participatory process of decision-making that is conducive to development for all. Thus, for the purpose of complementing our conceptual framework and before delving into Mexico's response to HIV/AIDS, in this chapter's two remaining sections, we will look at some of the key factors associated with the current global environment within which Mexico's quest for development is taking place, as well as at the centrality of a policy networks analysis.

THE CURRENT GLOBAL ENVIRONMENT

In the implementation of developmental and social policies, the Mexican State – as a national boundary-setting institution - is not alone regarding the need to confront a series of challenges that arise from the ever changing circumstances of the international system. Under these set of conditions, referred to by many as the process of globalization, the nature of state sovereignty and its decision-making autonomy are changing in fundamental ways (See Cohen 2001). Thus, in order to incorporate the international dimension to the current analysis, the following section will help us define globalization and its significance for what will also be defined as increasingly global or internationalized policy environments. The aim is to understand how today's international environment and actors affect public policymaking and implementation, particularly in the case of HIV/AIDS and health. In looking at increasingly influential actors, we will underline the role that organized civil society groups play, and briefly refer to the effect that their professionalization is having, as well as the centrality that the international human rights discourse and regime have played in their struggles against the pandemic.

Globalization vs. Globalism

It is imperative to start by saying that, as is the case with most popularized concepts, globalization can mean many things for different people. In fact, there are opposing views and even some confusion on the meaning of this concept, even amongst academics. Thus, in an attempt to shed light and due to its implications for the Mexican case, a distinction will be made between globalization as a broader phenomenon and globalism as a narrower agenda.

In an interesting magazine's article, entitled "The Collapse of Globalism," John Ralston Saul (2004)[31] provides a provocative discussion of globalization for an audience beyond academia. Unfortunately, although his analysis is engaging, the overall argument is weakened by the author's interchangeable use of the two terms, that is globalism and globalization, which is also not such an uncommon error in scholarly literature. Therefore, triggered by the need to underline the distinction between them, and as a reaction to some of Ralston Saul's provocative ideas, *the present analysis refers to the neo-classical economics agenda that defined the so-called "Washington Consensus" and the economic processes triggered by it as globalism.* Defining it as a new "-ism" (a system of beliefs, a set of principles, or an ideological movement; e.g. conservatism, jingoism, feminism)[32] will facilitate the exercise of depicting it as an agenda that is based on a new type of 'religiosity.' In contrast, by globalization we refer here to the broader global phenomenon defined by a greater variety of actors, ideas, and trends.

As a phenomenon, *globalization represents the ongoing historical process of increasing cultural, economic, political, social and technological interconnectedness that characterizes the world today.* In a seminal work on the subject, Held (1997) argues that "globalization is not a singular condition, a linear process or a final end-point of social change" (Held et al. 1997, p. 258; See also Held et al. 1999). Similarly, for Anthony Giddens (1990) globalization is characterized by "the intensification of world-wide social relations, which link distant realities in such a way that local happenings are shaped by events occurring many miles away" (p. 64). Globalization is also defined by the world-wide spread of modern technologies of industrial production and communication of all kinds across frontiers – affecting trade, capital, production and information (Gray 1998, p. 55). And although, as Gray (1998) goes on to say, almost all economies are interconnected with other economies throughout the world, globalization does not represent an end-state towards which all economies must converge. On the contrary, in some cases (and especially between North and South) it accentuates uneven development between countries.

Culturally, globalization is often perceived as an equivalent to the spread of values originating in the United States (U.S.). (See Barber 1995) - or as it is often and misguidedly termed "Americanization"; given that America represents a whole continent and not only the U.S. Yet in reality there is little evidence to prove that this process is making U.S. values universal. Quite the contrary, it can be argued that this process makes some people more aware of the plural nature of an interconnected world. Or as maintained by Gray (1998; 2003), reality suggests that a modus vivendi will have to be found among cultures and nations that are likely to remain different.

In contrast with Ralston Saul's analysis and as stated above, the current analysis puts emphasis on the need to distinguish globalization from globalism. Thus, globalism is equated with the economic discourse stemming from international financial institutions and trade associations such as the International Monetary Fund

---

[31] Ralston Saul, who is considered by most scholars a non-academic thinker and a public intellectual in Canada, provides a very insightful discussion on globalization.
[32] See definition of "-ism" in the Canadian Oxford Dictionary.

(IMF), the World Bank, the United States (U.S.) Treasury, the World Trade Organization, or agreements such as NAFTA.[33] To different degrees, other powerful international actors (e.g. National governments and trans-national corporations) have further supported this neo-liberal economic agenda and the policies emanating from it, which is associated with the economic side of globalization based on the so-called "Washington Consensus." Admittedly, there have been some adjustments to the more orthodox initial "consensus", which have been reflected in the so-called post-Washington Consensus. However, as suggested by Ralston Saul (2004), there is a set of clear motivations that explains the ongoing predominance of the neoliberal hegemonic discourse, such as the need of some members of the economic and political élites to maintain their ideological power, economic benefits, and their position in the international system.[34] This is not to say that the international system is perceived as a monolithic and static structure. Yet it is argued here that although the global arena is conceived as a loose and heterogeneous constellation of interwoven political and economic interests, as well as cultural and ideological traits, the globalist agenda continues to have sufficient momentum to steer the globalization process and to deter other alternatives.

O'Brien (2003) calls the current process of globalization (which again has been dominated by globalism) "uncivilized" due to the fact that all values (i.e. those related to the protection of the environment, national cultures, labour standards, and social policies) seem to be subordinated to the values of economic efficiency and the creation of wealth (See also Rajaee 2000, and Barber 1995). In fact, these critical views of the dominant agenda driving the process of globalization serve as a reminder of a warning put forward by Polany, back in 1957 in *The Great Transformation*. In it, Polany pointed to the risks of allowing unregulated markets to be set up for their impact on people's lives.

It is important to remind ourselves that globalism and its subscribers owe a great deal to the well-known report published in 1975, elaborated by The Trilateral Commission (Michel J. Crozier, Joji Watanuki, and Samuel P. Huntington), entitled "The Crisis of Democracy: Report on the Governability of Democracies." As is widely known, this report has had a major impact at the global level. In it, its authors "explained" the increasing problems that the industrialized economies were facing through the "excesses" of democracy, and it gave entrance to the basis of the neo-liberal agenda, or as it is called here, the globalist agenda. The task for the supporters of this agenda was to fashion a framework of regulations within which market economies could flourish. In turn, University of Chicago professors Friedrich Hayek and Milton Friedman (who, interestingly enough, happened to be tenured professors and therefore foreign to the uncertainties and insecurity associated with the

---

[33] The North-American Free Trade Agreement signed between Canada, Mexico, and the United States.

[34] Unsurprisingly, the main advocates of globalist policies have been the governments of wealthy countries, banks, corporations, investors, and technocratic élites in LMICs, who have profited the most from their implementation. For example, at the height of the neo-liberal agenda, 46.3 percent of exports and 46.4 percent of imports took place between the European Union, the U.S., and Japan alone (WTO 1998, p. 12).

"flexibilization" of labour laws) took up the challenge. Friedman, a neo-classical economist, developed the theoretical formulas such as reducing salaries and incomes, strengthening the private sector, deregulating the economy, restoring the market, and curbing the influence of unions, all of which would serve as the basis of the "Washington Consensus;" known also as 'neo-liberalism,' 'Reaganomics,' or the economic agenda of the 'New Right.' This ideology has been responsible for the promotion of a vision of economic growth and free trade as intrinsically good, and has shaped the development discourse and policy choices among key international institutions since the late 1970s. As we all know, the turning point occurred in 1989 with the fall of the Soviet Union, giving globalist reformers a decisive paradigmatic advantage over their opponents. Since then, this wave of economic ideology has been the predominant discourse vis-à-vis other key features for the maintenance of a stable international system: namely state sovereignty, people's welfare, and democratic values.

The so-called consensus behind globalism is based on the belief that there is a single truth, an endpoint, similar to the now mostly discredited 'End of History' thesis of Fukuyama's (1992). Economists in institutions such as the IMF and the World Bank, as well as government technocrats sympathetic to the globalist agenda throughout the world, seem to believe that they have a comparative advantage in knowledge. This knowledge, they claim, allows them to come up with the right vision on how to model the international system. This explains one of the major problems with globalism, in the sense that it limits the capacity of the world's manifold cultures to pursue development models that are adapted to their own histories, circumstances, and distinctive needs. After all, as argued by North (1990), we must not forget that visions are and will always be culture-bound, class-bound, time-specific, and path dependent.

For the most part, the economic arguments behind globalism are the reflection of political preferences of extremely powerful groups in favor of a capitalist and market-oriented economic system. As such, globalism is inevitably reductionist, resulting in its need to accommodate a set of practices dictated by the theory, which more often than not do not respond to the economic and political realities of actual countries and peoples. As pointed out by some scholars (Perrot, Rist and Sabelli 1992, p. 195), there is also almost a kind of religiosity behind some of the core beliefs of the globalist model, such as the universal necessity of unlimited and continuous economic growth. In this case, we do not see economic growth per se as a problem, but as Perroux (1961) once argued, the type of economic growth pursued should be the kind that is harmonious and which "leads to the development of the whole man within each man" (p. 170). In fact, one of Perroux's main contributions was to underline the need to always investigate the real economy, instead of trusting abstract models whose assumptions obscure our vision. Or as Seers (1963) clearly put it, the task of economists should be to study economies, rather than economic models that in some instances are quite distanced from varying realities. Thus, it is necessary to firmly express our serious reservations about the scientific character of the economics behind the globalist agenda, even more so given the fact that its defenders hardly ever recognize any reservations at all.

These reflections on the distinction between globalization and globalism lead us back to Ralston Saul's (2004) piece. The problem with his interchangeable use of the terms (although, once again, one must admit that he is not the only one who fails to clearly distinguish these two concepts) arises from the argument he makes, which consists of the claim that we have been witnessing the collapse of globalization. Although interesting and quite provocative, his argument is problematic – to say the least – and needs to be qualified, even if limited only to globalism. Globalism, the ideology that promotes a world-market economy, has not been defeated. On the one hand, it might be true that, as Ralston Saul argues, the terrorist attacks of Sep/11 of 2001 could have slowed down the process of economic liberalization and integration – as a consequence, mainly, of the so-called U.S 'War on Terror' and its increased 'homeland' security measures (See Colombani 2002; Kellner 2003).[35] Yet, on the other hand, strong globalist élites remain in power and the organizations (e.g. IMF, World Bank, WTO) put in place to support the international trade and financial system at the end of World War II – and more recently the globalist agenda - have shown a significant degree of adaptability.

Throughout the 1980s and 1990s, the globalist agenda was concretized in the IMF's and the World Bank's promotion of a series of policies under the banner of 'Structural Adjustment Programs' (SAPs). Although the debate around the impact of the implementation of SAPs continues, some argue that it accentuated the divide between the Global North (mostly HICs) and the Global South (mostly LMICs) (See Berry 2003).[36] One major negative effect that the dominant economic agenda behind the process of globalization – what we call globalism - has had on LMICs (Mexico included) is the diminishing of tax-collecting capacities of the state due to the lowering of taxes for foreign investors, privatization of formerly own corporations, and the introduction of more flexible labour laws. These pressures originated in the increasing global move towards market-oriented economies. This has left most of LMICs ill-equipped for taking a range of responsibilities necessary to meet the needs of their impoverished populations (Clapham 2002, p. 781). Under these circumstances, and in spite of the increasing pressures on them, however, as argued by Gray (1998, p. 77), states will remain decisive as mediating structures, which influential economic actors will compete to control. Moreover, the protective function of the state is likely to expand as more and more citizens demand shelter from the havoc caused by global capital speculation.

---

[35] For a varied analysis of the consequences of 9/11 see also Chomsky (2002), Friedman (2002), Daalder (2003).

[36] In his analysis of the gains and losses from globalization (which he defines in strictly economic terms, and which makes it closer to the current definition of globalism), Berry debunks various myths around this discussion. Amongst others, he renders false the idea that internationalization must be divorced from the defence of social programs (i.e. the Scandinavian countries), and points to some LMICs who have in fact benefited from trade (e.g. Taiwan and South Korea). Yet Berry (2003) also points out that in the last two decades – under the globalist model – "we have seen many cases of increasing inequality and few of the opposite trend" (p. 19).

Although some analysts point to the fact that the population in LMICs as a whole has experienced an increase in income, most of it is due to the cases of China and India (Berry 2003, p. 22).[37] Therefore, it has become clear that globalism benefits only a minority of LMICs, and as argued by Berry (2003, p. 22), the winners are likely to be those middle-income countries which are already competitive in some tradable goods markets. In most cases, the "winners" tend to be countries where the infant-industry approach has been used either with great (i.e. South East Asia) or relative success (i.e. Mexico and Brazil), before being removed from the tool kit under free trade (See Berry 2003).[38]

The materialization of the globalist agenda in a set of practices - which flow from economics research centres, or "think tanks," and the leading financial institutions to national governments – has had consequences beyond the realm of economics. For instance, although officially, the IMF and the World Bank support the democratic institutions of all countries, in reality they have imposed policies that undermine the democratic process and the state's claim to legitimacy in the eyes of many of its own citizens (See Walton 1989). For its part, the World Bank has continuously denied any intervention or influence on the political life of the states, based on its own Articles of Agreement. In article IV, section 10, it is stated that "… the bank and its officers shall not interfere in the political affairs of any member, nor shall they be influenced in their decisions by the political character of the member or members concerned. Only economic considerations shall be relevant to their decisions." In reality, however, it is clear that for both financial institutions market rules have been elevated beyond any possibility of revision through democratic choice (Gray 1998, p. 18). Moreover, as clearly put by Duquette (1999), the economic and philosophical speculations stemming from their "consensus" sounded like music "to the ears of the architects of authoritarian regimes" (p. 19) and were translated into stringent policies (i.e., Dictator Augusto Pinochet in Chile, or Mexico under Carlos Salinas de Gortari's government).[39] These policies gave more scope to an already wealthy corporate sector through the privatization of public assets sold off at bargain prices (See Duquette

---

[37] The reasons behind the reduction in poverty in these countries are still being debated and a full discussion of them falls beyond the scope of the current analysis. For a critique to some of the claims regarding the link between neo-liberal reforms and poverty reduction see Kiely (2004), who argues that "optimistic claims for poverty reduction in the era of globalization are based on selective and questionable data" (p. 17).

[38] In discussing the impact of globalist policies, development theory cannot ignore the South East Asian cases – which have been repeatedly used as examples of successful integration to the global markets. In this regard, Berry (2003) argues that although they benefited from export booms, which in turn produced wage gains that contributed to falling inequality, their experiences are unlikely to be replicated and their models generalized. For globalism believers, however, especially before the Asian financial crisis of the late 1990s, the South East Asian countries represented a few miracles to be reported. This should not come as a surprise, since, as put by Rist (1996, p. 239), although most people catch themselves doubting, the need to hang on to one's beliefs forces people to pray with one voice when taking part in collective rites. Moreover, even if financial crises force globalist institutions to pour billions of dollars in order to keep the international monetary and financial system from collapse, the essential goal is to keep the faith in the economic model going.

[39] The recent history neoliberal policies under PRI and PAN federal administrations in Mexico will be discussed in chapter three.

1999; Teichman 2001). More troublesome is the fact that today's world-wide free market lacks the necessary political checks and balances. Consequently, towards the end of the 1990s, which represented the height of the neoliberal agenda, some scholars argued that the most important reform was to democratize globalization (See Amin 2000; Sen 2000).

Initially, the defenders of SAPs tended to deny or ignore the positive effect of social policies on economic efficiency. Apparently, in their view of the world, efficiency and productivity seemed to be disconnected from human wellbeing. Soon after their implementation, however, some of the negative consequences arising from SAPs became evident. In 1987, for example, analysts associated with UNICEF published the first major critique of adjustment entitled "Adjustment with a Human Face." It focused on how the poor, particularly women and children bore a disproportionate share of the cost of adjustment. Although not necessarily unique or original, since other voices had been pointing to the same problems, their critique stirred heated debates. Three years later, the costs of structural adjustment were also underscored by the UNDP's first *Human Development Report* (1990).

Fortunately, some of the criticisms directed toward SAPs did not go unheard, which resulted in some economists at the World Bank gathering empirical data from a number of case studies and identifying the 'flaws' of the first wave of adjustment experiments. They ended up engineering a somewhat hybrid model, one which called for adjustment reforms that ought to include social concerns (See Birdsall 1993; Psacharopoulos 1993; Hausman 1994; Fishlow 1995). Officially, they also recognized the central role of the state in the promotion of development. In the World Bank's 1997 Development Report ("The State in a Changing World") they declared that: "[c]ertainly, the state-dominated development has failed. But so has stateless development ... History has repeatedly shown that good government is not a luxury but a vital necessity. Without an effective state, sustainable development, both economic and social, is impossible" (In Gray 1998, p. 202).

Eventually, some World Bank economists became critical of the Bank's policies. Amongst them, Joseph Stiglitz (1999, 2002) -now a former Bank official- and a faculty member at Columbia University, in New York, has declared that if there is a factor that can make the current international economic system explode it is the poverty and the big gap that SAPs seem to have generated between rich and poor. In his critiques, Stiglitz included, as other Bank members did later, a reconsideration of the importance of civil society. These concerns have been incorporated into the World Bank's discourse in the form of social capital. Yet, as some critics of this discourse point out (Standing 2000, p. 754), the elasticity of the definition of social capital is problematic. Standing argues that by not pinpointing what destroyed some social capital in the first place they miss a crucial point. As a result of the expressed concerns, the Bank has come up with the idea of partnerships in order to bring in civil society and address the social shortcomings of SAPs. The idea of partnerships is not free of potential problems either. The involvement of civil society or more concretely some Non-Governmental Organizations (NGOs) brings with it the moral hazard of NGOs adapting their behaviour to increase the probability of being involved and getting funded. Additionally, there is also the question of which civil society groups are involved and the nature of their participation. In spite of one's reservations regarding the Bank's official discourse, if one's vision of sustainable human development includes democracy, sooner or later one needs to incorporate interest representation in decision-making. These are central questions in the analysis of development and democratization and will be dealt with more concretely, in the following chapters, for the analysis of health and HIV/AIDS.

In Latin America as elsewhere, social groups as diverse as women's organizations, labour unions, Church-led communities, rural workers, ecologists, and sexual minorities have swiftly mobilized in response to the undemocratic practices associated with the globalists agenda and the unbearable costs associated with it and structural adjustment programs (See Przeworski 1991; 1995, 2000; Korzeniewicz and Smith 2000; Friedman, Hochstetler, and Clark 2001; Stahler-Sholk, Vanden, and Kuecker 2002). In fact, more than knowledge stemming from the World Bank and IMF headquarters, or the change of heart of former officials, it was external pressure that forced them to reconsider some of their policies. Thus, not surprisingly, it can be argued that the discourse of adjustment with a human face has been a response to the increasing pressures on policymakers from the excluded fringes of the population. And as mentioned in the introduction, it is clear that contrary to former Mexican president Ernesto Zedillo's statements at the 2000 World Economic Forum (Davos, Switzerland [40]) about "globaliphobics," civil society activists have expressed dissatisfaction with neo-liberal globalism, not with globalization. Once again, one can see significant differences between the Global North and South with regards to the consequences of neo-liberal economic reforms. In HICs ways have been and may more easily be found to mitigate the risks imposed on citizens by world markets, through the availability of better instruments for social protection. In poorer countries, however, with weaker states, global laissez-faire can produce violent reactions (i.e. the rise of fundamentalist religious groups and/or the formation of terrorist networks) and work as a catalyst for the disintegration of the modern state (Gray 1998, p. 21; See also Reno 1998).

After the first wave of neo-liberal oriented SAPs, and still under the auspices of both the World Bank and the IMF, governments throughout the globe adopted a series of so-called second-generation reforms. In some cases, these reforms represented a move beyond macroeconomic policy to address institutional and social policy issues, and involved more detailed conditions, specifying policy and implementation, but also endorsing – at least rhetorically - principles such as participation and accountability in public life. For Schmitter et al. (1993) the new emphasis on social policies was considered as a consequence to the work of the moderates within international financial institutions and local government officials. Health is a key example of these second-generation reforms that involved both elements of adjustment and compensation to targeted sectors of the poor. This attention to health is due in part to the growing evidence that globalism has had an adverse effect on the state's primary

---

[40] http://zedillo.presidencia.gob.mx/pages/disc/ene00/28ene00nmultipleforms.html

responsibility for public health (See Buse et al. 2002; Fidler 2003). As a result, and for the purposes of the present analysis, there is a need to emphasize the centrality of health in understanding the interaction between globalization and development. Interestingly, and as a response to the overwhelming evidence of the negative impact of globalist policies on income distribution, there was a sudden explosion of recommendations, injunctions, and advice on how to "overcome" poverty. Somehow belatedly, as put by Rist (1996, p. 255), the new concern for the poor and their health had the strange virtue of making the world suddenly look more complex.

In sum, much current debate confuses globalization (a historical process that has been underway for centuries) with globalism (a more ephemeral political and economic project). In the last couple of decades, however, the latter has dominated the former, which has made spatial segregation and exclusion become integral parts of the process of globalization. In disentangling the misconceptions around globalization, the obvious must be emphasized; a global capitalist and free-market economy is not a law of historical development but a political project, whose flaws have already caused much unnecessary suffering. Among the human needs that free markets neglect are the needs for human security and social identity. Paraphrasing Bauman (1998, p.3), it is contended here that in some cases and to some degree, neo-tribal and fundamentalist tendencies might reflect and articulate the experience of people on the receiving end of globalism and might be its legitimate offspring as much as the widely acclaimed "hybridization" of top culture. Under these circumstances, as put by Gray (1998) in reference to Schumpeter, capitalism must be tamed for if left to itself it can destroy the cohesion of society and liberal civilization altogether.

Based on the above characterization of the phenomenon, the following sections and chapters will show that the current process of globalization represents both a threat and an opportunity for development; some of its features can be conducive to or hinder development. Not surprisingly, the interaction between the two – that is, globalization and development - increasingly became the focus of analysis amongst development scholars (See Cerny 1995; Rajaee 2000; Sandbrook 2003), and has forced them to rethink the relation between the state and civil society. Fortunately, and in spite of the strength and influence of the globalist agenda, the analysis of the global fight against HIV/AIDS provides us with examples of new efforts from different governments and civil society groups around the globe to assert state power and autonomy. Two good examples of this are the decisions made by the South African and Brazilian governments to secure the availability of drugs (some of them produced in India) for their respective populations affected by HIV/AIDS (under circumstances that will be briefly discussed in chapter two). Their actions and the international support they gathered from various state and civil society actors, in opposing the interests of the multinational pharmaceutical industry and the globalist agenda, represent a case in point regarding the changing and varied nature of globalization. Moreover, the learning and cooperation that characterizes the interactions among civil society actors, as part of the current phase of globalization, have led to their increasing professionalization and the establishment of more formal structures (i.e., Non-Governmental Organizations or NGOs), which has allowed them to be able to exercise more effective influences on the policymaking process.

Civil Society's Professionalization or NGOization

As core elements of the phenomenon of globalization, domestic and international NGOs have managed to forge political alliances among very diverse actors around specific issues. In linking locally-based groups with global actors, they have helped placing issues such as child labour, land mines, environmental protection, human rights, and HIV/AIDS on the global agenda. They formed trans-national coalitions to reform the World Bank (See Fox and Brown 1998), and to resist the free trade agenda, giving shape to what some have called the 'non-governmental order' (*The Economist*, December 11, 1999, p. 20-22). NGOs also act as watchdogs of the pharmaceutical industry, advocate on behalf of primary health care, and women's and sexual minorities' health, and ensure that continuing attention is paid to community involvement and human rights in health matters around the globe (See Keck and Sikkink 1998; Korzeniewicz and Smith 2000; Friedman, Hochstetler, and Clark 2001; Stahler-Sholk, Vanden, and Kuecker 2002). In general, regardless of whether or not NGOs have a specific organized constituency, the domestic-international divide does not represent an obstacle for co-operation for most of them. On the contrary, most of these groups are quite effective and at ease at the global level. And as we will see in some of the cases presented below for the case of HIV/AIDS, they have become active participants at different United Nation (UN) fora, in engagements with multilateral institutions, and in the forging of new international norms and demands. Some of their concerns centre on how to democratize the global arena, and how to more effectively participate in it.

The task for the observer of those groups that are strong enough to gain access to the decision-making bodies, and able to sit at the respective tables, is to identify the proposals and ideas they present and to assess how effective they are at influencing policy (Brooks and Fox 2002, p. 426). In their efforts, NGOs face various challenges, some of which are clearly recognized by them. As acknowledged by some members of civil society groups, "while scholars may be too distant and detached, those of us who work on the ground with impoverished communities in crisis often have the opposite problem. We have noted in our own work that it is easy for us to lose perspective through our very closeness to local situations. Our intense loyalties to the people we seek to serve and to the organizations within which we work can prompt us to dismiss wider structural questions and global or theoretical perspectives as irrelevant – or we may simply find no time left to consider them" (Quoted in Millen at al., in Yong Kim et al. 2000, p. 386). In contrast, there are other civil society actors who have the resources, particularly those think tanks or research university centres that often produce large numbers of studies to support a specific agenda (i.e. health care financing), whose work is translated into what some call the non-governmental policy transfer (See Stone 2000). In her analysis, Stone shows, for instance, how think tanks promote the spread of policy ideas about privatization, and further discusses their involvement in domestic and trans-national policy networks.

Most analyses of the process of professionalization, or NGOization of civil society groups and activists, emphasize its effects on the relations between civil society and the state, and warn us about three main risks; the shrinking distance between the two, the resulting lack of autonomy for the former, and the detrimental impact on a vibrant public sphere. In contrast, the current analysis intends to show that there should be a more nuanced assessment, by way of providing some optimistic insights to counter such warnings, which are based on a close analysis of the NGOization of HIV/AIDS activism, both internationally and in Mexico.

NGOization is taking place both at the domestic and the international levels, and it represents not just the spontaneous proliferation of NGOs (with specialized staff, structured funding, and salaries) but also the active promotion of their formalization by governments, international institutions, and donors. In fact, and in line with the neoliberal globalist agenda, the preferred NGOs are expected to be rhetorically restrained, politically collaborative, and technically proficient in their practices. That is precisely why, under these circumstances, most critics have pointed to the detrimental impact of this phenomenon on the autonomy of social movements, vis-à-vis the state. As a good example of the increasing attention paid to this phenomenon, George Yúdice, in *The Expediency of Culture* (2003) states that; "NGOization is not scandalous, but nevertheless contributes to the weakening of the public sphere, precisely the opposite of the intent of the social movements. That institutionalization resulted in activism giving way to bureaucratic administration. Those movements have been permeated by international discourses on cultural citizenship, where identity is the lynchpin of rights claims. To be sure, how identity is deployed depends on the performative possibilities holding in different societies. In such contexts, there is little to be gained by deploying identity or disidentity if there is no juridical or other institutional uptake to transform rights claims into material changes. This question of uptake is crucial and it has confounded many a study that has presumed the receptivity to identity rights claims on the basis of experiences in other contexts" (pp. 77-78).

As stressed by Yúdice, it is undeniable that in most instances institutional channeling tempers activism and can favor the assertion, in public, of certain identities. This can force social movements to dovetail with the agendas set by NGOs and funders, whereby funding patterns often lead to a shift away from the construction of ideological or transformational alternatives to project-based and often limited developmental activities. Furthermore, some smaller organizations, which ultimately depend on the same pull of grant providers, risk their continuing existence due to the lack of professional means to sell their projects and activities like their bigger sisters. For their part, some of those more 'successful' NGOs end up becoming social service providers to governments, global institutions and even businesses, thereby undermining their autonomy and social activism. Ultimately, there is often less room for organizations to be actively engaged in the ideological construction and promotion of alternative forms of global political organization, wider social inclusion, and democratization.

Nevertheless, and despite those warnings, the actual effects of civil society groups and activists' institutionalization have been positively surprising in some cases, with great effectiveness shown in engaging with the state and international institutions while maintaining a significant degree of autonomy. Thus, based on the analysis of various networks of HIV/AIDS and sexual minorities activists in Latin America that, it has been argued that the effects of professionalization are more nuanced (See Torres-Ruiz 2013). Furthermore, the following section and chapters will show the ways in which the adoption of a human rights discourse by many of those activists and NGOs, within the process of democratization in Mexico, has served as a strong discursive and political tool for the emancipation of previously excluded and marginalized groups. In fact, the creation of HIV/AIDS NGOs and policy networks has allowed them to engage in some transformational practices that take place at several points in those networks, which has made social action possible. Although this has resulted in their growing visibility, positioning, and influence on the policymaking process, some concrete challenges regarding the continuity and broadening of their agenda will also be addressed.

Human Rights and HIV/AIDS Activism

Before defining policy networks, it is essential to underline the centrality of a human rights approach in the pursuit of sexual health for all, especially so when it comes to sexual minorities activism. In fact, the adoption of a human rights discourse has been at the center of the fight against the pandemic, both globally and locally. First of all, sexual health has been defined as a state of physical, emotional, mental, and social well-being in relation to sexuality; it is not merely the absence of disease, dysfunction, or infirmity. Therefore, the right to sexual health requires a positive and respectful approach to sexuality and sexual relationships, as well as the possibility of pleasurable and safe sexual experiences, free of coercion, discrimination, and violence (Asher 2004; Chen, Leaning, and Narasimhan 2003). Thus, successful promotion of sexual health goes hand in hand with the protection and enforcement of human rights for all, and it requires a comprehensive program of activities that encompasses the health and education sectors, as well as the broader political, economic, and legal domains. In turn, the entitlements created by a human rights approach to health lead to governments' corresponding obligations under the respective international regimes, and to the resetting of priorities. As a result, governments find it far more difficult to justify the withholding of basic provisions and services on account of alleged financial constraints or because of certain (often discriminatory) priorities. In this context, a central advocacy principle for civil society groups or NGOs, with a human rights approach to health, is that governments are accountable for their obligations under international law and within the framework of national constitutions and legislation. This entails ensuring the incorporation of international treaty provisions into domestic legislation and the access of individuals and communities to effective judicial or other appropriate remedies in the face of their rights violations. In summary, the right to health has empowered civil society groups that are politically engaged in the fight against HIV/AIDS. Ultimately, under a human rights approach, becoming healthy and remaining so is regarded not merely as a medical, technical, or economic problem but also as a question of social justice and concrete government obligations.

It has become increasingly clear that the adoption of a human rights discourse by activists and NGOs, in the struggle against HIV/AIDS, turned out to be a very effective move in two major ways. First of all, it provided a common and widely accepted language in the definition of the circumstances faced by those affected, whose lives were threatened not only by the disease itself but by a multiple set of factors determining their vulnerabilities. Secondly, it facilitated the articulation of a powerful rationale to pressure governments and other institutions to respond with a clear set of public policies that would lead to fairer institutional arrangements. This has taken place within a context in which the international human rights regime is helping define a system of international relations that seems to be moving in the direction of multi-level governance.

Indeed, globalization and the aforementioned internationalized policy environments have opened up new avenues for marginalized communities to test the accountability of different key actors, not just when it comes to HIV/AIDS (See Benedek et al. 2007; Halbert 2005; Manokha 2008; Ostergard 2007) but more generally in claiming basic rights for all (See Gibney 2003). However, and in contrast to the case of national or local governments, we know that direct accountability of intergovernmental organizations to populations is unusual. Traditionally, they are accountable only to their member-states. World Bank officials, for example, have repeatedly stated that political decisions are irrelevant to loan allocations, and have rejected the idea of being bound by human rights law. Yet since the 1990s, the Bank has been willing to finance human rights projects and has adopted internal instructions that touch upon them, such as the Inspection Panel.[41] And although such panel is not a mechanism that allows holding it responsible for complicity in human rights violations, its acceptance of some - if limited - accountability implies recognition of the impact that its financing has on the quality of life and human rights of affected people. This is an important step forward in enabling marginalized communities to question the legitimacy of an actor whose interventions are otherwise largely immune to legal challenges. Additionally, the fact that the international human rights regime is quite fragmented has forced activists and NGOs to make strategic choices on their point of entry. Thus, forum shopping and switching has been essential. In other words, the best practices in achieving recognition of human rights violations require an ability to identify the optimal forum, with options varying according to the targeted perpetrator; different bodies deal with the responsibilities of states, the corporate sector, health care providers, international financial institutions, etc. (See De Feyter 2005; De Gaay Fortman 2011). Sometimes, it is a matter of appealing to

---

[41] See http://www.accountabilitycounsel.org/wp-content/uploads/2013/05/HRGM_WWW_WB.pdf

intergovernmental organizations or international courts, while others times, it is about using domestic legal systems and the extraterritorial reach of some laws.

Social monitoring and other activist support provided by international organizations such as Human Rights Watch (HRW), Amnesty International (AI), the Oxford Committee for Famine Relief (OXFAM), Médecines sans Frontières (MSF), Free the Children, the Red Cross, and many others, help to advance the effective reach of acknowledged human rights. Together with monitoring of violations, the use of non-legal means such as public campaigns focusing on "naming and shaming" to force Multi-National Corporations (MNCs) and governments to act are central in the wide range of available avenues. The fact that some of these actions can be effective (at least, in putting the violators on the defensive) is an indication of the reach of public reasoning when information becomes available and ethical arguments are allowed rather than suppressed. The importance of communication, advocacy, exposure and informed public discussion intimately relate to a more open and democratic environment and show that human rights can have influence without necessarily depending on coercive legislation.

When looking at the current economic order and its negative effects on human rights, it could be argued that one of the main problems is the propensity by economic and political elites to overvalue destructive things – such as financial derivatives and crude oil – and undervalue truly valuable things – such as sustainable food production, quality public health care, education for all, our global climate, and other so-called externalities that the capitalist market society has often neglected (See Benedek et al. 2007; Branco 2009; De Gaay Fortman 2011). This results in huge inequalities in power, for example, between Multinational Corporations (MNCs) and individual citizens or local communities. A big challenge is to come up with the same kind of commitment to binding human rights treaties as there is to trade and economic agreements, both at the global and intergovernmental level. In fact, since its formal creation, more than twenty years ago, the WTO dangerously unbalanced the emerging system of global governance (See Manokha 2008). This is because the WTO gave concrete expression to mankind's yearning for universal rights and the global rule of law, speaking also the language of freedom (market freedom that is). The catch lay not in its logic but in its asymmetry. Fully enforceable rights were proclaimed for corporations but not for citizens, as part of the rules to promote an open and global marketplace. As a result, the international economic regime has supra-national clout in the sense that its principles and rules prevail over its member nation-states' domestic constitutions, in what Clarkson (2014) refers to as a kind of external constitution (See also Torres-Ruiz and Clarkson 2009). Under the WTO rules, arbitration allows for strong transnational judicial processes between governments and corporations, which are effectively enforced. So that there is an imbalance between the hard-law nature of this "supra-national constitution" and the soft-law character of most other multilateral regimes, especially those on human rights. Under these circumstances, it is very easy to sign and ratify all sorts of human rights, labour-standards, developmental goals, and environmental conventions without feeling obliged to respect their commitments. In the case of HIV/AIDS, free-market fundamentalism's or neo-liberal globalism's emphasis on the protection of the pharmaceutical industry's drug patents for profiting represents a major challenge for guaranteeing universal access to treatment for all those in need (See Halbert 2005). Admittedly though, the responsibility is not solely that of an industry, but governments too fail to enforce rights for different reasons; lack of political will in some cases, conflicting interests that are often explained by the economic model and the ideology behind it, the institutional structures in place, lobbying and electoral campaign's funding by the pharmaceutical industry itself, etc.

Understandably, and a result of globalism's constraining effect on state action, civil society and human rights activists have mobilized in an attempt to correct the constitutional imbalance that is constraining the regulatory state. They are pressuring governments to get in step with their citizenry to give clear priority to human emancipation rather than market liberation. Here, it is important to re-state that efforts in favour of human rights enforcement need not be confined only to making new laws. After all, although legislation might turn out to be the right way to proceed, human rights also function as powerful moral claims. As argued by Amartya Sen (2009), who draws from Immanuel Kant, moral obligations can be both perfect and imperfect. In fact, the struggle for the enforcement of economic, social, and cultural rights has to do with the recognition of 'imperfect' global obligations in this respect. This means that human rights are strong ethical pronouncements as to what should be done; what is being articulated or ratified is an ethical assertion – not a proposition about what is already legally guaranteed. Admittedly, these public articulations of human rights are sometimes invitations to initiate some fresh legislation, and they represent a kind of template for new laws that could be enacted to legalize those human rights across the world. Often, the challenge is to sustain a sense of urgency and solidarity in the face of the atomizing effects of neo-liberal economic policies, knowing that although human rights regimes cannot do away with unequal experiences, they can be a guide in efforts to secure a dignified human existence for all. If freedoms and rights are seen as important, people have good reasons to ask what they should do to help and defend each other from injustice. It is important to remember also that, in moving from the observation of a tragedy to the diagnosis of injustice, reasoning (in all its diverse cultural manifestations) must be involved. Thus, we must acknowledge that a calamity would be a case of injustice if it could have been prevented. We can also conclude that it is useful to preserve the common language of human rights, particularly in the context of globalization, since it helps to identify common causes of violations that are not just domestic or regional, but global. And as such, we can also see that human rights represent living instruments, and thus have the potential to provide protection against the adverse consequences of the current globalist agenda, and other future models driving globalization.

Another important challenge, of a more theoretical nature that is also associated with the legitimacy of the international human rights discourse, concerns its universality. We are all familiar with the recent history of the international human rights regime; from the drafting and promulgation of the Universal Declaration of Human Rights in 1948, which was followed by different covenants and agreements, global and regional, and its increasing worldwide recognition and acceptance by state and non-state actors alike. However, we are also aware of the critical questioning of its cultural relevance, the epistemological challenges it poses, and its global legitimacy (See Beuchot 2005; Sharma 2006; De Sousa Santos 2014). And although we associate the conception of those rights with historical events originated in the so-called West, it has been argued that civil society and social movements around the world have appropriated them in more recent years, considering them as a "Last Utopia" in their own struggles for freedom and justice (See Moyn 2010; Parekh 2008; Vincent 2010). In fact, there seems to be a general agreement, if not a true consensus, on the fact that human rights are directly related to the idea of democracy and human dignity, in the sense that it is through open dialogue and participation of all that respect for the freedom and equality of every human being can be truly realized (See Vincent 2010). Even more important, there is an increasing awareness of the changing nature of cultures and the conception or definitions of rights as well (See Merry 2001).

However, when looking at the global economy and human rights violations, we become acutely aware of the Western bias and the prioritization of civil and political rights (first generation rights) over the rest (See De Gaay Fortman 2011; Manokha 2008). Thus, there is an ongoing struggle for the full recognition of economic, social, cultural, and collective rights (second and third-generation rights), based on the argument that only then would it be possible to integrate ethical issues underlying general ideas of global development and justice with the demands of democracy. Yet as human rights' advocates struggle for the recognition of the importance of such claims and the acceptance of some social obligations to safeguard them, they are often quite impatient with intellectual skepticism, because most of them are concerned with changing the world rather than interpreting it. And we have to acknowledge that this proactive stance has had its rewards, since it has allowed the immediate use of the generally appealing idea of human rights to confront intense oppression or great misery, without having to wait for the theoretical air to clear. In this context, a globalized world can be described as conducive to or as a hindrance for human rights, depending on whether individuals and institutions fulfill their moral obligations to respect those rights. But it is necessary to acknowledge that in its current form, the international human rights regime has come to reflect the aspirations of a variety of peoples and issues put forward by all UN member states and some civil society groups as well.

We also have to acknowledge that human rights remain, for the most part, a general agreement on the ethical basis for the need to recognize the equality of all human beings, regardless of their gender, sexual orientation, class, citizenship, place of residence, caste, ethnicity, culture, religion, age, language, or any other characteristics that might help define their own identities. There is something very appealing about the idea of universal human rights, in spite of the fact that some people see them as just loose talk, attractive as a general belief or even as politically effective rhetoric (See Moyn 2010; Sen 2009). As stated above, the fact of the matter is that most UN member states have, at least officially, agreed upon the legitimacy of such rights and have put in place an international regime for their protection. This just goes to show that we may be quite close to a general agreement on their relevance, without necessarily achieving universal consensus and enforcement.

GLOBALIZATION AND POLICY NETWORKS

The changing nature and increasing influence of globalization has augmented the need for a better understanding of the dynamics between the domestic and the international dimensions of public policymaking processes. Especially when as we will see below, in the case of Mexico, membership in regional and world trade agreements such as NAFTA and the WTO represents a central determining factor in the definition of an international environment within which the government's autonomy to formulate public policies is increasingly limited. Similarly, external variables and actors have steadly influenced the process of democratization and civil society participation in Mexico in recent decades. Thus, the following two sections will provide an overview of the meaning and significance of internationalized policy environments and policy networks, both of which are central for our analysis of HIV/AIDS policies in Mexico.

Internationalized Policy Environments

Similar to the case of globalization, it must be underlined that the significance of the interaction between domestic and international realities is nothing new.[42] Yet what concerns us here is to show the degree to which this interaction is generating a new set of circumstances for public policymaking and implementation in specific issue areas. Furthermore, the type of linkages that are being established between domestic and international actors in the case of HIV/AIDS provide a good example of this new dynamics. As such, it will be argued that this new dynamics goes beyond the more dichotomous division between the domestic and the international that are characteristic of the International Relations literature (See Putnam 1988; Evans et al. 1993).

In fact, globalization has led to a set of circumstances that could be defined as internationalized policy environments. These new environments are giving rise to complex processes of international lesson-drawing, policy convergence, policy diffusion and policy transfer (See Coleman and Perl 1999; Dolowitz and Marsh 2000), and they tend to have a varying impact on the range of public policy choices available to LMICs vis-à-vis HICs. Similarly, different public policymaking approaches inform the analysis of internationalized policy environments. According to some scholars, for example, the level of socio-economic development of a country is more significant in determining public policy than factors such as the ideological orientation or the organizational structure of a specific political regime (See Cutright

---

[42] In the International Relations literature this has been widely discussed; see for example the concept of interdependence in Keohane and Nye (1977), Gourevitch's (1978) 'second image reversed', and Putnam's (1988) 'two-level games'.

1965; Jackman 1974). For others, the world-wide spread of social development programs can also be explained not so much as the result of nations independently responding in a similar way to similar problems (See Spalding 1980), but rather, they should be seen as the product of the diffusion of models and concepts from "innovative" centres to other nations throughout the world, or as the imposition of development models and economic agendas – of which globalism is a prime example. Under this perspective, Spalding (1980, p. 433) argues that the need to secure the symbols of "modernity" may be behind some of the imitative policy actions of LMICs.

Policy Networks Analysis

The current analysis of HIV/AIDS and health-related policies, which we consider as fundamental components of the democratization and development process in Mexico, adopts and adapts the concept of policy networks. The adoption and use of this concept will allow us to determine the extent to which traditionally closed political cliques ('camarillas') have gone through a process of transformation, allowing for a more inclusive process of public policymaking.

As briefly mentioned at the very outset, the relatively new global phenomenon characterized by the formation and consolidation of diverse sets of networks has been defined by Manuel Castells (1996 and 2010) as the network society. According to him, it represents a new social structure that could be seen as a reaction to the double global crisis of state legitimacy and economic/social instability. And although Castells' analysis mostly refers to civil society or social movements networks, his work and insights are central to our own reflections on the global reality within which HIV/AIDS and health-related activism has organized/mobilized and policies have been articulated. As pointed out by Castells, social movements often require an emotional trigger by outrage against blatant injustice, while at the same time examples of successful mobilization or uprisings in other parts of the world gives them a strong sense of hope and possibility (Castells 2010, p. 220), creating a kind of viral effect. This has clearly been the case among sexual minorities and HIV/AIDS activism, whose actions have been linked through following by example, as well as through personal contacts and new networking technologies. Castells refers to this as a hybrid of cyber and physical space that leads to a third space of autonomy. In turn, this so-called third space provides the platform for their continuing expansive networking practices.

Furthermore, and in relation to our previous analysis of NGOization, these networked movements analyzed by Castells are local and global at the same time, with a split between local communal identity and global individual networking. In most cases, they are generally leaderless, and their togetherness is a work in progress, while their sense of community is defined by Castells as rather a commonality in the practice of the movement. Not unlike HIV/AIDS activists and NGOs, most of these social movements are networked in multiple forms, and their different structures afford them flexibility and protection against bureaucratization and manipulation.

However, there are some critical differences between strictly social movement networks and what we will define as policy networks bellow. For instance, although the former are strongly and openly aimed at changing the values of society and at projecting a new utopia of networked democracy based on local and virtual communities in interaction (Castells 2010, p. 228), it is mostly the latter that do recognize the feasibility of fair participation in the institutional channels (Torres-Ruiz 2006; 2011; 2013). Although it is fair to say that, along with Castells' reasoning, the critical passage from hope to implementation of change depends on the permeability of political institutions to the demands of the movement and on the willingness of the movement to engage in a process of negotiation. Another important difference between the two is that whereas social movement networks are rarely programmatic, policy networks do focus on a clear, single issue (i.e., HIV/AIDS policymaking). And in contrast with movement networks that do not have a core or a centre as such (Castells 2010, p. 221), policy networks do have one, which allows them to effect change and influence policymaking directly. Yet success for all of them is often measured in terms of their capacity to set policy agendas and the broadening of channels of political participation.

It is within the context of internationalized policy environments and a networked society that we move on now to the introduction of policy networks. Thus, and based on the examination of the Mexican reality, we define a *policy network* as follows: a *permeable cluster of interdependent organizations and individual actors (public and private), with frequent interactions and a set of common interests and goals, connected to each other by resource dependencies, with a core and a periphery, whose members participate in the formulation and implementation of a set of policies*. This definition draws from the works of a variety of scholars (See Coleman and Perl 1999; Hass 1992; Hassenteufel 1995; Jordan 1990; Marsh and Rhodes 1992, among others).

As such, the idea of policy networks originates in the British and the U.S. public policy analysis literature (See Moore 1978; Richardson and Jordan 1979). Originally, the notion of policy networks was used to describe continuity in many fields, given the limited number of interests that were involved in the policymaking process. This continuity did not necessarily refer to policy outcomes, but more often to the groups involved in the process. Moreover, usually, the existence of a common interest – which according to some can reduce transaction costs (See Jordan 1990) – and the common values among members, further contributed to the stability and continuity of some forms of policy networks (See Haas 1992). For their part, and based on their empirical analyses Marsh and Rhodes (1992) have defined these networks as non-exclusive. In fact, the network can be permeable depending on the extent to which different groups are consulted.

Similar to the case of Marsh and Rhodes's (1992) definition of a policy network, the current division of the network between core and periphery indicates a distinction among the network's members based on access to financial resources and actual political power or influence on it.[43] Thus, in examining networks, and as suggested by Knoke et al.'s (1996) work, we will also be looking at the institutionalization of power relations within both the network and the broader socio-economic and political context. For the purposes of the current analysis, power is defined as a relational concept between individuals, groups or agencies. Although there are various definitions of power, we adopt the widely held view that a power relationship exists where A is able to get B to do something that the latter would not otherwise do (See Weber 1948; Dahl 1957). Power can also be defined in a negative sense, that is the ability to thwart B's wishes by preventing some issues from entering the political agenda (See Bachrach and Baratz 1970). Force, of course, can be one way of bringing about change or effecting action, but there are subtler ways as well. Therefore, in the analysis that follows, we will be looking for manifestations of dominance, manipulation or persuasion in the process of HIV/AIDS policymaking. Additionally, in a situation such as the transition to democracy in Mexico, it is expected that the distribution of power might be changing. Very concretely, one would expect the distribution of power to change from being more concentrated in a few state actors to being more dispersed among a greater number of individuals, groups, and agencies.

In adopting a policy network approach, it is important to say that although it does not represent an entirely new analytical framework, it does help in softening the opposition between pluralism[44] and corporatism,[45] placing them at the two extremes of a continuum (Hassenteufel 1995, p.94).[46] In fact, Marsh and Rhodes (1992, p. 3-4) argue that the recent interest in policy networks is partly due to some of the limitations of the pluralist and corporatist models. They also underline the fact that this type of analysis facilitates the study of varying government-interest group

---

[43] Given that policy network analysis has traditionally helped to explain continuity in public policies, Wilks and Wright (1995) recognize that some efforts are needed in order to allow the policy network analysis to be able to explain change and its effects on policies. Therefore, it is necessary to pay attention to the effects of macro variables on policy networks and of these networks' impact on policies at the macro level.

[44] Under the 'pluralist' approach the state is seen as a product of society (See Dahl and Lindblom 1953; Dahl 1971), emphasizing the role of interest groups in initiating and pressing for policy outputs (See also Truman 1951). Interest groups use various mechanisms -such as parties, the legislature, bureaucracies, and the press, etc.- to express competing demands and preferences. Policy is then the reflection of the shifting alliances and coalitions of the more powerful pressure groups.

[45] Corporatism is defined as a formal relationship between selected groups or institutions and the government (See Schmitter 1974). Under corporatism, welfare policy is seen as initiated by a small and closed elite that operates in entrepreneurial fashion to anticipate or even consciously mould the demands of various sectors of society. Furthermore, policy is the product of elite groups that play a relatively autonomous, architectural role. This elite sponsors welfare programs as means by which to undermine and/or co-opt opposition forces and to strengthen the loyalty of beneficiary groups to the state (See Malloy 1979; Rimlinger 1971).

[46] Amongst its critics, Robinson (1997) argues that policy network analysis is not adequate to studying agenda setting. He maintains that the advocacy coalition framework of Paul Sabatier's (1988, 1991, Sabatier and Smith 1993) constitutes a scheme capable of incorporating multiple levels of government, policy networks and dynamic systemic events, and that it contributes to explaining the factors that slowdown change and assure the independence of the network. For our analysis though, we prefer to adopt Robert Watt's (1997) position. He says that we can either reject one by one the community networks, the policy networks and the advocacy coalition approaches, or else combine them in order to deepen our knowledge and understanding of the policy making process.

relations across different policy areas (See also Le Gales and Thatcher 1995). Traditionally, the emphasis has been on the middle-level of analysis that this concept allows for.[47] Yet it is important to remember that the middle-level cannot be separated from the macro and micro levels, without which it simply loses explanatory capabilities.[48] As suggested by Marsh (1995, p. 161), it must provide a link between the micro-level analysis, which deals with the role of interests and government in relation to particular policy decisions, and the macro-level analysis, which is concerned with broader questions concerning the distribution of power within contemporary society. For most pioneering analysts of policy networks (See Coleman and Perl 1999; Hass 1992; Hassenteufel 1995; Jordan 1990; Marsh and Rhodes 1992), major changes in public policies are triggered by economic or political transformations, variations in party or government ideology, knowledge evolution or the influence of international actors and institutions. This way of conceptualizing change in public policies is crucial for the study of HIV/AIDS and health–related policies in Mexico, given the recent alternation in power at the federal level through electoral democracy and the increasing influence of external factors associated with globalization.

In order to complete our definition of policy networks, it is also necessary to make an explicit distinction between these and policy communities. At first, the two concepts were interchangeable and served to describe the close links or ties that existed between public officials and organizations of interest groups that were somehow favoured. Along with Coleman and Perl (1999), however, we argue that there is considerable value in treating policy communities and policy networks as two separate, albeit interdependent, phenomena. Thus, we propose using the term *policy community* in reference to *all the stakeholders in a policy arena or domain.*[49] For its part, the policy network includes only those members of the larger policy community who share public power and financial resources.[50] In fact, some subset of actors within a policy community will be directly participating in the making of policy choices, becoming part of the policy network, while others will inevitably remain at the edge or outside of it. Those actors who become members of the policy network

---

[47] It has been used to analyze national elite networks working at the transnational level (Moore 1978), as well as in the elaboration of sub-sectoral policies in different areas in the European Union (Peterson 1994, 1995). Additionally, other works have focused on the analysis of central policies (Marsh and Rhodes 1992), as well as intergovernmental (Rhodes 1988) and local ones (Wilks and Wright 1995, Evans and Davies 1997).

[48] The use of the concept has been adopted in the analysis of public policy making -agenda setting, evaluation of alternatives, policy formulation, policy implementation, and policy evaluation - in different regions. In particular, "the German and the Dutch literatures seem to be more ambitious, treating networks as a new form of governance; in this sense as an alternative to markets and hierarchies" (Marsh and Smith, 2000, p.4). In contrast, the British and the U.S. literatures are narrower in focus, and they tend to concentrate more on the role networks play in the development and implementation of policy.

[49] As indicated in Coleman and Perl's (1999) analysis, policy communities form around policy problems that involve complex political, economic and technical tasks.

[50] See Knoke et al (1996), for the analysis of power relations within policy networks.

engage in more intimate and frequent exchanges involving the sharing of information, expertise, and political support.

There are other important features that distinguish the policy network analysis from others, such as the fact that it does not approach the state as an abstract and homogeneous entity, but as a set of concrete state actors (some of whom, together with non-state actors, are members of the policy network). It emphasizes the importance of learning more about the internal processes of decision making within organizations. It also downplays the linear and sequential vision of the process of public policymaking, and it emphasizes the importance of the implementation stage, in which decisions are made and problems reformulated (Hassenteufel 1995, p. 96). Furthermore, the policy network approach facilitates the analysis of specific sectors or policy arenas, given that most of these networks are established within the core of issue domains such as education and health. In the analysis of sectoral networks, however, one must avoid the risk of overestimating the separation of policy domains, and take into account the interdependencies between them (i.e. economic vis-à-vis health policies). Additionally, the policy network approach facilitates the understanding of how institutions evolve over time in response to emergent social problems, in periods where the institutions themselves are re-organized, and when institutions are competing for control over important public policies (Baumgartner and Jones 2002, p. 5). In contrast to the use of advocacy networks by Keck and Sikkink (1998) and others, the concept of policy networks incorporates both private and public actors as essential members of the network. In their analysis, the policy network would represent what they call an "action network": that is, the moment when advocacy networks become more strategic and are most likely to achieve their goals (Keck and Sikkink, 1998, p. 5).

For the analysis of Latin America, Judith Teichman (2001, p. 16) has adapted the concept of policy networks - to the study of structural adjustment reforms - to be a set of personalistic relationships among international and domestic actors that functions as the conduits of policy influence. According to Teichman's analysis, "personal relationships and loyalties are key factors in the recruitment and cohesion of policy networks in Latin America" (Teichman 2001, p. 160), which further distinguishes it from its original definition, and adapts it to the realities of the Latin American context. In contrast to her use of the term, and as will be shown in chapter four, the current definition of policy networks significantly differs from Teichman's, mostly regarding the non-exclusionary character of the HIV/AIDS policy network. However, her use of the concept is limited the analysis of market reform, and as such it facilitates the contrast of these networks with those in the health sector. Additionally, Teichman argues that in Latin America, "individuals may (and often do) constitute a policy network before they obtain formal positions in the state, and networks may even survive after governmental network participants have lost their official positions" (Teichman 2001, p. 17). As highlighted by Teichman, in Latin America, the access of a wide variety of societal groups has been restricted in market-reform policies. Also, even though technocrats are often the predominant actors in policy networks, the involvement of non-technocrats (caudillo-type leaders and members of the private sector) distinguishes Teichman's (2001, p. 18) use of the concept of policy network from that of epistemic community (See Haas 1992). As such, the policy network analysis facilitates the "identification of the actors involved, their political calculations, and their responses to powerful constituencies and to policy ideas" (Teichman 2001, p. 18). According to Teichman, another special feature of the Latin American market-reform policy networks is that initially they aimed to break down resistance and lead policy change. Similarly, and in support of her use of policy networks analysis, the aim here is not to substitute the use of shifting coalitions— which has been more commonly used in the analysis of market reforms. The goal is to deepen our understanding of policymaking by way of going inside some of these coalitions.

Additionally, it will be shown that in the context of internationalized policy environments, where different policy domains feature institutionalized connections between sub-national, national, regional and international levels, domestic policymaking is increasingly constrained by international economic, political, and cultural forces (See Coleman and Perl 1999; Cerny 1995). [51] Under these circumstances, the use of middle-level approaches that draw on the policy community/networks analysis provides a promising avenue for explaining policy change induced by globalization.[52] As such, globalization can be expected to vary in its impact on different policy domains and in the undermining of state autonomy. After all, as Coleman and Perl (1999, p. 693) pointed out, "environmental policy, macroeconomic management, the regulation of financial services, international trade rules- all are areas in which effectiveness depends upon states 'pooling' sovereignty or working with autonomous supranational institutions."[53]

Lastly, a central feature of the policy networks approach is that it allows one to look beyond the public-private divide and consider the informal norms and networks that, as pointed out by Evans (1996), make people collectively productive. This, Evans argues, allows one to look at norms of trust and reciprocity that result from networks of repeated interaction and "forces [one to think] about development outside old models" (p. 2).[54] Here, it is important to underline that these norms and the trust

---

[51] In the International Relations literature this has also been discussed; see for example the concept of interdependence in Keohane and Nye (1977), Gourevitch's (1978) 'second image reversed', and Putnam's (1988) 'two-level games'.

[52] Again, in the International Relations literature, the use of the notion of epistemic communities is more common. These are defined by shared beliefs, a set of causal axioms, notions of validity and a common set of policy goals or a policy enterprise, which are often rooted in a specialized discipline or science. All these characteristics often give the epistemic community a transnational membership base.

[53] Yet, as Garrett and Lange (1996) emphasize, it is important to remember that domestic institutions mediate between internationally induced changes in the preferences of domestic actors and policy outcomes. Hence, as the number of veto points in the political regime increases, internationalization pressures will have a more muted effect. Therefore, the changing nature of the state-civil society relations forces us to redefine governance in relation to the analysis of domestic and international policy communities/networks (See Tsebelis 2000).

[54] In his analysis Evans draws from Robert Putnam's (1995) work, and points out that labelling such norms and networks "social capital" allows contemporary theorists to "project primary ties as potentially valuable economic assets" (Evans 1996, p. 2). It is significant also to look at Judith Tendler's (1997) work on

built up from intimate interactions are not restricted to relations within civil society groups (Evans 1996, p. 204), but it extends to state-civil society ones as well. This feature, at the core of the policy networks approach, is key for the current analysis, given that it aims at capturing some of the complex formal and informal interactions among members of the HIV/AIDS networks.

CONCLUDING REMARKS

So far, we have argued that any serious consideration of Mexico's elusive quest for development must incorporate democracy, as well as human rights promotion and enforcement into our analysis, as these phenomena are inextricably intertwined. Furthermore, to look at democracy as an integral part of an elusive quest for development is of particular relevance for a country like Mexico, which has been undergoing a difficult and profound process of economic, political, and social transformations in the last few decades.

On the one hand, democracy is essential for the implementation of social policies that can effectively address the most urgent needs of the population, including an effective response to HIV/AIDS and access to health care. Moreover, the democratic exercise of political and civil rights, particularly those related to the guaranteeing of open discussion, debate, criticism, and dissent, is central to the process of generating informed choices and essential for inducing social responses to economic and social needs. On the other hand, the discussion of development allows us to emphasize the fact that as a middle-income country, Mexico presents significant levels of extreme poverty, inequality, income polarization, and the lack of a consolidated welfare state. And as such, these factors limit the state's capacity to respond to some of the new global health challenges such as the HIV/AIDS pandemic.

When it comes to the global context, and in spite of the strength and the persistent dominance of the globalist agenda, it is possible to find evidence of the broader nature of the phenomenon defined as globalization. The latter process has facilitated the rise of new and the strengthening of old civil society networks, as active social and political actors at the national and international levels. Additionally, the global adoption of the human rights discourse, especially by civil society actors, and their appeal to governments for the fulfilment of their obligations within the international regime, provide some further evidence of globalization's more positive side.

For its part, the adoption and use of the policy networks approach will facilitate the analysis of the process of HIV/AIDS and health-related policymaking and implementation, as part of the broader processes of democratization and development In fact, any attempt to understand the complexities of the changing Mexican reality, and to address the gap between the theory behind development, democratization, and

---

blurred public and private boundaries, in which she argues that there are significant benefits from networks that span the divide between state and civil society, where synergy is produced by the intimate entanglement of public agents and engaged citizens.

human rights promotion on one hand, and the reality of an overwhelming number of people living under dire conditions, on the other, must go beyond the national level of analysis. Increasingly, it has become essential to look at the international environment and the ways in which it influences domestic policies today. Therefore, before moving on to the specifics of the Mexican case, the following chapter will engage in the discussion of the interaction between various domestic and international factors and their impact on health and policy options in the context of globalization and HIV/AIDS.

CHAPTER 2

Globalization, HIV/AIDS, and Human Rights

As argued in the previous chapter, any serious attempt to analyze the evolution of HIV/AIDS and health-related policies in Mexico must be framed within the broader processes of development and globalization. This becomes even more important when one realizes that the recent transformations have been significantly influenced by actors and ideas associated with the latter, and by the dominance of the hegemonic economic discourse and policies associated with both of them. Furthermore, the examination of globalization is essential for the analysis of the impact of HIV/AIDS and the public policies implemented as a response. This facilitates a better understanding of a world reality in which most health matters have become global; both in terms of their reach and in the way they impact on the formulation of national policies.

It is in the context of globalization that the growing links between external and domestic actors have become central to the process of democratization, and to public health policymaking in Mexico and most other countries. On the one hand, the globalist economic agenda has been translated into economic reforms that limit the options for public health policy. On the other, the broader process of globalization has opened up opportunities for transnational co-operation and contributed to the inclusion of a more diverse set of actors in the making of HIV/AIDS policies, and for the visibility of traditionally marginalized sexual minorities. These openings have been further facilitated by the adoption and promotion of a human rights discourse that shows increasing world-wide acceptance and legitimation.

GLOBAL HEALTH AND HIV/AIDS

As we have seen, globalization has accentuated the importance of the international sphere for domestic public health policymaking. Thus, it is necessary to discuss some of the effects that the aforementioned economic and political transformations associated with globalization and globalism have had on health in many LMICs. Among the many factors contributing to the deterioration of health, one can list the increased poverty, rapid urbanization, environmental degradation, inequitable access to health services, and reduced public expenditure on public health infrastructure - some of which have been the result of the implementation of the globalist agenda.

As a consequence of the increasing vulnerability of people in LMICs, some diseases have made a comeback in some of the poorest countries among them - such as cholera and tuberculosis - while others, like HIV/AIDS, have taken a greater toll on their populations. In fact, the HIV/AIDS pandemic can be seen as both a product of and a cause for globalization, linking all regions of the world. As put by David Altman (2001), "HIV/AIDS fits the common understanding of globalization in a number of ways, including its epidemiology, the mobilization against its spread, and the dominance of certain discourses in the understanding of the epidemic" (p. 69). And in a globalized context, the global human rights discourse has proven to be a very effective tool in the struggle against the pandemic, especially in how national and international activists and organizations have strategically framed their agendas.

Global Health

Unfortunately, in spite of the commitment to health care in the official discourse of international development agencies and national governments, figures tell a different story. As we all know, 2015 was the final year for the United Nations (UN) Millennium Development Goals (MDGs), which had been set by all 194 UN government members in 2000, to guide global efforts to end poverty. Among them, health-related goals were central. Yet given the mixed results, in September of that same year countries agreed on new and more ambitious global goals for 2030 at the General Assembly in New York. In addition to committing to accomplish the remaining MDGs, members agreed that the post-2015 agenda needs to tackle emerging challenges including the changing social and environmental determinants that affect public health worldwide.

Among some the achievements reached, however, by the end of 2015 the world was able to turn around the epidemics of HIV, malaria, and tuberculosis, while increasing access to safe drinking water. In particular, when it comes to HIV, new infections reported in 2013 were about 2.1 million people, down from 3.4 million in 2001 (See WHO 2015). Similarly, more than 13 million people received antiretroviral therapy (ARTs) globally. Of these, 11.7 million lived in LMICs (representing 37% of people living with HIV/AIDS there). Although the target of achieving universal access to treatment for HIV will be more challenging. Among other shortcomings, the world failed to meet the MDGs target on access to basic sanitation for all. In fact, around 1 billion people have no access to it and are forced to defecate in open spaces such as fields and near water sources. This puts many people at high risk of diarrheal diseases (including cholera), trachoma and hepatitis.

Admittedly, the proportion of people in good health today is greater than 50 years ago, and some improvements were also made in reducing child undernutrition, maternal and child deaths, and in increasing access to basic sanitation. However, as recognized by the WHO's Director-General, Dr. Margaret Chan, there are wide gaps between and within countries, with large numbers of the world's most vulnerable people without access to quality health services (about one fifth of the global population). Thus, the gap between the Global North and South with regards to health indicators cannot be ignored and must be repeatedly and constantly underlined. For instance, although the overall life expectancy in the world has increased by 17 years over the last half century, in several African countries it has been falling dramatically. This fall is due to the linked pandemics of HIV/AIDS and tuberculosis - exacerbated by the negative effects that the implementation of SAPs had on poverty and health infrastructure (See Yong Kim et al. 2000). Additionally, by the year 2015, in some

LMICs less than 5% of total government expenditure was on health, ranging from an average of 4.4 to 6.7 per cent, compared to a 10.2 per cent in HICs - for Latin America and the Caribbean the average was 7.4 per cent. In the Mexican case, public spending in health represented only 2.8 percent of the GDP (6.9 in Canada; 6.5 in the U.S.; 2.3 in Chile; and 4.3 in Argentina) (UNDP 2015).

Health has always been related to the familiar challenges of poverty, inequality, and resource constraints. Yet an increasingly global dimension on these challenges is becoming more and more apparent, arising from the extensity (geographical reach), density, and intensity of the interconnectedness that characterizes globalization (See Buse et al. 2002). The various global economic crises of the 1980s and 1990s and the economic policies that ensued, for instance, are recognized to have had a profound negative impact on public sector expenditure on health programs such as family planning and basic health services (See Lee et al. 2002). This, in turn, has led to the generalized agreement among public health scholars on the need to re-conceptualize international health in a way that recognizes the effects that both globalization and neo-liberal economic reforms (globalism) have had on peoples' health. For Lee at al. (2002), for example, "international health becomes global health when the causes or consequences of a health issue circumvent, undermine or are oblivious to the capacity of states to address [them] effectively through state institutions alone" (p. 5). Thus, in a context where trans-border externalities in the form of health risks increasingly defy state-centric approaches, global health is concerned with factors that contribute to changes in the capacity of states to deal with the determinants of health (See Buse et al. 2002; Lee and Dodgson 2000). In other words, global health can thus be understood as a concept that refers to the ways in which globalization impacts public health policy and, alternatively, the policies needed to respond to the challenges raised by this phenomenon (Lee et al. 2002, p. 10). As such, the adoption of a global health approach goes beyond the state and incorporates non-state actors in its analysis, including Trans-National Corporations (TNCs), especially pharmaceuticals and private health providers, and civil society groups.

For Fidler (2003), there is a central problem to be dealt with in the discussion of global health, namely the need to provide a rationale for making public health a higher priority on the global diplomatic agenda. With similar preoccupations as the focus of their analysis, Buse et al. (2002) argue that "[t]he foremost challenge [in thinking about health policy in a globalizing world] is the need to define the analytical boundaries of global health more clearly in terms of the particular policy issues raised by globalization" (p. 270). For their part, and back in the last decade of the Twentieth Century, Chen and colleagues (1996) stressed the fact that we were entering an era of global health 'interdependence', the health parallel to economic interdependence, which raises complex questions regarding the additional functions that could be entrusted to international health organizations. In an increasingly globalized world, however, as a matter of law sovereignty remains primarily in individual nation states. As such, national governments retain principal responsibility for the health of their populations. This makes it clear that the success of current health reforms "will depend largely on the building of consensus in the world community about the essential functions of international health organizations, and about a coordinated division of labour among them," including state governments (Jamison et al. 1998, p. 514). The fact is that technical co-operation and development financing for health are increasingly provided in an integrated way between the national and international levels. This trend is particularly evident in the redefinition of some international governmental organizations' missions (e.g., the World Bank and other regional development banks), as they direct growing amounts of their portfolios to health and education.

Obviously, the attention given to health on the international agenda of states is not new. In fact, the nineteenth century brought the initiation of bilateral and regional health agreements, giving way from 1851 onwards to periodic International Sanitary Conferences to promote intergovernmental cooperation on infectious diseases' control. For its part, the creation of the World Health Organization (WHO) in 1946 was fueled by the post-war faith in scientific and technical solutions to defeat ill-health. More recently, however, this strong faith would be seriously shaken by the uncertainty and challenges that accompanied the new phase of globalization of the last few decades (See Lee and Dodgson 2000).

Since its creation, the WHO has been the directing and coordinating body on international health work. Its objective is "the attainment by all peoples of the highest possible level of health", health being defined as "a state of complete physical, mental, and social well-being and not merely the absence of disease or infirmity" (WHO Constitution, 1948, p. 1). Throughout the years, and based on the WHO's founding act, international regimes on public health have been charged with the collection, analysis, and dissemination of information, knowledge, and technical expertise for the member states' benefit (See WHO founding act, 1946). More recently, the WHO launched a new policy, called "Health for All in the 21st Century," the aim of which is to deal with persistent inequalities, both with respect to primary health care[1] and relatively new health challenges (See WHO 1998).

An important reason for explicitly incorporating the analysis of globalization and global health, to the study of HIV/AIDS and health in Mexico, is to bring home the message that the health sector is directly and indirectly affected by other sectors such as trade and finance, the environment, labour, communications and transportation, to name a few. In this context, not only the WHO, but other organizations such as the World Bank and the WTO have also become increasingly important players, and their decisions have a growing influence on public health (See World Bank 1993, 1997; WTO 2001).[2] Similarly, there is an increasing interest on a wide range of determinants of health such as housing, education, water, sanitation, nutrition, energy, health-related services, industrial and agricultural policies (See Bhargava et al. 2000). There are also a growing number of micro and macroeconomic studies establishing

---

[1] Primary health care by the WHO consists of maternal and child care, family planning, immunization, treatment of common diseases, essential drugs, safe water and sanitation, and access to trained personnel, with regular supply of twenty essential drugs, within one hour's travel.
[2] The role of some of these other organizations will be furthered discussed below.

the links between health, productivity, and GDP levels in cross-country comparisons (See Merson et al. 2001).

Ironically, the World Bank, one of the foremost architects of SAPs, is now the single largest lender for HIV/AIDS prevention efforts in Africa and other regions. Somewhat belatedly, the Bank acknowledged the centrality of health and HIV/AIDS for development. During the SAPs era, however, governments were pressured to cut spending and found it easy to reduce expenditures on services for those with little political influence, increasing the vulnerability of marginalized groups to various diseases. Among those diseases, cholera and tuberculosis are other prime examples of the ills of globalist policies; thriving in the midst of increased poverty, and widening inequalities within and across countries as a result of the public sector's shrinking (Lee and Dodgson 2000, p. 214).

It should also be noted that although increased trade has been behind the adoption of new health-related technologies throughout the world, some of them lifesaving, this is not necessarily working to improve human security for all or to reduce the vulnerability of the poor. Instead, it has often resulted in the emancipation of market forces from social and political control, which has come to define the privatization of health care systems for the benefit of mostly better-off individuals (Gray 1998, p. 208). Additionally, world-wide health care reform has focused heavily on enhancing private sources of financing; favouring privately managed individual pensions systems versus policies of collective social responsibility for the aged (See Lee and Goodman, in Buse et al. 2002).

There are other general trends, which have defined health sector reforms at the global level. For its part, the World Bank (1993) has promoted a series of very concrete measures in this area, based in an important way on the experiences of HICs. Three waves of health care reforms have been identified so far (See Cutler 1998; Cutler and Richardson 1998). The first wave took place from the early 1950s until the early 1980s, when most country-members of the Organization for Economic Co-operation and Development (OECD) built their health insurance systems (See Cutler 1998). The growing cost of medical care led to the second wave of reform, which focused on cost containment. Thus, in the midst of the globalist reforms, large-scale limits were imposed on medical spending in the 1980s: pre-determined budgets for hospitals, volume reductions on physicians, and spending limits in public sector institutions. Tight budget constraints led to inefficient provision of services (i.e., long waiting lists) and a growing role for the private sector. As a result, many OECD countries initiated reforms designed to improve the efficiency and responsiveness of their health systems throughout the 1990s (See Hurst 2000; Cutler and Richardson 1998). Some countries concluded that what was necessary was to encourage more of a market rule in medical care provision. Cutler and Richardson (1998) refer to this trend as the third wave of health care reform, which was followed suit by many LMICs' as a response to the "recommendations"/conditionalities of the World Bank (1993). An important question to be asked, for the purposes of our analysis of development and HIV/AIDS, is whether these reforms have been implemented after a thorough analysis of the particular circumstances prevailing in each nation. This is essential if we are to consider the big gap between the Global North and the South mentioned above, and in order to be able to assess the consequences of health-care reforms for the health status of LMICs' populations.

Two other elements characterize the reform of the health sector in LMICs: decentralization and participation. The World Bank has integrated the notion of decentralization as a core element of its own recommendations to LMICs[3] (See Bossert 1997a, 1997b; Mills et al. 1990; Segall 1983). Social or community participation were also introduced as a central element in the process of health care systems reforms (See Ottawa 1986; Jakarta 1997). However, as it relates to the discussion on globalization and globalism, critics have raised some concerns regarding the notion of participation, arguing that, as stated by De Keijzer (1992), states with constrained budgets have been forced to cut back on social spending. This has also forced them to look at participation and self-care as new ways to unload state responsibility and extend coverage at lower costs often charged to communities.

In spite of some of the cautionary considerations that the whole 'participatory' or partnership approach deserves, there are instances where the influence of global social movements has proved to be positive. One such case is the women's health movement, which has positively contributed to the democratization of some policy issues (i.e., family planning and birth control) (Lee and Dodgson 2000, p. 222). Examples like this one show that health policy is not simply a matter of technical knowledge, but the product of political struggles. After all, as put by Farmer and Bertrand in what they call the hypocrisies of development (in Yong Kim et al. 2000, p. 107), "public health action takes place on a terrain of contested meanings and unequal power, where different forms of knowledge struggle for control" (p. 107). It should be clear by now that, as pointed out before, health - as an integral part of social welfare policies - is a key factor for the achievement of sustainable human development. Similarly, for a state to satisfy the needs of its population regarding the promotion and protection of health (which are part of a world-wide consensus) (See PAHO-WHO 1993) it is necessary to address equity issues in the establishment of a national health-care system (See Berman 1995). Reform efforts must incorporate local communities, not with the main intention of unloading responsibilities on them and reducing costs, but in order to incorporate their knowledge and concerns in the very same process of policymaking (See Paul 1995).

In sum, privatization, decentralization, and participation have been essential components of the new global orientation of public policymaking in health. These notions and the implementation of associated reforms have important implications for political economy analyses, due to the increasing interaction of different levels of government, international governmental organizations, national and international civil society groups, and the continuing central role of the state. Admittedly, while the influence of economic, political, and social forces on health has long been recognized, the actual practice of documenting these connections remains rare. Therefore, in order

---

[3] As of July 1999, health reforms were in progress in sixteen Latin American countries—including Mexico—with World Bank and Inter-American Development Bank funding (Tussie and Casaburi 2000, p. 400).

to contribute to filling this gap in knowledge, the present analysis engages in the examination of the specifics of HIV/AIDS and health-related policies.

HIV/AIDS: The Complexities of a Pandemic

The prevailing optimism that characterized the decades after the creation of the WHO was based on the increasing successes at controlling infectious diseases, and culminated in 1978 when its members signed the *Health for All, 2000* accord. The relative success of international efforts such as the expanded program for childhood immunization mounted by the UN Children's Fund (UNICEF), and the WHO's smallpox eradication campaign contributed to this optimism (See Garret 1996). This self-congratulatory mood, however, came to a dramatic end in the 1980s, when an obscure micro-organism that caused an unknown disease (at that time) started to make it to the news. With the discovery of HIV, which causes AIDS, a new era in the fight against infectious diseases came to light. In fact, the HIV/AIDS epidemic has been described as one of the greatest scientific, political, and moral challenges of the last decades. Without any doubt, it can be said that HIV/AIDS has become a central challenge for global health today, since it brought to the fore the need for vigorous international action, and forced the international community to engage in the development of a comprehensive cooperation strategy.

There is a clear association between poverty and HIV/AIDS (See Whiteside and Barnett 2002), and the divide between North and South manifests itself dramatically with respect to the prevalence and effects of the pandemic. As stated at the very outset, as of 2016, 90 per cent of the people with HIV/AIDS were living in LMICs (UNAIDS),[4] and up to this day many of them do not know that they are HIV carriers. Therefore, governments in these countries confront the difficult task of meeting the needs of the population that has been affected by HIV/AIDS without neglecting the needs of those who suffer from other diseases related to poverty. So that on top of the ethical challenges that it poses to the global community, HIV/AIDS entails an enormous loss of human and economic resources and represents a substantial threat to sustainable human development in many LMICs. The accumulated direct (medical) and indirect (loss of productivity) quantifiable global costs of the disease were estimated to amount to US$500 billion by the year 2000 (Garret 1996, p.72). This is partly explained by the fact that HIV/AIDS requires expensive and long-term health care; it mainly affects adults in the most productive years; it raises complex legal and ethical issues; it reaches all segments of society; and it has grown rapidly.

At this point, it is important to remind the reader of some of the figures presented above and expand on the numbers behind the pandemic for the Latin American region. According to the latest data available, since the first cases were identified more than three decades ago, an estimated 34 million people have died from AIDS-related causes so far.[5] An estimated 36.7 million people were living with the Human

---

[4] http://www.unaids.org/en/resources/fact-sheet
[5] See http://www.who.int/features/factfiles/hiv/facts/en/index3.html

Immunodeficiency Virus (HIV) in 2016, with 1.8 million persons being infected that same year and another 1 million losing their lives to Acquired Immune Deficiency Syndrome (AIDS)-related illnesses (UNAIDS [6]). The numbers are particularly staggering for Sub-Saharan Africa, where an estimated 25.8 million people live with HIV, while around 790,000 died due to HIV/AIDS-related causes in 2016 alone. Some countries experience a prevalence rate that exceeds 5 per cent of the total adult population, and some areas have close to 30 per cent of pregnant women infected with HIV. Although the figures for Latin America are far from reaching those levels of infection, there is an increasing concern regarding the need to act promptly to prevent a similar situation among marginalized groups. In recent years, for instance, there has been an important increase in the spread of the disease among the poorer and the least educated sectors of society, although the greater impact has been mainly concentrated in homosexual men, or men who have sex with men (MSM) (See Izazola and Siqueiros 1999; Fórum 2000; Foro 2003, Notiese 2017). According to the epidemiology of HIV/AIDS, in Latin America, which represents 8.4 per cent of the world population, we find 5 per cent of all the people currently infected with HIV in the world. Of this population, 80 per cent is concentrated in 9 countries (Brazil, Mexico, Argentina, Colombia, Venezuela, Honduras, Dominican Republic, Peru, and El Salvador, with Guyana, Haiti, and Honduras being the hardest hit in the hemisphere), of which 18 per cent are women. AIDS has caused approximately 150,000 deaths and has become the most important cause of death among men between the ages of 25 to 44 (which represents a major proportion of the region's productive force) (See UNAIDS; See also Smallman 2007) (More specific figures for Mexico will be presented and discussed in chapter four).

For Latin America, and more particularly for the Mexican case, there is a need to underline the effect that the epidemic has had on sexual minorities and women. These are places – as a region and a country - where the lack of control over the sex behaviour of women's partners, and the role of conservative groups and the Catholic Church regarding sexual behaviour, have had a great negative impact on women's capacity to protect themselves (Hernández Avila et al. 1995, p. 116-117; See also González Ruiz 2002). Similarly, sexual minorities, especially homosexual and bisexual men, or MSM, have faced overt hostility from conservative groups and large sectors of society, which has resulted in discrimination and the violation of their basic human rights (See Galván Díaz et al. 1991; Pecheny 2003; Parker et al. 2003).

At first, nearly every country in the world denied or covered up the presence of HIV within their borders and in some cases, and up to recently, some governments refused to co-operate with the WHO, manipulating incidence reports or denying access to statistics (Garret 1996, p. 74). Thus, misinformation and ignorance have been some of the greatest obstacles for a broad mobilization against HIV/AIDS, breeding passivity, pessimism, resignation, or a sense that the disease is someone else's problem (See Irwin et al. 2003). Significantly, in LMICs, the combination of

---

[6] As we all know, the latest United Nations AIDS (UNAIDS) program's report offers figures for the previous year, but the agency updates its figures more regularly online: http://www.unaids.org/en/resources/fact-sheet.

entrenched poverty, economic inequality, racial discrimination, the subordination of women, discrimination based on sexual orientation, religious prejudices, and other forms of structural injustice (or vulnerability) contribute overwhelmingly to the spread of the HIV infection. The mix of all these factors have rendered prevention efforts less effective than they have been in other settings – namely countries in the Global North (See Farmer 2001, 2003; Whiteside and Barnett 2002).

Under the aforementioned circumstances, it is clear that to educate for the prevention of new infections is not enough; social, political, cultural and economic determinants must be considered and addressed. Admittedly, in recent years, some of the social and political dimensions of issues like discrimination against people based on sexual orientation, the consequences that gender relations have on the negotiation of safe sex, and the correlation between poverty and vulnerability have been increasingly, although not sufficiently, acknowledged. However, it is also important to highlight the fact that at the International HIV/AIDS Conferences[7] there continues to be a limited number of works analyzing social, economic, and cultural variables. And although early on there was a scarce presence and participation of groups representing those living with HIV/AIDS at these conferences, their increasing contributions have been critical. These groups have called the attention - of the international community gathered at those meetings - to the need for holistic approaches in the consideration of proposals to deal with the pandemic. And as a response to some of these demands, the world approach to the disease has gone through three major stages. At the beginning the emphasis was on information for the prevention of new infections. Later on, attention was directed to the significance of reproductive and sexual rights in dealing with the disease. While more recently, after continuous fights by different groups and the learning process itself of the world community working in this area, a more holistic analysis has started to develop.

It is widely known that HIV/AIDS directly affects sexual minorities, who have been highly stigmatized and marginalized in most societies. This explains the fact that the fight against the pandemic has become a catalyst for political mobilization and increased political participation world-wide, and not just in Latin America (See Rayside 1998). Programs around HIV/AIDS have often made use of identities such as sex worker (male and female), or gay/bisexual men/ men who have sex with men, and thus play a part in the further globalization of movements based on such identities (See Altman 2001). Moreover, in some cases, the support and acceptance from international bodies given to HIV/AIDS activists and organizations have allowed them to become firmly established at the national level as well (See Parker et al. 2000). Furthermore, the convergence of a very diverse set of actors, all working together against the pandemic, has been critical for the establishment of official national and international programs on HIV/AIDS. On July 26 of 1994, UNAIDS, for example, a joint and Co-sponsored United Nations Program on HIV/AIDS was established to provide an internationally co-ordinated response to the pandemic. The goal has been to provide global leadership and promote global consensus on policy

---

[7] Annual International Conferences on HIV/AIDS started in Atlanta in 1985.

and programmatic approaches to the fight against HIV/AIDS. As such, UNAIDS is guided by a Programme Co-ordinating Board (PCB) which serves as its governing body. The PCB has representatives of 22 governments from all regions of the world, the 7 UNAIDS Co-sponsors (UNICEF, UNDP, UNFPA, UNDCP, UNESCO, WHO and the World Bank), and 5 NGOs (which rotate yearly), including associations of people living with HIV/AIDS.[8] As such, UNAIDS was the first UN programme to include NGOs in its governing body. Its PCB holds a regular session once a year in Geneva, and it holds thematic sessions outside Geneva in alternate years, as requested by the members. And since its creation, the programme has promoted broad-based political and social mobilization to prevent and respond to HIV/AIDS within countries. Its stated mission is to ensure that national responses incorporate a wide range of sectors and institutions, and to advocate for greater political commitment in responding to the pandemic at the global and country levels, including the mobilization and allocation of adequate resources for HIV/AIDS and health-related activities. Its aim is to help mount and support an expanded response; one that engages the efforts of many sectors and partners from governments and civil society groups.[9]

More recently, at its 37th meeting (26-28 October, 2015), the UNAIDS PCB adopted a new strategy to end the HIV/AIDS epidemic as a public health threat by 2030. Their 2016-2021 strategy is in line with the broader UN Sustainable Development Goals, which also aim at ending the HIV/AIDS pandemic by 2030. The goal is to reach people left behind so far, and it represents an urgent call to front-load investments and to reach the 90–90–90 treatment targets by 2020; 90% of all people living with HIV will know their HIV status, 90% of all people with diagnosed HIV infection will receive sustained antiretroviral therapy, and 90% of all people receiving antiretroviral therapy will have viral suppression.[10]

For its part, the WHO, through its initiative on HIV/AIDS and sexually transmitted infections (STIs) and as a co-sponsor of UNAIDS, strengthens the response of the health sector through the development of norms, standards and guidelines for research, advocacy, technology development, and technical cooperation with countries. The areas covered by its initiative include the following: prevention of HIV and STIs, particularly for those vulnerable and/or at increased 'risk'; ensuring safe blood supplies; vaccine development; surveillance of HIV, AIDS and STIs; and the development and evaluation of STIs/HIV/AIDS policies and programs (See WHO 2003).

As a response to the increasing need for additional efforts, just between 1986 and early 1999, the World Bank committed over US$ 750 million for more than 75

---

[8] For a list of the NGOs that were part of the PCB in 2016, see Appendix 2.1.

[9] The first HIV/AIDS WHO program was the Special Program on AIDS, established in 1986 in order to respond to the emerging HIV/AIDS epidemic. In 1987 the program became the Global Program on AIDS (GPA), which was ultimately dismantled with the creation of UNAIDS. Throughout its 10-year existence, the GPA advocated the need for multi-sectoral response to the epidemic, which the WHO continues to support.

[10] See: http://www.unaids.org/en/aboutunaids/unaidsprogrammecoordinatingboard/PCB37_26-28October2015.

HIV/AIDS projects worldwide, with an ongoing commitment to provide funds for HIV/AIDS (which for the case of Mexico will be later discussed in chapter four).[11] Most of the resources have been provided on highly concessional terms through the Bank's International Development Association. In its policy dialogue with borrowing countries, the World Bank stresses that HIV/AIDS is a development priority and highlights the need for top-level political commitment. Yet, as discussed before, the Bank's commitments to health improvement is often seen to be at odds with its requests for systematic health care reforms.[12]

Unfortunately, in many LMICs there does not seem to be any sustained commitment from public authorities in the fight against the pandemic. In that sense, there is a great need for explicit government commitments for the allocation of financial resources, and more initiatives for the development of national and international collaborative programs. Moreover, obstacles to prevention remain constant in various areas, such as; social inequality, cultural and economic differences, neo-liberal economic reforms, as well as the violation of basic rights in the area of sexuality (See Fórum 2000; Foro 2004; Irwin et al. 2003; Smallman 2007, Torres-Ruiz 2013). Additionally, the refusal of power holders to provide life saving AIDS treatment to poor people has also become an obstacle for the realization of the commitment to 'Health for All' (See Irwin et al. 2003). Not surprisingly then, power relations and their impact on society reveal themselves through the generalized tendency of the pandemic to evolve towards the steady spread into groups that have been highly marginalized and socially disadvantaged; women, children, sexual minorities, migrants, drug users, and the poor in general (See Whiteside and Barnett 2002; Truby 2014). In other words, HIV/AIDS works somehow almost as a highlighter of social vulnerability or lack of human security. Furthermore, the response to the pandemic has confronted the opposition of political actors to some of the measures that need to be taken for its prevention. For instance, in countries such as Mexico, as will be discussed in more detail in chapter four, condom advertising has been a bitterly contested issue. This has brought conservative groups and the Catholic Church into direct conflict with HIV/AIDS activists and the State (Altman 2001, p. 76; See also González Ruiz 2002; Lumsden 1991; Torres-Ruiz 2011, 2013). In order to understand some of these social-power relations and their significance for our analysis, it is necessary to elaborate on the distinction made before between vulnerability and risk. This distinction is central to the analysis of development and health, since risk is generally associated with probability and individual choice, whereas vulnerability is a social concept that reflects structural inequalities; differences based on power and control, as well as socio-economic status, determine social vulnerability. It is evident that by allowing certain groups access to health and health care services, the degree of vulnerability can be reduced. However, it is not surprising to find obstacles to these efforts, given that in most cases access implies

---

[11] See the World Bank's web site: http://www.worldbank.org.

[12] This point is of particular interest for the present analysis, given that the World Bank's agenda on health has also favoured the privatization of the health sector, which some argue goes against concerns such as treatment for all and the strengthening of governments' effective responses to the pandemic.

redistributive strategies. In fact, much of what could be done to control the spread of HIV/AIDS depends on political decisions at the highest levels of governments and international governmental organizations, and is related to the distribution of resources and the setting of priorities.

The fact is that, up to this day, governments are directly responsible for controlling the spread of HIV and for mitigating the impact of AIDS. However, social norms and political interests hinder to a large extent the formulation and implementation of adequate policies. It is therefore necessary that governments and civil society at large acknowledge that measures designed to protect the defenseless against prejudice, intolerance and exploitation will also help to protect the entire population from HIV/AIDS and other sexually transmitted infections. Unfortunately, despite the fact that the HIV/AIDS pandemic had already caused too many deaths, as pointed out by Izazola and Siqueiros (1999, p. 35), there were and still are some public officials, experts, and academics who question whether this epidemic does represent one of the most serious health problems countries around the world face today. The stigma and discrimination associated with the infection contribute to the explanation of some of these attitudes.

For Latin America, international co-operation has represented a fundamental tool in the construction of national responses to the HIV/AIDS pandemic. Throughout the region, international agencies have been developing collaborative efforts with governments and national HIV/AIDS programs (See Fórum 2000; Foro 2003; Turby 2014). Compared to national governments, from very early on in the spread of the pandemic, there seemed to be a greater diversity in the proposals of international agencies, which have also been very active in establishing partnerships with local and national governments and civil society groups (See Child 1999). We have to acknowledge, however, that in some cases the increased economic resources from international institutions have also been a source of difficulties, such as competition and bitter disagreements over funds and their appropriate use among civil society groups (Roberts 1995, p. 260).[13] Similarly, trans-national civil society organizations have also played central roles in the fight against the epidemic. Global groups such as ACT UP,[14] the AIDS Alliance, and the International Lesbian and Gay Association (ILGA), as well as regional and local groups (i.e., 'The Latin American League of People Living with HIV/AIDS'[15]) have actively engaged in the formulation of responses to the disease.

In addition to the urgency that arises from its current and future impact on development, the analysis of the global fight against HIV/AIDS contributes to the understanding of some ongoing transformations of diverse political and social realities. And the study of HIV/AIDS and related policies allows for a discussion of the need to establish a more inclusive process of public policymaking that better

---

[13] More details and current conditions will be provided in this regard for the case of Mexican NGOs in chapter four.

[14] Which was formed in New York in 1987 as an activist group largely concerned with access to treatments for HIV/AIDS.

[15] Liga Latinoamericana de Grupos de Personas Viviendo con SIDA.

responds to the challenges imposed by globalization, further highlighting the links between democracy, vulnerability, health, and sustainable human development. It is under these circumstances that LMICs' officials, Mexico included, are forced to resolve the tension and find the balance between prevention and care, in order to guarantee access to services for the entire population, including those affected by HIV/AIDS, and in accordance to their human rights obligations.

THE NEED FOR A GLOBAL RESPONSE TO THE PANDEMIC

As stated above, globalization can be regarded as both a threat and an opportunity for the pursuit of sustainable human development. On the positive side, and as will be contended in chapter four the Mexican case, globalization has allowed for a growing trans-national co-operation that has resulted in the emergence of a more inclusive HIV/AIDS policy network. On the negative side, however, the globalist agenda has come to represent a set of limitations on the available options for public health policies and the capacity of the Global South to respond to new and old health challenges. Hence, the need to look at the opportunities and limitations associated with globalization, and the importance of understanding the nature of the relationships between international actors and national governments and civil society groups. It is through the identification of the main features of these relationships and the channels through which these develop that it will be possible to assess the impact they have on the formulation of HIV/AIDS policies in Mexico.

Thus, the purpose of this section is to show which external actors and variables influence HIV/AIDS and health-related policies in the present context of globalization. Similar to the subsequent analysis of the domestic arena, attention will be paid here to the role of a variety of actors, from international governmental organizations and trans-national civil society groups, to the private sector. As in the case of the domestic HIV/AIDS policy network, it will be argued that not all policy community actors are members of what is described as a cluster of individuals and groups that form an influential HIV/AIDS policy network or network of networks at the international level. In fact, although some civil society groups have gained access to a seat at the table, others seem to only have a foot in the door, while still others remain outside. It is also important to emphasize that not all external influences have democratic effects. The aim is to determine whether any of these external factors have contributed to an open competition among a set of realistic and functionally alternative policies that are meaningfully different and reflective of citizens' needs and preferences.

As outlined before, globalization has had a major impact on the internationalization of health issues – giving rise to what has been referred to as global health and internationalized policy environments. In discussing the challenges faced by most states with respect to health protection and promotion in the context of today's globalization, one has to keep in mind the effects that the increased mobility of people across borders has had on the spread of diseases around the globe. The recent global health scares associated with the inter-continental spread of the West-

Nile Virus (1999-2002/2003), SARS (2003), Ebola (1976/2014), Zika (2015/2016), the increasing presence of some drug-resistant strains of tuberculosis, and of course, HIV/AIDS itself are only some concrete and recent examples and reminders of this reality. In this new context, faster and cheaper means of transportation have accelerated the rates of dissemination of these and other diseases, increasing the need for international co-ordinated actions related to global health and the well-being of the world's population.

Not surprisingly, as it is the case with globalization and its impact on other aspects of today's national realities, the debate regarding its effects on health is also polarized. On the one hand, there are those who argue that globalization provides opportunities to create renewed commitments to global health (See Yatch and Bettcher 1998), whereas others put more weight on the damaging effects of global markets on health (See Abbasi 1999; Berman 1995; Chen, Evans, and Cash 1999; Commission on Macroeconomics and Health 2001; Navarro 1998; Shakow and Irwin 2000). For instance, in their analysis, Chen, Evans, and Cash (1999) illustrate the consequences and probable impact of some of the major factors of globalization on the health of individuals and nations (i.e., macroeconomic policies, travel and migration, environmental degradation, unfair trade, and drug patents). As part of the environment within which health policy networks operate, there is also an increasingly important regime framework based on trade agreements and organizations that significantly influence and condition HIV/AIDS and health-related policymaking. In the case of Mexico, for example, the North-American Free Trade Agreement (NAFTA) and the WTO are of particular significance, given their implications for the transformation of the health sector through a dominant globalist agenda and increasing private foreign investment.

For the purposes of the current analysis and under the present global circumstances, it will be argued that, regardless of the conclusions reached in our assessment of the impact of globalization on people's health, it has become more problematic to draw a dividing line between international and domestic health agendas. Among other reasons, this problem arises from the difficulty in defining a single legitimate authority with the ability to exercise public policy for a common purpose, be it at the global, regional, national, or local level. This difficulty originates in the various current responses to global health issues, which have been characterized by the creation of networks and partnerships involving a host of new and old actors. Thus, it is necessary to recognize that, as argued by Jamison, Frenk, and Knaul (1998), although the responsibility for health remains primarily national, the determinants of health and the means to fulfil that responsibility are increasingly global. Furthermore, in the context of countries like Mexico, where major political transformations are taking place, it has become even clearer that external societal and institutional support for change has to be considered as central in the context of globalization, and for all sorts of different issues, including health. As argued by Fox (in Evans 1997, p. 139), a good and to some extent extreme example of the centrality of external/global support for the search of a negotiated solution to local problems is the case of the Zapatista (EZLN) uprising of 1994 in Chiapas. In this case, the attention and support from international civil society groups, the media, and the global community at large were essential in order to maintain the necessary political space for the Zapatistas to survive and contain the immediate authoritarian backlash.[16]

In the case of a world health crisis such as HIV/AIDS, the global response has involved a diverse set of actors and has been central to the strengthening of local vulnerable groups. In fact, external support has served as a catalyst for the empowerment and inclusion of civil society groups in the process of public policymaking at the domestic level. As such, it will be argued too, that the formation of the domestic HIV/AIDS policy network would not have been possible without external support. Furthermore, it is highly probable that by way of establishing strong links with the international HIV/AIDS policy community and network(s), the domestic side has been able to secure its own survival in the long term. And as a consequence, the inclusion of a more diverse set of actors in the process of HIV/AIDS policymaking positively contributes to Mexico's elusive quest for human rights, democratization, and development.

INTERNATIONAL HEALTH POLICY NETWORKS

When domestic networks establish strong linkages with the international community, this can give rise to the formation of international policy networks as well, or to the incorporation to already existing ones. However, according to the present analysis, it will be argued that international policy networks are not very integrated yet, and they seem to be relatively less institutionalized than their domestic counterparts. In fact, domestic policy networks continue to retain the initiative in various stages of the policymaking process. Yet some of these domestic networks draw on advice and support from international or trans-national policy communities and networks when necessary. Thus, it is important to determine whether we have witnessed the formation of an international HIV/AIDS policy network, and the extent to which this has been a catalyst for further participation and democratization in this policy area in Mexico.

One of the main assumptions of the policy network analysis is that whenever international actors concur in the formation of international policy networks, they tend to exert significant influence on the formulation and implementation of policies at the domestic level. In doing so, they have an impact on the broader transition or transformation of a national political system (See figure 2.1, below), beyond their influence on specific policy domains (e.g., HIV/AIDS or market reforms). And one would expect the presence of various policy networks formed around different health issues (e.g., HIV/AIDS, health care financing, reproductive health, etc.) (See figure

---

[16] This refers to the immediate reaction of the then president Carlos Salinas de Gortari's government (hours after the uprising) – the bombing of some areas in Chiapas – and the subsequent military presence in the state, with the widely known actions of paramilitary cacique-supported killings (See González 1995; Womack 1999). Under a more 'closed' regime, with a more controlled media (See Hughes 2000) and a less interconnected world (i.e. Mexico during the 1968 Tlatelolco crisis), the Mexican government would have been able to act in a more violent and decisive way against the insurgents.

2.2, below). Furthermore, some members of the HIV/AIDS policy network have played a central role in the gains made regarding access to ARVs and other drugs essential for HIV/AIDS treatment.

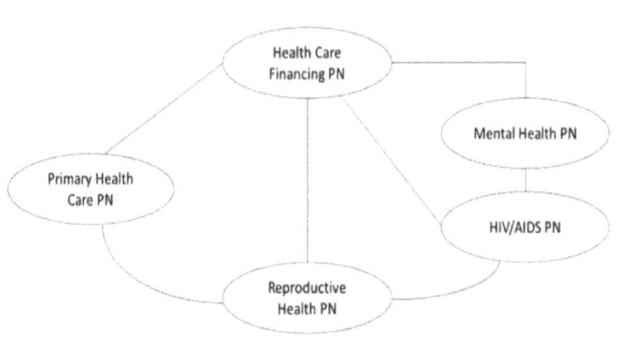

Figure 2.2 - International Health Policy Networks (PN)*

* Elaborated by the author, based on the current analysis

In fact, it will be argued, in chapter four, that the very same formation of a domestic network and its strengthening are explained by the establishment of strong linkages with external actors. In this sense, the transformation of the domestic process of policymaking in this area is directly explained by the presence of a domestic and an international policy network working together. It is important to emphasize, however, that the linkages between different members of the international HIV/AIDS network tend to be both formal and informal and, some could argue, somehow less institutionalized than at the domestic level. In contrast to the Mexican case where, as we will see, a defined group of NGOs – those with the expertise, long experience, and strong formal and informal links with public officials – remain at the core of the network, NGO membership on the Program Co-ordinating Board (PCB) of UNAIDS is of a rotating character. At the international level, some non-state actors play the role of interest groups and are situated outside the network (i.e., pharmaceuticals and socially conservative groups), while others participate in the creation and functioning of the policy network and are positioned at the core or the periphery (i.e., rotating NGO members of the UNAIDS PCB).

In the context of internationalized policy environments, there are relevant actors involved in the fight against HIV/AIDS that are considered as non-state actors: Trans-National Corporations (TNCs) and health NGOs, consultancy firms, research institutions, international philanthropists, religious and other social movements. In several areas of health policy, particular ideas and values have emerged from some or all of these different actors, concerning the role of the state and its perceived responsibilities to finance and provide health care (See Lee and Goodman, in Merson et al. 2001).[17] And domestic policymaking is increasingly constrained by international economic, political, and cultural forces. For instance, in international policy debates, universal access to health care and affordable drugs seems to be at odds with the globalist ideology of market fundamentalism and the privatization of health. Yet the orthodoxy of privatization exists alongside the growing recognition, by some, of the need to pay a closer look at the relationships among social justice, wealth, and health (See Sen 1997; Daniels, Kennedy and Kawachi 1999; Kapstein 1999). These different views are also reflected in the way alternatives are presented between more biomedical solutions and the urgently required actions to deal with the socio-economic determinants of health in LMICs. In fact, some analysts speak of the economization of the political state. However, states are trapped, says Rosecrance (in Kaul et al. 1999, p. 203), "in the international coils of economics," affecting all sorts of issues, including health and the response to HIV/AIDS.[18] This significantly explains governments' paradoxical behaviour in international organizations, witnessed in the debates on the floors of WHO's decision-making bodies on essential drugs, or at the discussions at the WTO's on TRIPS,[19] regarding tobacco control, and breast milk substitutes (Kickbusch and Buse 2002, p. 717).

The Health Care Financing Policy Network

A good and comparatively well-researched example of an international health policy network is the one formed around health-care financing; a brief discussion of which will help us to contrast it with the HIV/AIDS policy network. As such, the analysis of the health care financing policy network will contribute to the discussion of the globalist agenda's impact on health issues. It will also allow us to emphasize the contrast in the views and positions of organizations such as the World Bank and the World Health Organization.

Over the last two or three decades, health-care financing, or the mobilization and use of financial resources in the health sector, in countries at different levels of per capita income has been under close scrutiny. In fact, it was the publication of "Financing Health Services in Developing Countries: An agenda for reform" (World Bank 1987) that opened an active debate both within and outside the Bank on the role

---

[17] Significant efforts have been made to understand the international changing environment. The former Mexican Secretary of Health, Julio Frenk (1995), for example, has presented a comprehensive policy analysis, and pointed to the porous nature of national-level health policymaking, and the importance of actors and forces that cross over state borders. Similarly, Walt (In Merson et al. 2001) has extended pluralist theory to the international level in her description of international health policy networks.

[18] As discussed before with regards to globalization and globalism (chapter one), the preponderance of economics has been behind the shift of power in most nations, from the Ministries of Health to the Ministries of Finance (See Berlinguer 1999). This shift has been reflected in decisions made concerning the reforming of health care systems and public spending in health.

[19] Agreement on Trade-Related Aspects of Intellectual Property Rights.

of economics in health development. The discussions that followed laid the groundwork for the World Bank's World Development Report of 1993: "Investing in Health." In it, the Bank identified four major problems with several national health care systems: 1) the misallocation of funds to less cost-effective interventions; 2) inefficient use of funds; 3) inequity in access to basic health care, and; 4) the explosion of health care costs, which were outpacing GDP growth in most countries. Its policy recommendations included shifting the focus of government investment away from tertiary care toward public and primary health, introducing private or limited social insurance plans, and fostering competition in the delivery of health services (Abbasi 1999, p. 690).

At first, the undermining of the fundamental principle of universal access to basic and public health-care alarmed some health professionals. According to Lee and Goodman (in Merson et al. 2001), there was a significant debate even within the Bank regarding the predominance of public health concerns versus economic matters. Not surprisingly, whereas the World Bank's report of 1987 represented a more economics-defined agenda for health care financing reform, the World Development Report (1993) was a retreat from it. And although the World Bank's position on health remains a point of debate, there was a stronger emphasis on human capital and social sector lending, which suggested continued efforts at reconciling the different factions within the Bank (See Merson et al. 2001). Later on, other regional players became more active in the field of health care financing. For instance, some argue that the Inter-American Development Bank's incursions into health-care financing were due to former World Bank's economist Nancy Birdsall's moving to serve as director of health of the continental institution in 1993 (Lee and Goodman 2001, p. 113). For its part, the Pan-American Health Organization was not an active player until the mid-1990s, after boasting two or three health economists at its headquarters in Washington D.C., and at the country level throughout the region. In general, civil society groups were absent from this debate, with the exception of some academic institutions, which will be mentioned below.

In looking at the formation and functioning of the health-care financing policy network, the link between the training and research at certain institutions and the propagation of policy ideas becomes clearer. It also has some resemblance with the formation and operation of the market reform policy networks discussed before (See Teichman 2001). The health care financing policy network has been characterized by a relatively small and tightly integrated group of policy makers, technical advisers and scholars who have defined and shaped the content and process of policy reform. In the United States, the foreign Aid and Development Agency (USAID) took the lead by funding projects in a number of U.S. universities (e.g., Harvard and Johns Hopkins). These included influential work on community financing in Senegal (1978) and prepayment schemes in Bolivia (1984-5) (Lee and Goodman, in Merson et al. 2001, p. 105). As a consequence, the period between 1987 and 1993 saw a significant increase in policy work on health-care financing, with the World Bank substantially developing its technical expertise and taking a leading role in influencing policy debates, and in expanding the role of the market in the health sector. Despite its official role as a full partner of the World Bank, the WHO remained a relatively low-key player during that period. In fact, the WHO had limited expertise in health economics, which continued to be the case into the 1990s. This was partly a reflection of its lack of financial resources for health development relative to the World Bank. For example, the WHO increasingly relied on extra-budgetary funds from donors with short-term financial commitments, more significantly the U.S. and other European countries.[20]

The emergence of new challenges and the competing role of the World Bank fueled the growing dissatisfaction with the role that the WHO was playing. Consequently, the debate on health-care financing forced the WHO to shift its almost exclusive focus on the delivery of primary health-care to other areas, including the financing of health-care systems. Attempts to reform the organization were initiated in 1992, by the then Director General Hiroshi Nakayima. Yet the scope, nature, and pace of change were limited and deemed to be slow due to the continuing lack of international financial support (Walt, in Merson et al. 2001, p. 684). In 1998, with the appointment of Gro Bruntland, a prominent international figure, as the new Director General, there was a collective sigh of relief in the international health community. The WHO began to expand its links with other actors beyond states - looking for an increased and more diverse participation in health co-operation and new partnerships - such as civil society groups and the private sector (See Merson et al. 2001). Eventually, the WHO began working on the improvement of planning of health finances in collaboration with Brian Abel-Smith at the London School of Economics, as well as with Peter Mach and Anne Mills at the London School of Hygiene and Tropical Medicine. Some of the funding for this work came from the then United Kingdom's Overseas Development Administration (now Department for International Development) (Lee and Goodman, in Merson et al. 2001, p. 105). One of the WHO's main primary recommendations in the area of health-care financing was the introduction of a list of essential drugs to be guaranteed by the public sector, especially in primary health-care facilities (Walt, in Merson et al. 2001, p. 681).

With time, the health-care financing policy network extended and found its base on those two different hubs. The Washington hub of institutions (supported by the World Bank and USAID) focused on Latin America, the Philipines, Egypt and Francophone Africa, while the London hub's research (centred on the WHO) was especially directed to Southern and East Africa, and Thailand. As a result, there have been a series of promotions of students, who attended the respective academic institutions, to policy-making positions in LMICs or international health

---

[20] In the 1990s, 10 countries provided 90 per cent of these funds, increasing the risk of placing the organization in the thrall of those who gave it the money (Walt, in Merson et al. 2001, p. 683). This situation triggered an investigation on the role of such funds, which cautiously concluded that there was some truth in the assertion that a small number of donors to WHO were 'driving health policy' (See Walt, in Merson et al. 2001; Vaughan et al. 1996). As a result of its lack of economic "expertise," the WHO continued to focus on administration and management of health care at a time when the World Bank and even the UNICEF were exploring user fees and other sources of finance. Traditionally, for the WHO, primary health care was to be supported by public financing (Lee and Goodman, in Merson et al. 2001, p. 109).

organizations. From there, members of the policy network have built collaborative links with the institutions where they were trained (Lee and Goodman, in Merson et al. 2001, p. 115). And as it has been the case with other policy areas, a prominent feature of this global policy network has been the existence of a 'revolving door' of career progression, which has facilitated the movement of individuals between national and international institutions.

The study of the links among policy networks' members helps us to understand the way in which policy ideas and practice are being propagated. One question that emerges from this analysis is whether the leadership (individual and institutional) is representative of the various interests affected by policy changes. The case of health-care financing, for instance, suggests that world-wide reform in this area has been fostered by the emergence of a policy elite rather than a rational convergence of health needs and solutions. In this case, it can be argued that there is little evidence of a major opening up in the decision-making space for a wider range of individuals and groups. In fact, a central and missing debate is the one regarding the boundaries of collective responsibility for health, which would allow different LMICs to indicate what parts of health care should be financed by society at large. Yet, as it is structured today, the health-care financing policy network resembles more an epistemic community: a network of professionals with recognized expertise and competence in a particular domain and an authoritative claim to policy-relevant knowledge within that domain or issue-area.[21] This policy network is global in the sense that it includes a broad range of state and non-state actors across high, middle, and lower-income countries, and like Cox's (1987) definition of a trans-national managerial class, it encompasses public officials in national and international agencies involved with economic management. Together, and in most cases as defenders of the globalist agenda, they serve as the foci for generating the policy consensus for the maintenance and defense of the system.

By looking at the global health-care financing policy networks, we become aware that their emergence should not be automatically equated with wider participation and representation in decision-making, as has also been shown in the case of market-reform networks in Latin America (See Teichman 2001). Yet the same network analysis can help us to uncover cases of policy domains in which there are signs of emerging policy networks that are relatively more inclusive and responsive to a broader set of interests and actors. Thus, the need to turn now to the formation of international HIV/AIDS policy networks, as a contrasting case that presents us with a situation in which globalization has allowed the formation of a different and more diverse type of association.

---

[21] Individuals in an epistemic community usually have a shared set of (a) normative and principled beliefs; (b) causal beliefs; (c) notions of validity; and (d) a common policy enterprise.

The Emergence and Operation of International HIV/AIDS Policy Networks

It is in the context of global health policy debates that the case of HIV/AIDS is unique in the establishment of partnerships, alliances, and networks of a different nature. It is important to clarify that as such, partnerships and alliances tend to involve more formalized agreements and at times sporadic or temporary coalitions, while networks represent a looser grouping of parties (individuals, organizations, and agencies) organized generally on a non-hierarchical basis around some common and long-term issues or concerns. The prototype partnership in the health sector was established by the pharmaceutical Merck & Company for the donation of its drug Mectizan (ivermectin) to treat onchoceriasis (river blindness) (Kickbusch and Buse 2002, p. 721). For its part, the 'International AIDS Vaccine Initiative' represents a partnership between the World Bank, UNAIDS, private sector sponsors (e.g., Levi Strauss), private laboratories, the development agencies of the Swiss and British governments, numerous foundations (i.e., The Gates Foundation) and academia (Buse and Walt, in Merson et al. 2001, p. 45).[22] As argued by Kickbusch and Buse (in Buse et al. 2002), these new partnerships and alliances, which have been created around a single disease, raise the hopes for other NGO initiatives and policy networks to follow the same pattern. They further argue that these types of alliances seem to be more successful when they address a single high-profile issue; when their goals are clearly specified, time-bound, and measurable, and can be well presented in the media (Kickbusch and Buse, in Buse et al. 2002, p. 722). After all, as put by Walt (in Merson et al. 2001, p. 677), all countries seem to have a direct stake in the health of people around the world, either due to the enduring traditions of humanitarian concern or to the compelling reasons of "enlightened" political self-interest.

It is under circumstances of state and civil society groups engagement with international actors in the fight against HIV/AIDS that we have seen the emergence of at least one clearly identifiable international HIV/AIDS policy network (or a network of networks), that is: a cluster or set of clusters of interdependent domestic and international organizations and individual actors connected to each other by resource dependencies, with a core (UNAIDS – including NGO members of its Programme Co-ordinating Board -, and two of its sponsors; the WHO, and the World Bank) and a periphery (National HIV/AIDS programs and various other International NGOs and local networks), who participate in the formulation and implementation of a set of policies, with frequent interactions and a common interest (See figure 2.3, below). Here, it is important to underline one of the components of the definition, namely the fact that a network is formed by a cluster or a set of clusters of individuals and groups.

---

[22] The International AIDS Vaccine Initiative (IAVI) was established in 1996. It aims to ensure the development of safe, effective, accessible, preventive HIV vaccines for use throughout the world. As such, IAVI is an international non-profit NGO governed by a board of 12 members representing scientists, public sector member organizations, policy-makers and industry leaders. In 1999 the Global Alliance for Vaccines and Immunization (GAVI) was set up to fulfill the right of every child to be protected against vaccine-preventable diseases of public health concern. GAVI is a partnership between multilateral and bilateral agencies, the private sector, philanthropic foundations, the research and development community, and LMICs (Walt in Merson et al. 2001, p. 689).

As such, although we do refer to an international HIV/AIDS policy network in the singular, it can also be argued that what we have is a set of various HIV/AIDS policy networks with strong links among them. Based on the analysis of the international reality, however, and in order to facilitate the analysis of the interaction between the domestic and the international level, it will be argued that there is a network that is particularly influential.

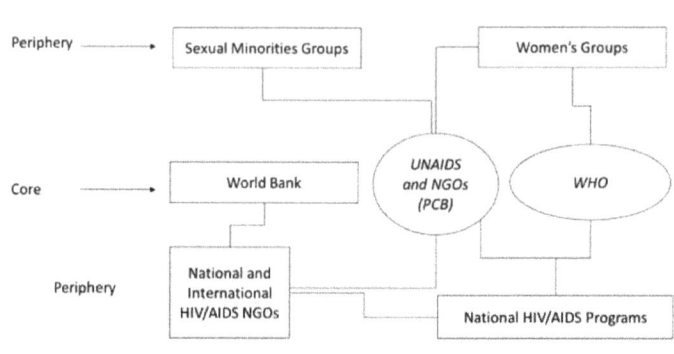

Figure 2.3 - International HIV/AIDS Policy Network*

Elaborated by the author, based on the current analysis

This is a network that is relatively less institutionalized than the domestic ones (i.e. the one in Mexico), which is characterized not so much by its policymaking power but more as being a source of guidelines, recommendations, and financial support for domestic policy networks to succeed in their endeavors. One of the challenges faced in the analysis of the international HIV/AIDS policy community and network is the difficulty in assessing or quantifying the degree of collaboration between the state, civil society groups, and international actors, given that it is defined by various formal and informal coordination mechanisms. What has become clear in the case of HIV/AIDS, however, is the presence of increasingly significant global interconnections, where the state and civil society groups have engaged in new forms of co-operation. For its part, the state, as one of the central actors, is entangled in a complex set of relationships with many different organizations at international, regional, and national levels.

For their part, civil society groups working on HIV/AIDS have also increasingly engaged in the establishment of complex relationships with their counterparts and intergovernmental organizations at the global level. This has been the result of two different forces. On the one hand, we have the actions taken by major donors, throughout the 1990s and into the 2000s, to broaden their focus on NGOs and the funding of a wider range of civil society groups, whose members often participated in lobbying and other political activities. In some cases, support for such groups was seen as a way to build up democracy (Walt, in Merson et al. 2001, p. 687). In fact, some bilateral organizations, such as USAID, decided to provide all their funding through NGOs, rather than governments, leading to an explosion of NGO activity at both the country level and internationally. Other institutions, such UNAIDS, have worked through co-operation with both state programs and civil society organizations. On the other hand, as will be discussed below, civil society organizations have actively sought increased participation in decision making at the national and international level.

Of major significance for the current analysis is the fact that the UNAIDS Programme Co-ordinating Board (PCB), which serves as its governing body, includes at least 5 different NGOs every year. NGO representatives from national and international organizations working on HIV/AIDS and associations of people living with HIV/AIDS are elected, by all members present at one of the two biannual meetings of the general assembly, based on their expertise and long-term engagement in the fight against the pandemic.[23] At least one organization from each of the five major geographic regions (Africa, Asia/Pacific, Europe, Latin America/Caribbean, and North America) must be elected each time. Thus, through its PCB, UNAIDS has allowed a significant number of NGOs to position themselves at the core of the policy network (See figure 2.4, above). Furthermore, and as will be shown in chapter four, the incorporation of the NGO community within the UNAIDS structure served as an example and as leverage for the efforts of domestic civil society groups that resulted in the creation of the NGO Department within Mexico's HIV/AIDS program (CENSIDA). It is possible then to establish significant parallels between the domestic and the international policy network, both in terms of the establishment and

Figure 2.4 - Linkages between Domestic and International Policy Networks*

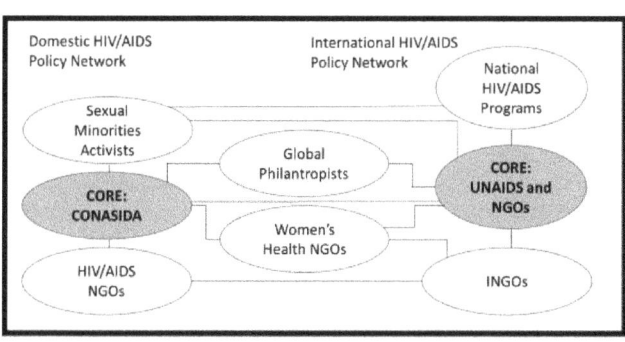

* Elaborated by the author, based on the current analysis of the interaction between the domestic and the international environments.

institutionalization of the linkages between civil society groups and governmental bodies (See figure 2.4, above).

---

[23] Of the two biannual meetings, one of them takes place in Geneva, while the other one changes location, trying to cover all regions in cycles of five years.

It is necessary to underline that the nature and strength of the linkages between domestic and international actors working on HIV/AIDS in Mexico make it very difficult to disentangle the domestic from the international policy network. In fact, as we will see below, civil society groups as much as state actors have established a very strong network of relationships with their international counterparts. Therefore, it is mainly for analytical purposes that the analyses of the domestic and the international are presented separately. In this case, and in contrast to the previously mentioned two-level game analysis of Putnam's (1988; See also Evans et al. 1993), and the more limited win-sets that derive from it, the HIV/AIDS policy network analysis portrays a different set of dynamics. As such, it represents a relatively new reality in which domestic actors have firmly positioned themselves in this policy domain, through the establishment of institutionalized linkages, both domestically and internationally. Furthermore, often these linkages represent horizontal partnerships between many different actors, including the state, UN agencies, industry, and NGOs, which make them of a different and more inclusive nature than past experiences in Mexico. What is characteristic of this set of circumstances, which Castells (1996 and 2010; 1998) calls "the age of the network," is the fact that in spite of the globalization of some issues, this has been paralleled by the localization of polity. In other words, we are witnessing the participation of civil society groups locally and an increasing activism at the global level.[24]

For their part, and as the two main sponsors of UNAIDS with the required expertise in health issues and their respective programs on HIV/AIDS, the WHO and the World Bank find themselves at the core of the various international clusters of actors that are part of the policy network. As key actors in an increasingly globalized reality and as providers of funding, these International Governmental Organizations (IGOs) play a major role in facilitating or hindering the dialogue and exchange of experiences among different nations, especially regarding the health-care conditions prevailing within their own borders and the possible solutions to their existing problems. Thus, it is necessary to refer to some major differences in their approach to health. On the one hand, and until recently, as a strong supporter and promoter of the globalist agenda, the World Bank's policy recommendations had a negative impact on access to health-care services, and have put access to treatment at risk (particularly for HIV/AIDS patients dependent on public funds and services). In contrast to the World Bank, the WHO and UNAIDS do not share the same view regarding a declining role of the state in the health sector, therefore counterbalancing - at the core of the policy network - the privatizing proposals of the Bank and their effects on the formulation of

---

[24] For an interesting and non-academic take on these issues see the article "Could this be the new world?" by R.D. Kaplan (Op ed.), in *The New York Times*, September 27, 1999. The incorporation of civil society groups into the formation and functioning of the HIV/AIDS policy network can also be seen as a response to the tension between globalism and globalization. At an event such as the protest at the WTO meeting in Seattle in 1999, and at the various world conferences on HIV/AIDS ever since, the message has been clear: the international system has a significant democratic deficit and a disregard for people's concerns about their livelihood and the welfare of the planet. This has motivated a significant number of civil society groups to engage in the endeavour to make multilateral organizations more deliberately democratic (See Verweij and Josling 2003).

HIV/AIDS and health-related policies at the domestic level. Fr the longest time the problem with many of the recommendations emanating from the World Bank had to do with the lack of political considerations and the required sensibility to address social concerns. And as a consequence, some of the economic reforms supported by the Bank's globalist agenda have had a negative impact on family income, restricted access to public services, and forced local businesses to collapse under the sudden pressure of foreign competition. Although it is hard to tell how much of the negative effects are explained by the globalist agenda itself, or by the way globalist policies were carried out in specific countries like Mexico, the fact is that these reforms were followed by major job-losses, the lack of job-generation and, the weakening effect that these two factors have on the work-based social security system. What can be said with more confidence is that the World Bank's policy recommendations and actions have had mixed consequences for public policymaking at the domestic level.

As we saw before, the World Bank spearheaded a new health development paradigm for the health sector (See World Bank 1993), soon to be implemented in LMICs as an approach to health-care reform. Yet, partly as a response to some of the criticisms and pressures previously discussed in the section on globalization and globalism, as well as to some changing in priorities, the World Bank has gone through a sort of identity crisis, and has questioned some of its previous policy recommendations. Under increasing criticism, the Bank's mandate, operations, and areas of intervention have become moving targets. The new demands from global civil society groups have put it under increased visibility and constant fire. This can be seen as early as 1992, in the Bank's report on effective implementation (the Wapenhas Report[25]) (See World Bank 1992), which tried to respond to the internal pressures to achieve better "development results." "The State in a Changing World" (World Bank 1997) reinforced these themes.

Somehow reluctantly, after being a central target of NGO environmental, human rights, and antipoverty campaigns for more than two decades, the World Bank had to undergo an important revision of its policies and approach to development. In terms of involving civil society groups, its management has, at times, initiated co-operation with NGOs that goes beyond what some member governments are prepared to support.[26] Additionally, as part of its incipient but growing efforts to promote civil society participation, its inspection panel opened in September of 1994, and as of January of 2003 it had received twenty-eight claims from around the world requesting an independent investigation into various World Bank-financed projects (Clark et al.

[25] See World Bank 1992, "Effective Implementation: Key to Development Impact", Washington, D.C., World Bank, Portfolio Management Task Force.

[26] The Structural Adjustment Participatory Review Initiative (SAPRI), for example, is a joint review of national adjustment programs by the Bank, NGOs, and borrowers, proposed by US-based NGOs and authorized in 1996 by the Bank's President Wolfenson (Nelson 2000, p. 418). This, of course, was not very welcomed by many borrowing governments. In the Mexican case, Teichman (2004, p. 55) also reminds us that participation was largely uninvited by the Bank, with some key documents not made available to Congress and civil society organizations.

2003, p. 1).[27] As put by Clark et al. (2003, p. 283), these precedents opened up new possibilities for civil society actors to hold the Bank accountable, both to its poverty alleviation mandate and to the negative consequences of its macroeconomic development model. Although they represent relatively small gains, one has to admit that some of these efforts have also come to represent some changes in the way the institution views and establishes relationships with civil society actors. After all, as argued by Fox and Brown (1998), the failure to effect any change would have seen as a total lack of effectiveness and success of NGOs' campaigns mounted over the last fifteen to twenty years. What we have witnessed is a small and uneven degree of new public accountability as a result of protest, urging public scrutiny, and the empowering effect on insider reformists (Fox and Brown 1998, p.2). For some, these small successes should be regarded as getting a 'foot in the door' as opposed to a 'seat at the table' for civil society organizations (Clark et al. 2003, p. 285). Of the three HIV/AIDS policy network core institutions, however, the World Bank remains the less inclusive. In fact, governments retain a good deal of discretion in their negotiations with the Bank. Yet, as a result of the ongoing reforms, at least stakeholder participation has become a catchword, making it "easier" for civil society organizations to insist on their right to participate in development programs and policies.[28] Of course, there is always the risk associated with the uncertainty of what will happen if the door gets stuck or slammed shut, as a result of the tension between insider reformists and pro-status quo Bank managers.

In a case like Mexico's, it is necessary to underline the Bank's role and influence, given the country's significant dependence on outside capital and foreign trade (Camp 2003, p.13). Although the World Bank's loans have not traditionally represented a large proportion of Mexico's federal revenue or expenditures (See Fernández and Adelson 2000), it does play an important role in policy development. The Bank provides macroeconomic policy advice and participates in a large number of compensatory and sectoral reform programs.[29] Even if we limit our assessment of the Bank's impact to health, some scholars argue that the World Bank has had a negative

---

[27] The function of the inspection panel is to determine if the Bank has violated its own policy framework, and it provides local people with access to an international forum (See http://inspectionpanel.org). While most claims have focused on infrastructure, some have addressed also sustainable development issues and SAPs. As a consequence of these claims the Bank has given legitimacy to some claims regarding the negative, direct and tangible impact that macroeconomic policies can have.

[28] Translation of official documents has been very rare though, which represents a clear obstacle to disclosure. In 1995 and 1996, more than sixty Mexican NGOs organized a campaign to convince the World Bank and the Inter-American Development Bank (IDB) to open in-country public information centres. The campaign called for the translation into Spanish of project documents and environmental and social impact assessments. After a long exchange of letters, both the World Bank and the IDB opened in-country public information centres with project documents available to the public (See Fox 1997).

[29] In the 1990s, the relations between the World Bank and Mexico strengthened. The World Bank itself stated that "a confluence of circumstances and new actors with new approaches on both sides in the eighties has served to make relations [with the Mexican government] closer and more comfortable" (World Bank 1994, p. x). By the end of 1996, Mexico was the World Bank's largest debtor, holding 12 percent of the World Bank portfolio, the same year the Bank began to put more emphasis on second-generation reforms. By 1997, the Bank had conceded 160 loans for a total of $27.29 billion. In 1998, the portfolio included three compensatory projects for a total of $342.2 million and $1.4 billion in loans for reform projects.

influence in persuading Mexican public authorities to implement policies that might not be in the best interest of its population, such as the privatization of pensions and health insurance (Laurell 1997; Leal 2000).[30] In its role as a central member of the health policy community and the health care financing policy network, the Bank has been particularly influential in the health sector reform, and has encouraged the Mexican government in the introduction of further reforms to the Social Security Institute (IMSS). As will be underlined in the discussion of the Mexican health care system (chapter three), these reforms faced great opposition from the National Union of Social Security Workers.[31] Yet, against widespread resistance to the reforms, the World Bank continued to support the government in its reform efforts, and by 1997 it had offices inside the social security institution (See Laurell 1997).

In spite of the globalist tendencies that characterize the World Bank, it has also been a central player in the fight against HIV/AIDS, and it made a public commitment – through its then HIV/AIDS Program Director, Debrework Zewdie- in the sense that no country with a national program would go unfunded (See *Notiese* 2003). Its Latin American and Caribbean Program (SIDALAC[32]) is also of central importance and has served as a driving force for some of the major moves forward in the fight against the pandemic in Mexico. The World Bank has also represented an enormous supporting force for the implementation of prevention campaigns amongst Men who have Sex with Men (MSM). In fact, to this day, the most important external source of funding for the HIV/AIDS prevention program in Mexico has been the Bank's loan of US$350 million negotiated by key members of the domestic HIV/AIDS policy network under President Zedillo's administration (1994-2000) (See discussion of the program in chapter four). Additionally, the key role played by the then head of the SIDALAC, José Antonio Izazola, in engaging civil society actors during negotiations with the Bank, generated windows of opportunity for the increasing participation of NGOs. Operational directives, for instance, mandate civil society groups' participation in the implementation of the Bank's HIV/AIDS projects, thus offering an opening not previously available under the old political regime in Mexico. This has allowed informed civil society groups – most of them with a long history of activism among sexual minority groups - with the required expertise and personal contacts to use World Bank's projects and funds as tools to claim their right to participate. To some extent, and being extremely optimistic, one could argue that the renaissance of market policies (the globalist agenda associated with individual agency and competition), and the world-wide expansion of liberal political systems have contributed to civil society groups being gradually accepted as legitimate international actors. It is interesting to see that, in the context of globalization and under the

---

[30] In analyzing the relationships between the Mexican government and the Bank, it is important to distinguish between, what Killick (1998, p. 11) refers to as, 'pro forma' and 'hard core' policy conditionality, and underline that as we saw in the case of market reform, the "conversion" and agreement on the part of the Mexican technocracy has certainly been a facilitator for the adoption of globalist policies.

[31] The national Union of Social Security Workers has undergone an internal democratization process itself and strongly opposed this second-generation reform.

[32] The World Bank's initiative for Latin American and the Caribbean for the control of AIDS and Sexually Transmitted Diseases (See discussion in chapter four).

globalist agenda, although NGOs are seen as vehicles for maximizing the effectiveness of international funds and the reign of market forces, paradoxically, some of them have also become the main challenge to the globalist agenda of international financial institutions. Put it another way, the increasing density of international networks of the kind seen around the fight against HIV/AIDS might contribute to generate growing pressure for global reforms.

At the regional level, and although the Inter-American Development Bank (IDB) does not play a formal role in the HIV/AIDS policy network, it is important to point to its special significance at the informal and not so informal level. Some of the IDB top officials have put pressure on national governments for the advancement of policies dealing with MSM (Confidential interviews with IDB officials, Rio de Janeiro 2000, Havana 2003, Mexico City 2008). Although not publicly identified as such, some gay men officials attend the regional conferences and strengthen personal links with gay and HIV/AIDS activists. This is translated into institutional support (financial resources) [33] and pressure on national authorities for the inclusion of prevention campaigns for MSM into the national programs (See Fórum 2000; Foro 2003; Mexico 2008).

For its part, the WHO has also been a central actor in the emergence and operation of the HIV/AIDS policy network. Since the creation of the first HIV/AIDS Global Program, in 1986, the WHO has been a prime advocate for the need to adopt a multi-dimensional response to the pandemic. A key figure in these efforts was Jonathan Mann, who according to other key actors involved in struggle against HIV/AIDS was a man with vision, and someone who was able to bring er all parties together (Interview with Stefano Bertozzi, Mexico City, December 13, 2001; Interview with José Antonio Izazola, November 27, 2001). After his sudden death, which was regarded by most as a great loss for the HIV/AIDS cause, Michael Merson became WHO's leading force in this area. Critics argue that since then the global response became more technically focused, and the HIV/AIDS policy network ran the risk of becoming as exclusive as its health-care financing counterpart (Confidential Interview with UNAIDS official, Rio de Janeiro, November 9, 2000). In fact, between 1993 and 1994, before the creation of UNAIDS and the appointment of Dr. Peter Piot as its director, people perceived a looming crisis in the management of the program. These fears gave rise to new alternatives to the global program, such as the World Bank sponsored SIDALAC for Latin America and the Caribbean, and other regional programs. Additionally, the appointment of Gro Harlem Bruntland[34] (1998-2002) as the new Director General of WHO provided the health agency with new leadership,

---

[33] See the declarations by the then IDB's President, Enrique V. Iglesias, in support of HIV/AIDS programs, and the various reports documenting the regional bank's financial support: http://iadb.org.
[34] A medical doctor, with a Master of Public Health (MPH), Dr. Brundtland spent 10 years as a physician and scientist in the Norwegian public health system. For more than 20 years she was in public office, 10 of them as Prime Minister. In the 1980s she gained international recognition, championing the principle of sustainable development as the chair of the World Commission for the Environment and Development, otherwise known as the Brundtland Commission).

and added to its legitimacy to initiate new policies as well as to carry on and reinforce others, including and especially HIV/AIDS related ones.

For its part, and as repeatedly stated above, UNAIDS, with a central role in the gathering and distribution of financial resources and together with its main sponsoring organizations, is at the core of the international HIV/AIDS policy network. The fact that UNAIDS became the first international program/organization to incorporate civil society groups into its governing body reinforced its position and legitimacy among the HIV/AIDS international policy community. Its Executive Director Under-Secretary-General of the United Nations from 1994 to 2008, Dr. Peter Piot, whose personal commitment and role was determinant in the incorporation of civil society members at the core of the HIV/AIDS policy network, also became a central figure within the community and the network (Interview with Stefano Bertozzi, Mexico City, December 13, 2001; Interview with José Antonio Izazola, November 27, 2001; Interview with Arturo Díaz Betancourt, Rio de Janeiro, November 9, 2000). Furthermore, Dr. Piot worked closely together with those NGOs that have sat on the UNAIDS PCB and many others. These NGOs have had strong links with their domestic counterparts, including Mexico, which has been of central importance to the work of the domestic policy network. Dr. Piot's successor, Dr. Michel Sidibé, who took office in January 2009, has followed on his predecessor's steps and shown leadership, working to ensure that no one is left behind in the response to HIV, and that everyone in need has access to life-saving HIV services. He initiated the global call to eliminate HIV infections among children, and his global advocacy has firmly secured HIV/AIDS at the top of political agendas. His idea of shared responsibility and global solidarity has been embraced by the international community, and it has encouraged increased ownership of their epidemics by some of the most affected countries.

To a certain extent, the differences in approaches between International Governmental Organizations are explained by what some define as the tension between inter-governmentalism and trans-nationalism within the UN system (See Cronin 2002).[35] In fact, the UN system and its various agencies symbolize not only inter-governmental but also trans-national entities, often representing a "common good" that transcends the sum of individual states' interests. Often, such concerns are promoted by NGOs and by the UN's specialized agencies, affiliated organizations,

---

[35] These two concepts refer to two different forces that encompass different sets of interests and reflect distinct constituencies (Cronin 2002, p. 53). As such, trans-nationalism refers to relations maintained by clearly identifiable actors linking at least two societies or sub-units of national governments. The literature on trans-national relations discusses at least three related but distinct understandings. First, it refers to the activities conducted regularly by non-state actors across juridical borders (Risse-Kappan 1995, p. xii) including Trans-National Corporations, civil society groups, advocacy networks, or cultural groups. Second, it can be used to refer to contacts between government bureaucracies charged with similar tasks who act on their own in the absence of national decisions (Keohane and Nye 1977, p. 34). This includes state officials within sub-units of national governments, international organizations, and regimes; these individuals often pursue common agendas independent of their governments. As pointed out by Cronin (2002, p. 56), Risse and Kappan (1995) refer to this as trans-governmental coalitions. For its part, the literature on epistemic communities explains how trans-national networks of knowledge-based experts develop, transmit, and legitimize a set of ideas and beliefs across national borders (Cronin 2002, p. 56).

bureaucracy, and the office of the Secretary General itself. Sometimes trans-national concerns conflict with the more traditional intergovernmental ones, such as security or economic "efficiency." The task then is to discern which constituency is being served at different times.[36] Moreover, the involvement of NGOs in the UN networks through Article 71, and through the 'subcontracting' of services, has helped to expand the organization's identity from a strictly intergovernmental to a trans-national organization.[37] As such, UNAIDS and the WHO represent prime examples of international organizations with a trans-national mandate that have established strong links with NGOs and incorporated some of them into their efforts to combat HIV/AIDS. And as will be further discussed below, they have provided civil society groups with both policy access and financial support, and their actions have been bolstered by key individual actors, such as Peter Piot or Michel Sidibé, who together with many other individuals and civil society groups have been central in the formation and strengthening of the HIV/AIDS policy network.

The commitment of the World Bank, the strengthening of the WHO, and the new leadership of UNAIDS were behind the momentum reached in June of 2001, at the UN General Assembly special meeting organized around HIV/AIDS. At that point in time, the Global Fund for Malaria, Tuberculosis, and HIV/AIDS was created. Yet the momentum reached at the special meeting was overshadowed by the events that took place on September 11 of that same year in New York City, and other sites in the U.S. Furthermore, in spite of the decisive political support and endorsement received at the World HIV/AIDS Conference in Barcelona in 2002 by world figures such as former U.S. president Bill Clinton, and South-African leader Nelson Mandela, of the required 10 billion dollars per year less than 8 billion have been committed since 2001. Interestingly, and in spite of the prevalence and influence of the globalist agenda, the fight against HIV/AIDS has shown some resistance to the exclusionary nature of other policy networks. Both globally and locally, civil society groups such as Médecins Sans Frontières (MSF) and others have been successful in positioning themselves at the core (See figures 2.4 above and 2.5 below) of the policy network and in negotiating access to treatment for AIDS patients and the promotion of prevention campaigns among sexual minorities.

---

[36] As declared by the former UN Secretary General (1982-1992), Javier Pérez de Cuellar, his office had to serve two constituencies: the governments of the member states and the people for whom the governments act (Pérez de Cuellar, "The Role of the UN Secretary General," 1994, pp. 138-141, UN).

[37] Article 71 of the UN Charter empowers the Economic and Social Council to "make suitable arrangements for consultation with non-governmental organizations which are concerned with matters within its competence." In Cronin (2002), p. 62.

Figure 2.5 - International HIV/AIDS Policy Network*

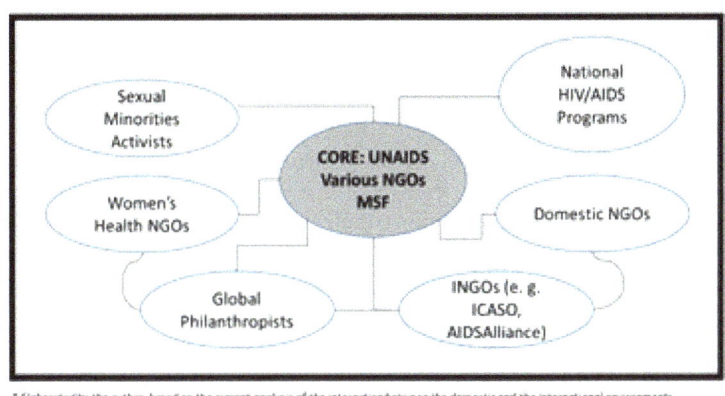

* Elaborated by the author, based on the current analysis of the interaction between the domestic and the international environments.

MSF is among some of the most influential international NGOs, and spite of the fact that it does not have a seat on the PCB, it finds itself at the core of the HIV/AIDS policy network. In fact, it can be argued that in some ways, it has surpassed an organization like the WHO and has positioned itself at the leading edge of some policy developments, such as price reductions for some essential medicines. In 2001, for instance, MSF's spoke person - Eric Goemaere – publicly denounced as a scandal the fact that TNCs could place economic profits above human lives (*Milenio*, March 13, 2001). Subsequently, MSF activists pressured 39 pharmaceutical companies to withdraw their demand against the South African Government for its purchase of imported generic ARVs from India (Interview with former MSF's president James Orbinsky, Toronto, April 28, 2004). MSF actions at the international level had major effects at the domestic level in various countries. In Mexico, the federal government initially argued that ARVs were not essential and that it did not have the resources to pay for them and provide access for all. However, as a consequence of the pressure exercised from within the policy network by MSF and other NGOs on UNAIDS and the World Bank, from 2000 onwards the Mexican government softened its position. Additionally, civil society organizations had threatened to sue the Secretariat of Health and IMSS, following the example of activists in Costa Rica, Venezuela, and Brazil (See *Notiese* 2000). At that point in time, domestic and international health authorities saw a major problem looming, which forced UNAIDS and the World Bank to seriously look into the negotiation of the costs of medications with pharmaceuticals. Thus, in the case of Mexico, the combined effect of the work of domestic NGOs and the external pressure resulted in the government's decision to provide full coverage of ARVs for all those in need of treatment.

In the fight against the pandemic, much is expected in terms of resources from the new global philanthropists, who are located at the periphery of the policy network (See figure 2.5, above) and some of whom, paradoxically, have profited the most from the dominance of the capitalist markets in a globalized world. Big profit makers in different areas, from the capital market (e.g., George Soros and the Soros Foundation

Network) to the global media (e.g., Ted Turner and his Foundation), and the computer software industry (e.g., Bill Gates and the Bill and Melinda Gates Foundation[38]), have contributed with some funds to varying degrees (See Kickbusch and Buse 2002). Some of these foundations have increasingly engaged in the fight against HIV/AIDS and have been a significant source of funding for many NGOs and some government programs. Like the World Bank, they have increasingly channeled funds through HIV/AIDS NGOs, allowing them to inform policy and to engage in advocacy. In fact, most NGOs prefer money from the World Bank and international foundations, and accept only a certain proportion of their funding directly from their own governments. This resource inter-dependency between the various governmental and non-governmental members of the network on international or global funds, as opposed to governmental ones, reinforces their linkages and guarantees their mutual support.

With regards to the historical links between globalization, democratization and HIV/AIDS, and the formation of the HIV/AIDS policy network, it is also necessary to look at the struggle for sexual minorities' rights. First of all, more "consolidated" democracies, which tend to be also economically powerful and internationally influential countries, were first in recognizing the rights of sexual minorities in the contemporary era (See Rayside 1998). Secondly, together with other values such as democracy, equality, and women's rights, globalization has also promoted the spread of a gay identity (See Altman 2001). And thirdly, and particularly important for the formation of the policy network, from the beginning there has been a strong world-wide involvement of sexual minorities and gay activists in the fight against HIV/AIDS (See Altman 2001; Rayside 1998). Paradoxically, however, it must be mentioned that in some cases people have questioned whether HIV/AIDS has delayed the age of "coming out," due to the stigmatization of gays and the fear of contracting HIV (Roberts 1995, p. 253).

Other Countries' Experiences

In Latin America, the largest numbers of people with HIV/AIDS are in the two most populated countries, Mexico and Brazil. Yet the most serious situations are under way in small ones such as Belize and Honduras, with more than 1.5 percent of those countries' respective adult populations living with HIV in 2015 (UNAIDS 2015). Similar to the Mexican case, in countries such as Guatemala, Honduras, Nicaragua, and Panama, there is high HIV/AIDS prevalence among MSM —between 9 percent and 13 percent among them is infected with the virus. In El Salvador, that figure reaches 18 percent. In most cases, this population group reported having female sexual partners as well. Although significant gains have been made in terms of access to treatment in countries such as Argentina, Brazil, Chile, Costa Rica, Mexico, Panama, Uruguay, and Venezuela, poorer countries in Central America and those in

---

[38] Currently, the Gates Foundation has HIV/AIDS programs for Cambodia, Mexico and Thailand, in the amount of five million dollars each.

the Andean region have struggled to expand treatment access in the face of persistent barriers to affordability.

When it comes to the links between the democratic character of a state and the actual governmental policies or results concerning HIV/AIDS prevention and treatment, and based on some more closely studied cases, conclusions are not so clear (for analyses of sub-Saharan Africa, see Goyer 2001; for insights into Uganda and South Africa, see Morisky 2006; Thornton 2008; and for a global overview see Smith 2013). Regarding the Americas, the responsiveness of governments has been associated with the general mobilization of civil society and social movements throughout the region, and as part of the regional processes of democratization (See Friedman, Hochstetler, and Clark 2001; Stahler-Sholk, Vanden, and Kuecker 2002). However, Cuba is an often-cited case, where mandatory confinement of HIV carriers and compulsory HIV testing characterized the often-controversial beginnings of Cuba's approach (See Farmer 2003; Fink 2003). Although most regarded this as an authoritarian set of policies and a source of human rights violations, their earlier policy did help contain the epidemic. In fact, today, Cuba serves as an example of a strong commitment by the state to the health and protection of all its citizens, including sexual minorities, with successful results (Leiner 1994; Lumsden 1996; Smallman 2007). While Dr. Jorge Pérez, the long-time director of the national AIDS program, is well respected at home and abroad, the program itself has been a target of both praise and sharp criticism (Fink 2003). It has been praised because Cuba has the lowest prevalence of HIV in the hemisphere (Farmer 2003); according to Ministry of Public Health statistics, there were only 4214 HIV-positive patients detected between 1985 and July 2002. Criticism, though, has been directed at some of the controversial policies that Pérez and others insist have contributed to keeping HIV infection rates so low. As put by Scheper-Hughes (1993), "it's a strong version of medicine and public health that would be a problem for Americans to swallow." For his part, Dr. Pérez says that the U.S. embargo on Cuba has made his job both easier and harder. Easier, because Cuba's initial isolation helped shield it from the spread of AIDS. Harder, because obtaining medications and diagnostic machines - such as a flow cytometer and viral load and CD4 detector - has been difficult and subject to delays (Fink 2003). "A more aggressive public health response at the very start of the epidemic might have saved countless lives," Scheper-Hughes wrote in a 1993 article for the medical journal *Lancet,* "a strong and humane public health system has just as often protected the lives of socially vulnerable groups as it has violated their personal liberties."[39]

In contrast, the cases of Brazil and Mexico serve as examples of the positive correlation between democracy - or democratization - and more effective and responsive HIV/AIDS policies. In both countries, the similarly positive changes in the state's approach to the epidemic are part and parcel of the democratization process and the mobilization of civil society experienced over the past few decades (De la Dehesa 2010; Frasca 2005; Smallman 2007; Smith 2013). In the case of Brazil,

---

[39] For a more comprehensive analysis of Cuba's policies, including the health sector as a whole, during the Revolutionary Regime see Farber 2011.

similar to that of Mexico's, the fight against the pandemic was part of the broader struggle for recognition and inclusion of gays, lesbians, and *travestis* (GLTs) into Brazilian society and politics. That struggle involved attempts at gaining access to and influence over political parties in order to push forward a pro-LGBT agenda (Marsiaj 2006; 2010). Similar too, to the Mexican case, is the fact that although greater support has been found in leftist parties, a closer look at specific gains and strategies shows that there have been cases of support from right-wing parties as well (Marsiaj 2006; 2010).

As already discussed, the Latin American region as a whole has been significantly affected by globalist policies, such as privatization and pressures to reduce the role of the state, which have resulted in the underfunding of public services and the subsequent negative impact on health-care service delivery. In addition, the predominance of the global market economy, in which pharmaceutical companies operate, has meant relative neglect for the "unprofitable" "developing-world" diseases, such as malaria and several other mainly tropical diseases. For diseases that have long been treatable and for which there are effective remedies off-patent, governments have been able to meet many of their essential-medicines needs through the availability of generic products at competitive prices. However, the WTO recently moved to extend patent lifetimes, and recent years have also witnessed the emergence of new or more resistant diseases like AIDS, which requires new drugs such as ARVs. As a consequence, the expense of the new and patented products has made it more difficult for governments in LMICs to provide adequate supplies of essential medicines in accordance with their human rights obligations. Thus, the challenges the globalist agenda imposes on health have not gone unnoticed.

The negative impact of international trade regimes on the right to health has been the subject of much international attention, debate, and NGO advocacy for a couple of decades now (Ostergard 2007; Tarabusi and Vickery 1993). As a consequence, exceptions have been introduced to certain trade rules in favour of human rights protection. For example, the Brazilian government led the way in the struggle for access to treatment. As early as November 1996, the same year in which new ARV drugs were launched at the International AIDS Conference in Vancouver, a law came into effect that gave HIV-positive people the right to free medications through the public health system. Brazil's government was then determined to produce generic versions of ARVs to meet its commitments (Smallman 2007). As expected, there was intense opposition to its efforts to break international patents and make generic medications more affordable, which drew the country into confrontation with pharmaceutical companies and the U.S. government. The increasing international attention and support from various intergovernmental and international civil society actors—including the UN Human Rights Commission and MSF, among others—for the efforts of a growing network of Brazilian NGOs (originally from the gay community) in concert with their government, resulted in the U.S. government's retraction of a complaint filed with the WTO in the summer of 2001 (Frasca 2005). As such, the Brazilian success story can be understood only within the global context, and it represented a key policy lesson to be replicated by other countries in Latin

America and beyond. In fact, countries in other regions, such as Thailand and South Africa, followed suit. As a result of the sum of these countries' actions, although the WTO's agreement on Trade-Related Aspects of Intellectual Property Rights (TRIPS) protects international patents in favor of TNCs, it also contains provisions for bypassing patent restrictions in situations of public emergency. This aspect of TRIPS became a central point of focus between 1997 and 2001, in the highly publicized case between thirty-nine pharmaceutical TNCs and the South African government, which threatened to violate ARVs' patents. As a result of lobbying by international civil society organizations, there was the important formal clarification that public health emergencies could be invoked to bypass certain patent restrictions under TRIPS (personal interview with the former MSF's president James Orbinsky, Toronto, April 28, 2004). This led to the adoption in 2001 of the Declaration on the TRIPS Agreement and Public Health at the WTO's Fourth Ministerial Conference in Doha (the Doha Declaration) (WTO 2001). The Doha Declaration recognizes that patents can impede access to affordable medicines and affirms that governments are free to take all necessary measures to protect public health in medical emergencies. As such, this major breakthrough in compulsory licensing represented a clear victory for countries like Thailand, South Africa, and Brazil, and it enabled others to implement similar policies. By 2002, other countries in Latin America, such as Argentina, Costa Rica, and Uruguay, had adopted national policies for providing free medication for all HIV/AIDS patients (Smallman 2007).

PERSISTING STRUCTURAL CHALLENGES

With regards to the organization and activism of sexual minorities at the international level, one of the most difficult problems for the discussion of homosexuality has arisen from conceptual and ethical debates about definitions of sexuality, both behaviorally and cross-culturally. In their efforts to overcome some of these obstacles, HIV/AIDS activists have come up with the aforementioned notion of Men who have Sex with Men (MSM or MWM). For many, given that men do not always identify themselves as homosexual or gay, it is easier or safer to define them or define themselves as MSM for policy formulation reasons (Various interviews with activists in Havana, Mexico City, Rio de Janeiro, Toronto, 2000-2008). Yet for others, the notion of MSM can be obscuring, since for them it is clear that the gay identity is also political and is related to issues of liberation. This becomes very concrete in terms of having the human, civil, or legal rights to live openly as homosexuals, with the same rights of association and relations as other men and women. Notwithstanding the significance of these differences in views, it can certainly be argued that the increasing debates around identity issues have resulted from the growing contact and dialogue between homosexual men from different regions. Ultimately, in an increasingly globalized world, gay men from both the Global North and the Global South travel to other countries to provide and acquire technical assistance, to attend international conferences, and to share experiences and expertise with each other.

Since the emergence of the pandemic, it has become clear that the organizing around HIV/AIDS prevention has been the foundation of many emergent gay organizations in LMICs, including Mexico. This is partly due to the fact that compared to other gay groups, HIV/AIDS-related gay-based organizations have received the most support and acceptance from international bodies to become firmly established at the national and global levels. Particularly significant for the current analysis is the fact that it was in Rio de Janeiro, during the Fórum 2000, that activists (both members of the policy network and the policy community at large) were able to convince Dr. Peter Piot (then head of UNAIDS) to refer to the urgent need to implement prevention campaigns and treatment for MSM in his official speech at the opening ceremony. Furthermore, they were successful in pressing for the commitment of new funds, from the World Bank and UNAIDS, especially directed to the prevention campaigns among MSM (Interview with Jorge Huerdo Siqueiros and other activists, Rio de Janeiro, November, 2000). In the very concrete case of Mexican NGOs, this gave them and the domestic policy network as a whole more leverage for the negotiation of further support from the national government. Eventually, as we will see in more detail in chapter four, this was translated into renewed political and financial commitments for universal access to treatment and prevention campaigns among MSM, even after the election of a conservative PAN candidate as the first non-PRI president in more than seventy years.

As argued by Roberts (1995), the increased formalization of services for MSM and the more open and public discussion of MSM behavior challenged long-standing social contracts. Thus, not surprisingly, the relative success of HIV/AIDS activism has been accompanied by continuing discrimination and homophobia in Mexico as much as in other Latin American countries (See Foro 2003; Fórum 2000). Yet again, for the case of Mexico, the success of the HIV/AIDS policy network in the renewed support for HIV/AIDS prevention campaigns and the expansion of sexual minorities' rights has taken place in spite of the persistent opposition from socially conservative groups. For its part, at the global level, the international HIV/AIDS policy network was confronted with the renewed support of the then U.S. president George W. Bush's administration and its Christian base for international socially conservative and religious groups (Islamic and Christians alike), which teamed up to lobby the UN against various specific progressive policies, such as abortion and the use of condoms (Washington Post, June 17, 2002). Against those challenges though, international socially progressive activists have continued to rally together around key issues related to HIV/AIDS and health. For instance, during the first Global LGBT Summit, organized by the International Lesbian and Gay Association (ILGA) in Oakland, California, from August 28 to September 1st, 2001, many workshops focused on gay men and women's health, with special attention to HIV/AIDS. Several Mexican NGOs and individuals actively participated in this conference, strengthening their links with their foreign counterparts.[40]

---

[40] See http://www.ighhrc.org; http://www.ilga.org

It is especially significant for Latin America that some international networks, such as the 'Association for Citizenship and Integral Health for Latin America and the Caribbean' (ASICAL[41]) – which was founded in Rio de Janeiro at the Fórum 2000, by members of NGOs from several countries in the region - have attached the agenda for access to 'Health for All' to their fight against HIV/AIDS.[42] Moreover, ASICAL played a key role in the aforementioned lobbying efforts of some NGOs for the incorporation of prevention campaigns for MSM into the UNAIDS' and World Bank's discourses and programs. In ASICAL's own view, from very early on the challenges confronted in the fight against the pandemic included the struggle against discrimination, for equal sexual rights, for full citizenship, equality, and justice (Interview with Arturo Díaz Betancourt, Rio de Janeiro, November 9, 2000). As such, their activism goes beyond the more immediate concerns around HIV/AIDS and addresses broader issues related to human rights, democratization, and development.

As part of the process of formation of the HIV/AIDS policy network, NGOs have previously recurred to various tactics in order to consolidate their positions. One of them, is what Keck and Sikkink (1998) call the 'boomerang pattern or effect.' This was clearly the case in the way in which the domestic HIV/AIDS policy network secured UNAIDS and World Bank support for MSM prevention campaigns, previous to the change of government in Mexico in 2000 (See discussion of the negotiations of PROCEDES in chapter four). Under certain circumstances, if a government ignores a group's pleas (in this case, prevention campaigns among MSM), some domestic NGOs can pressure their government through the actions of a group of international NGOs and international governmental organizations (UNAIDS and the World Bank) and thus succeed where normal domestic political avenues have failed. In the case of Mexico, NGOs actions at the Fórum in Rio, and in the negotiations of the World Bank's loan facilitated the success of MSM groups' pleas on the government to address their concerns.

It must also be recognized that NGOs and international governmental organizations are not the only actors capable of influencing the process of policy formulation, nationally or globally. Corporate actors also have an increasingly significant influence over some decisions at many international governmental organizations. For instance, major corporations lobby the World Bank directly, through their own governments, or through their executive directors (See Sam Loewenberg 1999). Thus our attention will now turn to the influence of other members of the policy community at large, such as the corporate sector, with a special focus on international trade regimes and their effects on health care provision. Similar to the opposition faced from socially conservative groups to prevention campaigns for HIV/AIDS and against discrimination based on sexual orientation, there are a number of persisting structural challenges faced by the HIV/AIDS policy network in its fight for access to treatment for all. Therefore, the following paragraphs will address the

---

[41] Asociación para la Salud Integral y Ciudadanía en América Latina y el Caribe. Arturo Díaz Betancourt, from Mexican NGO Letra S, a central figure to whom we will refer in more detail in chapter four, was among the founders and the first president of the association.
[42] See http://www.asical.org

ways in which the globalist agenda, and corporate international actors that support it, determine the policy environment within which the HIV/AIDS policy network operates and health-related policies are defined.

Globally, TNCs realize their cost-cutting, market-expanding goals by pressing governments, trade organizations, and international institutions such as the WTO and the International Labour Organization (ILO) for increased de-regulation of free trade, investment, labour markets, and the environment. Corporate representatives "advise" the leaders of these organizations on complex scientific and technical matters, as well as on intricate trade deals by providing them with the "objective findings" of corporate-sponsored "scientific" research. In fact, European and U.S.-based pharmaceutical manufacturers, along with the film and music industries, have played an influential role within the WTO in its efforts and successes to harmonize trade-related intellectual property rights (Millen et al. in Yong Kim 2000, p. 228). And although some TNCs have improved their environmental records, labour practices and increased wages, sharing concerns with other actors for the future of society, some of their representatives have expressed dissatisfaction with civil society groups having increasing influence at the global level. For instance, speaking in an interview about the sway of environmental and human rights groups within the UN, International Chamber of Commerce's (ICC) President Maucher warned: "we have to be careful that they do not get too much influence" (In Millen et al. in Yong Kim 2000, p. 239).[43]

In analyzing the role of some TNCs as contributing to the persisting challenges faced in the fight against HIV/AIDS, it is important to explicitly state that without any intention to demonize them, it is necessary to recognize the fact that as put by globalist theorist Milton Friedman, "there is one and only one social responsibility of business – to use its resources and engage in activities designed to increase its profits" (In Merson at al. 2000, p.56). Furthermore, the modern corporation has become a central actor and, as once put by John Kenneth Galbraith (1977, p. 257), is becoming the institution that exercises a greater influence on our lives than unions, universities, politicians or the government. Through their substantial influence on international trade and development organizations, including the WHO, the WTO, and the World Bank, corporate leaders have lobbied for deregulation, privatization, and liberalization, so that TNCs can maximize profits and growth, largely unencumbered by the regulatory efforts of national governments. In this context, recent trade disputes over hormone-treated beef, genetically modified organisms, and the commercialization of ARVs reveal the intensifying tensions between public health policy and multilateral trade agreements guided by a globalist agenda. Thus, with regards to global health and health promotion, for example, problems emerge in terms of the conflict of interests between WHO or UNAIDS on the one hand, and the pharmaceutical and insurance companies on the other (See Hancock 1998).

---

[43] The International Chamber of Commerce consists of more than 7,000 member companies and business associations in more than 130 countries. Maria Cattaui, who was its Secretary General in 2002, argued that the same rules for private corporations must be applied globally, and for that global framework they look to the UN and its agencies (Kickbusch and Buse, in Buse et al. 2002, p. 720).

It is clear that TNCs are key players in the definition of the policy environment within which HIV/AIDS and health-related policies are made. Cases such as the promotion of risky infant formulas and the political, economic, and cultural manipulation by tobacco trans-nationals are only some concrete examples of their not so respectable role in the area of global health (Yong Kim et al. 2000, p. 207; See also Chen and Winder 1990). Thus, the role of big TNCs such as pharmaceutical companies, which are part of the broader HIV/AIDS and health policy community, must be further scrutinized. After all, and even though pharmaceuticals are not considered members of the HIV/AIDS policy network, they exercise a tremendous influential power over the decisions made, globally and nationally. This is an industry that shows a high degree of concentration, with the European, the Japanese, and the U.S. markets combined accounting for 75 per cent of the world's production of medicines and 90 per cent of global pharmaceutical research and development (See Appendix 2.2, for an overview of the world's pharmaceutical industry). This is also an industry that has a major interest in the expansion of markets at the global level, due to the fact that most of its research-based firms have realized that for innovation to be profitable new drugs must reach markets all over the world in as short a time as possible.[44]

As a way to respond to this global reality, efforts aimed at establishing common ground between the pharmaceutical industry and multilateral organizations has been taking place since the beginning of the 1990s (See Mitchell et al. 1993). These efforts have led to round-table discussions between the WHO and the International Federation of Pharmaceutical Manufacturers, which began in October 1998 (See Bruntland 1999). The mergers between various companies (See Appendix 2.2), however, have empowered individual mega-companies vis-à-vis states and inter-governmental organizations, with the establishment of new public-private partnerships considered by some as a form of global neo-corporatism (See Buse and Walt 2000). However, and as already discussed in the previous section, in spite of the growing power of big pharmaceuticals the HIV/AIDS policy network together with the generic industry have won some battles in the fight for access to treatment for HIV/AIDS patients. Another example is the case, under TRIPS, of an important exception regarding pharmaceutical drugs referred to as the Bolar exception. This exception has to do with the patent law permitting research and development, as well as the submission of information and samples required by generic drug manufacturers from regulatory authorities. The purpose is to facilitate approval of a generic product for marketing before patent expiration, thus permitting a prompt introduction of generic versions after that date at a lower price than the patented drugs (Ranson et al., in Merson et al. 2001, p. 23). Indian producers of generic drugs have been quite active in

---

[44] Further imbalances between North and South are reflected in the fact that 75 per cent of the world's population who live in LMICs consume only 14 per cent of the world's drug supply, and more than 80 per cent of drug production takes place in HICs (See Appendix 2.2). Furthermore, as recently as 2014, only about 0.2 per cent of the annual global health expenditure related to research and development is for pneumonia, diarrhoeal diseases and tuberculosis, despite the fact that they account for 18 per cent of the global disease burden (See UNDP 2015).

this area and are interested in capturing the market of those drugs whose patent will expire in the next few years (representing more than 40 million in sales) (Leal and Martínez 2001a, p. 100).[45] Hence, trans-national activists such as MSF and the International HIV/AIDS Alliance have actively encouraged countries with the necessary technology and scientific knowledge such as India, Thailand, and Brazil, to offer good quality drugs at much lower prices to poorer countries. Yet WTO's TRIPS protects the patents of big pharmaceuticals (See discussion on trade agreements and health in Mexico, chapter four). Therefore, most LMICs, which were still outside the patent system, had to make important decisions before the end of 2005, when TRIPS regulations came into effect for most of them.

Another interesting development in this area, at the global level, was the aforementioned case of the WTO's Doha meeting of 2001. Before the Anthrax emergency in the United States that followed the 2001 terrorist attacks, and the world-wide SARS crisis of 2003, it seemed that compared to conditions in countries with poor economies infectious diseases no longer posed a major threat to public health in HICs. Yet partly as a response to this new reality, and due to the activism of trans-national civil society groups, the most important result at the WTO ministerial meeting in Doha, in 2001, was the "heightened concern expressed ... with social issues and ... the ability of countries to address social problems" (Johnson 2002, p. 32). The Doha Declaration, under U.S. and Canadian pressures in response to the Anthrax threat, made it clear that the TRIPS agreement "can and should be interpreted in a manner supportive of WTO members' right to protect public health and, in particular, to promote access to medicines for all" (WTO 2001, 1).[46] Here we have to underline again the role and influence of Médecins Sans Frontières and the International HIV/AIDS Alliance in the fight for access to ARVs and the outcome at Doha. They were present at the negotiations and saw a window of opportunity opening up for putting forward their own agenda to include drugs that were required for global health threats other than Anthrax (Interview with the then MSF's president James Orbinsky, Toronto, April 28 2004). The declaration reflected the increasingly important role of some civil society members of the HIV/AIDS policy network in influencing some principles of global trade.[47]

---

[45] The Indian generic manufacturer 'Cipla,' for example, has been selling the equivalent of an anti-biotic produced and sold by 'Pfizer' at the price of 10 US dollars for only 25 cents (Leal and Martínez 2001a, p. 100).

[46] As a result of the Doha declaration, and in spite of the U.S. opposition to a watered-down compromise that every other country had accepted, at the end of August of 2003 the WTO reached an agreement relaxing international rules on patent protection for LMICs. As stated above, this was facilitated by the fact that in the wake of the Anthrax attacks in the United States, the Canadian and the U.S. governments threatened to violate patents themselves on an Anthrax antidote in order to get an affordable price. As put by Miller (2001, p. 40), the pressure was such that for those same countries to continue defending patents on treatment for HIV/AIDS – which has killed far more people than Anthrax – would have represented nothing more than open utter hypocrisy.

[47] In the United States, HIV/AIDS activists' dissatisfaction with the Food and Drug Administration's (FDA) slow drug rate approval became politically significant as they blamed the agency for the unavailability of any drugs that could be effective against the deadly virus (Vogel 1990, 458-461). As a response to their pressures, in 1989, the FDA took a highly unconventional step to accommodate AIDS patients, granting a

As part of the global struggle for access to treatment, it is also imperative to refer to the South African and Brazilian campaigns to violate the patent protection afforded to multinational drug companies that produce ARVs. Their actions should be regarded as responses triggered by the constraints imposed on each country to pursue policies that can respond to the specific needs of their respective populations. In the case of South Africa, the pharmaceutical industry (as represented by the International Federation of Pharmaceutical Manufacturers Association [IFPMA]), reflecting a more restrictive interpretation of the TRIPS Agreement, challenged the legality of South Africa's action (which asserted its rights under TRIPS, arguing that a responsible government must be able to produce its own generic medicines or import them at more affordable prices) (Kickbusch and Buse, in Buse et al. 2002, p. 713). After intense negotiations, and under pressure from the international community (particularly, from key members of the HIV/AIDS policy network such as MSF and the International HIV/AIDS Alliance), the pharmaceutical industry dropped its case against the South African government. For its part, after months of testy negotiations, Brazil threatened to break the patent on Swiss Roche's AIDS drug, 'Nelfinavir' (See Notiese 2003). Facing this ultimatum, Roche dropped its price per dosage. In this case, MSF and the International HIV/AIDS Alliance, with the strong support from Oxfam international, successfully pressured the US government to drop the lawsuit against the Brazilian government through the WTO (Letra S, in La Jornada, June 7, 2001). One could argue that these battles have given rise to a new kind of Western "philanthropy," the kind that is performed under duress. As Swiss drug-maker Roche discovered to its chagrin, LMICs are demanding that big drug companies match generic prices.

As discussed in the previous section, the actions of various members of the international HIV/AIDS policy network have had a direct impact on Mexico as well. As we will see in our discussion of the domestic side of the analysis in chapter four, in March of 2001, Merck, Sharp & Dohme felt the pressure and reduced the price of its AIDS drugs sold in the Mexican market by 82 per cent, which represented public savings of US$15 million dollars.[48] Admittedly, with only 15 percent of drug-industry revenues coming from LMICs, and just one percent from Africa, such concessions do not greatly affect Merck's world profits. Unfortunately, and in spite of the fact that pharmaceuticals could dramatically improve the health of poor people, the pre-

---

'personal use exemption' for individuals to bring a drug into the United States for their own use if it had been approved for use in another country. This led to widespread growth of 'buyers' clubs,' which import and distribute drugs, at lower prices, primarily but not limited to people with HIV/AIDS (See Lindermann 1994). Thus, under increasing domestic political pressure to expedite the drug approval process not only for AIDS drugs but for other medicines as well, U.S. regulators became more willing to co-operate with foreign regulatory agencies (Vogel 1998, p. 10).

[48] Under a newly politicized market, other companies launched pre-emptive discounts in the name of public health. For example, Swiss giant Novartis' CEO, Daniel Vasella, announced that after realizing that only US$30 million worth of treatment in his portfolio could eradicate leprosy, his company was giving away a concoction, a combination of three different drugs called MBT, through the WTO (See *Notiese* 2003). A new Malaria drug has also been priced 20 times less in LMICs, while in March 2001, Merck introduced a pricing policy for AIDS-fighting drugs, Crixivan and Stocrin, that is based on the United Nations Human Development Index: the less developed the country, the lower the price (See *Notiese* 2001).

eminence of hot-selling prescription drugs such as Viagra, Prozac, and Claritin (which only between 1996 and 1998 drove the Dow Jones pharmaceutical index to a climb of 110 percent – a rise more than double that of the Dow Jones Industrial Average (Yong Kim et al. 2000, p. 220)) makes it difficult to draw more of their attention to the needs of the poor. Similarly, although TNCs can potentially improve the health of the World's sick and poor, most of the corporations involved in health-related activities are in fact driving the medical field's attention from public health to commercial concerns. As put by Yong Kim (2000, p. 220), "health-care provision, biotechnology, medical therapies, and even human blood and organs for transplantation are considered among the last great profit frontiers: they are regarded as 'dynamic growth markets' for business." Some TNCs have joined forces with other globalist actors to design policies that shift the focus away from public and community health to private and individual health, with a strong reliance on medical technologies, constantly looking for new markets for their goods and services. This trend has enabled U.S.-based for-profit-managed-care and health-insurance companies to expand their operations in countries such as Mexico (See chapter four). In most cases, they do not seek to provide services to vulnerable groups. Instead, they seek healthier, wealthier patients and clients, which contributes to making the commitment to treat health as a fundamental human right (set forth in article 25 of the Universal Declaration of Human Rights) seem an ever more remote ideal.

Most of those people living with HIV/AIDS in LMICs, who are denied the access to life-saving medications, are in that situation partly due to monopolistic drug pricing by global pharmaceutical companies. As such, the globalist agenda undermines the right to health for all. Consequently, as individuals are increasingly subject to these enforced injustices, there is an urgent need for co-ordinated international strategizing to challenge the unfair practices of trans-national corporate domination as it threatens to destabilize global health. Under these circumstances, the increased and to some extent successful pressure for transparency in WTO procedures for dispute settlement, and the systematic recourse to expert advice by more inclusive panels, may enhance the sensitivity of the WTO system to public health concerns. However, given the diversity of groups affected by the WTO agreements, the push for reform in a health-sensitive direction is not likely to emerge from industry groups. Hence, the undeniable value of the roles played by actors such as government officials, domestic and international/trans-national NGOs, officials of international/trans-national governmental organizations, and health workers in general who have participated in the formation of domestic and international HIV/AIDS policy networks.

CONCLUDING REMARKS

For some international organizations, experiences of participation, albeit sometimes loosely defined, have come to be seen as part and parcel of welfare policy. As such, often the notion of participation has been romantically loaded and failed to fulfill the raised expectations. Thus in practice, the meaning of participation, its importance, and effects vary depending on policy area. For the case of HIV/AIDS, it has been shown that the participation of various actors in the formation of international policy networks has represented a real force for change. Yet as we saw in contrasting the case of health-care financing with that of HIV/AIDS, it is not always easy to discern who will benefit from the formation of policy networks in the present context of globalization. But once again, in the specific case of HIV/AIDS, it has become clear that the international/trans-national policy network in place has allowed vulnerable and marginalized groups, as well as human rights advocates, to create systemic openings for influence at the global and domestic levels. This is particularly true for those affected by the pandemic, and especially for sexual minorities, who have made significant gains due to the strengthening of the links between members of the domestic and international HIV/AIDS policy networks. In this case, activists must be given recognition for their efforts, since they have demanded more than what liberal representative democracy under a market-driven economy would offer, and have been pressing for direct participation in all decision making, locally and globally.

With respect to HIV/AIDS again, it can be argued that some international and trans-national governmental organizations are opening up new spaces for actors that may or may not be to the liking of the incumbent national governments or their constituencies. And as we will further discuss in chapter four, this is certainly the case for sexual minorities in Mexico. The novelty of this dynamics is that some civil society initiatives, such as the increased fund for prevention campaigns among MSM, originate within the policy network and to an extent are exogenous to the political parties in power, somehow questioning their established legitimacy to control the policy process. It is true though that these achievements have not followed a linear progression. In fact, as we have seen with health-care financing and market reforms, the new dynamics still coexists with the persistence of traditional top-down and exclusionary practices. It can also be argued that international actors (governmental and non-governmental alike) might be regarded as being increasingly 'domestic' participants in terms of their functions and influence. This raises further questions and considerations regarding issues of accountability in public-private relations that must be addressed in the future. Such questions are particularly important given that although international organizations as well as most NGOs might have some degree of legitimacy, they do not always have the established mechanisms for holding decision-makers accountable to the greater public. In fact, some of these organizations, such as the WTO or TNCs, seem to be even further removed from domestic democratic accountability than the local political parties, civil society groups, or the government. In fact, the increasing prominence of pharmaceuticals, which have special access to decision-making within and without the UN system, is not always balanced by the same kind of access for aid/loan-recipient countries or marginalized groups.

Furthermore, the fight against HIV/AIDS shows that innovative partnerships can effectively cross the public-private divide, both locally and globally. This is particularly true for social groups that have been highly marginalized, whose basic human rights have been traditionally violated, and who suffer from a notorious vulnerability due to their living conditions and identity. In that sense, the response to the HIV/AIDS pandemic might help to diffuse the idea that civil society-state synergy is a real possibility for LMICs trying to enhance the welfare of their citizens. As a matter of fact, the analysis of the formulation and implementation of HIV/AIDS and health-related initiatives helps to underscore the significance of direct citizen participation in the formulation and implementation of developmental policies. In other words, synergy in the fight against the pandemic might be based on what has been defined as embeddedness -that is, on the institutional ties that connect citizens and public officials across the public-private divide. The question of course would be whether these networks could effectively trigger sustainable human development rather than just being instruments of corruption or rent seeking. Additionally, the fight against HIV/AIDS has the attraction of having developed substantial international networks and contacts, among political activists, medical researchers, and policy makers. It is an area where considerable steps have been taken by international and national health organizations to model and project the future spread of HIV, in an effort to strategically design prevention programs.

With regards to a country's participation in the world economy and trade, and the challenges this poses for the protection of health for all and access to health-care for HIV/AIDS patients, the question is not so much whether to engage in strong international linkages or not. The challenge is to ensure that the increasing interdependence does not compromise the ability to make autonomous decisions, especially concerning economic and social policies that are more inclusive and responsive to the needs of the national population. In this context, it is illuminating to see the ways in which HIV/AIDS policy networks have responded to the increasing challenges of global health. And that they have acted to protect the rights of vulnerable groups from the impact of international trade agreements and TNCs looking for new profit-making opportunities.

Finally, the increasing participation of some civil society groups in project implementation represents both an opportunity and a catalyzing force for the democratization process and the creation of openings not traditionally available in a country like Mexico. Undeniably, this new local-global dynamics has come to represent a challenge to the traditional mechanisms of state-civil society relations, and to the public policymaking embedded in the Mexican political system. Thus, in the following chapter we will look at Mexico's economic, political, and social transformations of the last few decades, to identify the concrete national circumstances under which the struggle against HIV/AIDS has taken place.

CHAPTER 3

Political Liberalization and Health Policies in Mexico

This chapter will focus on Mexico's major economic, political, and social transformation of the last few decades, which has been widely characterized as a democratization process. Thus, the first section will provide an overview of the traditional features of the Mexican political system, and then proceed to a discussion of the process of democratization and civil society's participation in it, paying special attention to the role of sexual minorities. Section two will look at the ways in which the globalist Mexican agenda has impacted social policies in general and health in particular. In sections three and four, respectively, will present a discussion of economic and health cliques or "camarillas," and a description of some of the most important health sector reforms.[49] The analysis that follows will mostly focus on the actual transition from the uninterrupted 70-year PRI rule that came to an end in the federal elections of 2000, to the last two full presidential terms of PAN members Vicente Fox (2000-2006) and Felipe Calderón (2006-2012), with just a few comments on the first half of the most recently elected federal administration of Enrique Peña Nieto (2012-2018) from PRI. It will be argued that some of the political changes that the country experienced during this period are the result of increasing pressure and activism of a variety of civil society actors, some of whom were formerly excluded. In turn, their efforts have been translated into an increasing participation in the process of public policymaking for the case of HIV/AIDS and health-related policies (the focus of chapter four).

MEXICO'S POLITICAL SYSTEM

It is important to emphasize that some of the traits of Mexico's political system are not unique, and one can certainly find similarities with countries within and beyond the Latin American region. Yet the aim is to understand the ways in which the particular set of defining characteristics of the Mexican case have played out in the context of globalization and in response to the HIV/AIDS pandemic. It is equally important to recognize that even though significant changes have taken place and

---

[49] It is important to underline that one of the central features of the policymaking process to which we will pay special attention is the so-called 'camarilla' (a political clique with very concrete characteristics). Therefore, a description and discussion of camarillas will be provided below, with a more focused analysis of health camarillas in section.

others are occurring, some of the long-lived features of an authoritarian and centralist regime remain in place.

Traditional Features

Mexico's political system has had a long history of a very strong state presence, in which vertical forms of social relations have been developed, with a tendency to establish inter-mediation bodies between social groups and the state. This was translated into a very weak participatory tradition, where centralism, corporatism, and patron-clientelism became part of the mechanisms used to manipulate and define collective action (See Cabrero 2000). [50] Additionally, for many years, scholars described the Mexican political system as being semi-authoritarian, presidential, and plagued with electoral fraud (See Camp 1999a; Kaufman 1973; Linz 1973; Schmitter 1974). In the last few decades, however, Mexico experienced a profound process of transformation, especially with respect to its electoral structures and division of powers. Thus, since the 1990s, these changes led scholars to depict it as a country with a political system in transition to democracy (See Camp, 1999a, 2003; Cornelius 1996; Domínguez and McCann 1996).

Although Mexico's institutional arrangements suggest a constitutionally weak presidential system, in reality the country has a long history of a strong "presidentialism." This concentration of power in the executive branch has been a central feature in the definition of the process of policymaking, and it subsequently determined development policies for many decades (See Bailey 1988; Cornelius 1996; Whitehead 1994). Not all power remained in the hands of one individual though, in fact, it has been argued that political power in Mexico goes hand in hand with economic power, and as such, the country has been under the firm control of a united, purposeful, exclusive power elite which was identified as the "bourgeoisie" (Aguilar 1970, p. 311). As put by Smith (1986) in his analysis of Mexican elites and with reference to Wright Mills (1959) "by power elite, we refer to those political, economic, and military circles which as an intricate set of overlapping cliques share decisions having at least national consequences" (p. 18).

Traditionally, public policy in Mexico did not emerge from within the ranks of the official party – Institutional Revolutionary Party (PRI[51])-, nor did it originate in the legislature, but it was very much concentrated in the executive office (namely the president), and the negotiations that took place behind closed doors (See Bailey 1988; Camp 2002; 2003). As put by Camp (1999b, p. 162), for many years, societal groups

---

[50] Patron-clientelism has been defined as the reciprocal relationship of a personal nature between persons of higher social status known as patrons and those of lower status referred to as clients. In this relationship patrons provide clients with their needs, which may vary from money or material goods to physical protection, in return for services that may also vary in content and over time (See Fox 1994). A clientelist system generates an individualistic dynamics and prevents the formation of a pluralist one – one that is based on associational autonomy. On the other hand, corporatism represents a formal relationship between selected groups or institutions and the government, through which social demands are channelled and the government responds to them (Camp 2003, p. 12).

[51] Partido Revolucionario Institucional.

in Mexico who wanted some part in national policy decisions had to make their concerns and interests known to the executive branch at the highest possible level. As a consequence, due to the hierarchical decision-making structure, for most of the twentieth century the president's private secretary acted as a gatekeeper in denying or granting requests to see the president, performing a crucial role in the decision-making process (Camp 2003, p. 71). And as a result, as underlined by Spalding (1980, p. 430), policymaking in Mexico tended to be highly particularistic and dis-aggregated.

For its part, traditionally, the legislative branch of the government was dominated by the PRI and controlled by the Executive, and as such it played a very weak role as an initiator in the process of policymaking. Yet due to some of the recent changes in the political system – to which we will refer below - there has been an increasing interest in the role the Congress can play and the changes necessary to strengthen it (See Ugalde 2000; Lujambio 1995; 2000). Thus, constitutionalist in form, with a fixed electoral calendar, a federal structure, no re-election, and progressively civilian supremacy over the armed forces, for many years the Mexican state was characterized by its hyper-presidentialism and centralism (See Camp 1999b; Whitehead 1995). Presidentialism resulted in the absence of most checks and balances and the perpetuation of one state-party free to monopolize public office, which in turn systematically marginalized organized opposition. This was accompanied by centralism, that is the allocation of more decision-making authority to the national government, which in the case of Mexico meant one individual, namely the president (See Bailey 1988).

For the most part of the twentieth century, the apparatus of the one dominant party supported presidentialism. Yet it must be pointed out that the consolidation of the PRI was not at all smooth. After the "official" end of the Mexican Revolution (1910-1920), the country still experienced some factional fighting among the 'revolutionary family,' as well as the rebellion of Christian forces against the state – known as 'Guerras Cristeras'[52] (1927-29) (See Joseph and Nugent 1994; Knight 1986). By the end of his presidential term though, Lázaro Cárdenas (1934-40) was able to officially achieve peace, allowing his successor, Manuel Ávila Camacho (1940-6), to lead the new regime to its consolidation (See Hamilton 1982). The following two decades – the 1950s and most of the 1960s - have been described as the most stable and prosperous period in Mexican recent history, one in which the PRI prevailed as the one dominant party. However, this period of political stability came to an end in 1968, when the political system was shaken by a series of social and political events that ended with a massacre at the student protest in Mexico City, in the public square of Tlatelolco (See De Mora 1973; Scherer and Monsiváis 1999). Since then, the country has experienced a slow transition from an authoritarian dominant party rule to a more democratic regime.

---

[52] Known in English as the 'Cristero' Revolts. These revolts had a long-lasting impact in Mexican history, since they were the basis for the creation of several conservative and powerful political groups, some of which have gained influential power in recent years.

As mentioned, the PRI regime was also marked by its patron-clientelistic (See Camp 1996; Cornelius 1996) and corporatist structures, which defined most state-society relations (See Camp 2003; Grayson 1998). Not unlike other Latin American countries, corporatism was widely used in Mexico as an instrument of political control to quell actual and potential dissent, and it has been legally constructed, thus having an important institutional framework. Under the auspices of PRI, workers were organized and formed the Confederation of Mexican Workers (CTM), peasants marched under the banner of the National Confederation of Peasants (CNC), whereas other popular interests were officially "represented" by the National Confederation of Popular Organizations (CNOP) (See Bizberg 1990; Grayson 1989). For the purposes of the current analysis of HIV/AIDS and health–related policies, it must be underlined that in officially recognized trade unions were incorporated into the social security system, through corporatist arrangements that resulted in generous benefits (See Mesa-Lago 1978; Laurell 1997).

There are two other major central features of the Mexican political system that deserve special attention: the use of co-optation and the existence of political cliques referred to as 'camarillas.' Co-optation, which for many years was the favoured mechanism used by the government to weaken opposition, helped to explain the diminishing of resources and the expansion of the state that were characteristic of the PRI's s rule (Camp 2003, p. 153). For its part, the so-called 'camarilla, or 'camarillismo,' is a key trait for the present analysis, since it has significantly contributed to determine who participates in the process of policymaking, and is directly associated with the centralization of power and presidentialism. Furthermore, and as will be shown below, this feature of the Mexican political system is still relevant for the analysis of the formation of the HIV/AIDS policy network and the formulation of health-related policies. A camarilla has been defined as "a group of people who have political interests in common and rely on one another to improve their chances within the political leadership" (Camp 1999b, p.116). Furthermore, this group represents "a network of public officials bound by ties of strong personal loyalty to a camarilla leader" (Teichman 2001, p. 130), and has long been regarded as a key variable in explaining the recruitment process in the Mexican political system (See also Smith 1979). This political clique has determined more than any other of the features of the Mexican political system presented above who goes to the top of the political ladder, the paths taken and the posts assigned, as well as participation in the process of public policymaking.

In general, and as a consequence of the aforementioned characteristics of the Mexican political system, the government has not been seen as a facilitator of civil society's participation. On the contrary, the PRI regime afforded the government leadership firm political control. In this context, the Executive occupied the central stage of the policymaking process, determining sectoral policies (e.g., health and education) through interpersonal relationships ('camarillismo'), rather than through professional or policy networks.[53] In addition, policymaking was largely insulated from public pressure, due to the absence of autonomous publics ('limited pluralism') and low social participation (See Kaufman 1973; Teichman 1988). And although some elements of this undemocratic legacy still persist, as will see below, the country has experienced a process of democratization in the last few decades.

Some state institutions were susceptible to societal pressures. In fact, in some cases and in a limited way state managers did respond to societal conflict, political-bureaucratic interests, and, especially, to the concerns of the business community (See Bailey 1988; Teichman 1988). Although, for the longest time, the business community was influential, the state had an identifiable will and was able to enforce that will against the wishes of the latter (Smith 1979, p. 191-216; See also Bailey 1988; Story 1986). Traditionally, Mexico's industrialists and politicians differed in basic respects, since, as argued by Smith (1979), "members of the two elites came from separate segments of the upper-plus-middle class, if not from separate classes" (p. 214). In fact, for years, Mexico's authoritarian regime reflected the constant interplay between a relatively coherent state interest and a somewhat less coherent set of business interests (Smith 1979, p. 215). More recently, however, big business has gained greater access to the highest levels of political power (See Alba Vega 1996; Roett 1998). For their part, and as we will see below, other groups within civil society have also made important gains in positioning themselves at the centre of the policymaking process in some issue areas, such as HIV/AIDS.

In addition to being centralized and very much driven by the Executive, since the administration of President Carlos Salinas de Gortari (1988-1994), public policy became more and more the product of the globalist economic agenda. And the formulation of public policy – especially in the area of economics – was dominated by the so-called technocratic elite (See Camp 1990, 1999b; 2003; Teichman 1988). More recently, however, especially since the first non-PRI President Vicente Fox Quezada's (2000-2003) was elected, the Executive and its economic cabinet have faced increased challenges in dominating the economic agenda. But undoubtedly, the globalist agenda has significantly contributed, and still does today, to the imposition of constraints on social and health policy options.

Another peculiarity of policymaking in Mexico, in the past as much as in recent years, is what Teichman (1988, p. 9) refers to as the contradictions between official rhetoric and actual policy. This factor contributes to the difficulties, for the analysis of public policy, in defining or trying to understand what the "real objectives of the state" are. Paradoxically, as stated by Whitehead (1995), the 1917 Mexican Constitution was an advanced liberal democratic charter, given that some aspects of it

---

[53] For an analysis of the contrast between the concept of professional and policy networks see Mark Evans, "Análisis de redes de políticas públicas: una perspectiva británica", *Gestión y Política Pública*, vol. VII, n. 2, México, CIDE, 1998, as well as P. Dunleavy and B. O'Learly, Theories of the States, London, MacMillan, 1987, and; A. Smith, "Les idées en action: le référentiel, sa mobilisation et la notion de policy network", in Faure, Pollet and Warin, La construction du sens dans les politiques publiques, Paris, L'Harmattan, 1995.

offered a more advanced form of "democracy" than other liberal charters of the time. As a matter of law, democracy was viewed not just as a juridical structure and a political regime, but also as a system of life based on the constant improvement of the economic, social, and cultural conditions of the people (Whitehead 1995, p. 250). Similarly, although the constitutional basis of the regime is the municipality, in reality power has been traditionally centralized at the higher levels of government.[54]

As such, for many years, the political system showed extraordinary longevity and resilience. It was not until the federal elections of 1997 that, for the first time in close to 70 years of rule, the PRI did not obtain the majority in Congress. And three years later, the long and uninterrupted PRI rule came to an end with the victory of the right-of-centre presidential candidate, Vicente Fox Quezada from the National Action Party (PAN[55]), in the elections of July 2, 2000. Although it is impossible to deny the persistence of some of the highly entrenched features of the Mexican political system listed above, it is also important to emphasize the fact that there have been important transformations in the last few years.

A Tamed Transition to Democracy

Although the Mexican political system began a slow process of transition since 1968, it was not until 1997 that the opposition won the largest number of congressional seats ever, 136 of the 300 majority districts. Combined with their plurinominal (based on proportional representation) seats, the four opposition parties - PAN, the left-of-centre Democratic Revolution Party (PRD[56]), the leftist Labour Party (PT[57]), and the conservative Green Party (PVEM[58]) - controlled 262 of the 500 seats and, for the first time, the Chamber of Deputies. As we have seen, for the most part of the Twentieth century the system was characterized by the submissiveness of the Congress and the Judiciary to the Executive. Yet after PRI's loss of control of Congress, the opposition, consistently and more successfully, challenged presidential power. And in spite of some persistent constraints on congressional power, and a continuing Executive control over the Judiciary, this new reality represented a change in the way public policymaking was to be conducted. For the first time, and from then on, the Executive was really questioned and the bills sent to Congress underwent scrutiny and were subjected to debate (See Lujambio 2000; Ugalde 2000).

However, two important structural conditions still contribute to the Legislative power's weaker policy-making position compared to the Executive's. The first of these is the continued prohibition on consecutive re-election of Congress representatives (which limits the expertise that would accompany a legislative career)

---

[54] Unfortunately, as Whitehead points out, most of the principles endorsed by the constitution have represented more of a rhetorical discourse than real commitments, with more ambitious clauses being added to the constitution than the upholding of the original dispositions.

[55] Partido Acción Nacional.

[56] Partido de la Revolución Democrática.

[57] Partido del Trabajo.

[58] Partido Verde Ecologista de México.

(See Nacif 1997; Ugalde 2000). The second one is the limited budget devoted to congressional resources and staff, with the consequent lack of preparation to consistently and effectively participate in policy formulation (Camp 1999b, p. 169; Levy and Bruhn 2001, p. 275). Yet in spite of these limitations, and as a result of the electoral victories from the opposition, since the early 1990s Congressional representatives from different regions were and continue to be able to exert more influence and make their voices heard (See Lujambio 1995).

It must be pointed out that in spite of the multiple-party control in the Chamber of Deputies during the transition period, the percentage of legislation pieces passed initiated by the executive branch remained remarkably high. For example, the Executive had a success rate of 99 percent from 1994-1997, and 90 percent from 1997-2000 (Camp 2003, p. 172-173). At the same time, the number of legislative proposals increased dramatically – nearly 150 percent – from the 1994-1997 to the 1997-2000 session (Camp 2003, p. 173). As a consequence of this, different groups who used to focus all their efforts on the president now also lobby members of Congress (Camp 2003, p. 177; Sullivan 2001, p. 184). In turn, this made the holding of a national legislative post increasingly significant in the policymaking process.

The year 2000 elections represented the culmination of a more than a decade-long series of opposition victories that occurred both at the state and local levels. For example, in the elections of 1997, the left-of-centre PRD made a significant comeback, as did the party's standard-bearer, Cuauhtémoc Cárdenas. Cárdenas won with 48 percent of the vote and handily defeated both PRI and PAN as the first elected head of government of the then Federal District (Now officially and legally called the City of Mexico) since the 1920s (Camp 2003, p. 196). All opposition victories were possible due to the reforms introduced in the 1990s to the electoral laws and institutions. The country spent millions of dollars creating technologically sophisticated and credible electoral institutions, revamping voter ID cards and registration lists, and establishing the non-partisan, autonomous Federal Electoral Institute (IFE[59]).

In spite of the inertial forces and the remaining features of the old PRI regime, the gains made by the opposition and the inroads towards a more democratic regime have had a significant impact on some of the various traits of the political system. Clientelism and corporatism, for example, have undergone major changes, especially in the 1990s (Camp 1999b, p. 10; See also Fox 1994; Grayson 1998). In his analysis of the Mexican case, Fox (1994, p. 157) calls the attention to the patterns of state-society relations involved in the transition from clientelism to citizenship. Fox shows that although redoubts of persistent authoritarian-clientelism still remained in place, new enclaves of pluralist tolerance and large grey areas of 'semi-clientelism' in between have materialized. Fox (1994) argues that the emergence of what he calls associational autonomy has been politically constructed and is the product of iterative cycles of conflict among three key sets of actors: autonomous social movements, authoritarian elites reluctant to cede power, and reformist state managers - the latter

---

[59] Instituto Federal Electoral, more recently re-structured and renamed as Instituto Nacional Electoral (INE).

being defined as those governmental actors willing to accept increased associational autonomy (Fox 1994, p. 156). As a result, different conflict cycles have led to three distinct patterns of interaction between the state and social movements; continued clientelism, modernized semi-clientelism, and more pluralistic bargaining, distributed unevenly both geographically and socially (See Fox 1994). Additionally, the combination of opposition electoral gains, economic crises, the privatization of public enterprises, and the shrinking of the state (factors that will be discussed below) also contributed – due to the depletion of public resources - to the weakening of corporatist and clientelistic arrangements (See Camp 2003; Teichman 2001).

In the past, fraud and abstensionism characterized the periodic convocation to vote. And although, after the election of Vicente Fox in 2000, it seemed that the country had put the worst days of electoral fraud behind, in 2006 and 2012, yet again, some serious doubts were cast over the respective presidential elections. In 2006 the difference between the first and second place candidate was 0.56% of the national vote, which together with Vicente Fox's meddling in the campaign in favour of the PAN candidate, led to the discontent of many and accusations of fraud by the then leader of Mexico's leftist Party of the Democratic Revolution (PRD), Andrés Manuel López Obrador (See Crespo 2008). The latter unsuccessfully demanded the recount of the ballots, who then lead to a series of long-lasting protests and never actually accepted the results, even after Felipe Calderón (from PAN) took office in December of that same year. Among other Mexican scholars, José Antonio Crespo (2008) argues that the refusal to do the recount of the votes left a stain on the electoral process and had a negative impact on the public perception and the legitimacy of the process and its results (See also Ortega Ortíz and Somuano Ventura 2015). In 2012, once again, there were serious complaints about irregularities during the federal election, which was described as far from fair, marred by media bias and voter fraud in favour of the PRI candidate and today's president Enrique Peña Nieto.

Even before the two most recent federal elections, and in spite of some of the transformations mentioned above in state-society relations, the growing pattern of opposition party victories did not result in a significant growth of citizen confidence in political parties (Levy and Bruhn 2001, p. 275; Crespo 2008; Ortega Ortíz and Somuano Ventura 2015). After the 1994 elections, when there was an extraordinary turnout of 78 percent of registered voters - the highest ever recorded in Mexico (Camp 2003, p. 194) – citizens' confidence has been undermined due to incompetence, unfulfilled campaign pledges, and corruption. According to a 1998 survey, only about one-third of all Mexicans gave positive marks to the different political parties (Camp 1999a, p. 234). More recently, according to the annual survey conducted by the Latinobarómetro in 2015, almost 83% of people in Mexico have little to no trust at all in political parties. When asked about whether democracy is preferable to any other type of government, only 48.4% responded positively. [60] This is particularly worrisome for the future of democracy, especially if one adds this to the declining respect for judicial courts (73.8% has little to no trust on the judiciary), given that

---

[60] http://www.latinobarometro.org/latOnline.jsp

together with political parties they represent two sets of institutions that are crucial to democracy's success (See Prud'homme 2015). As we all know, although elections are only one of the necessary elements of a democratic regime, one of their central functions is to provide individuals and social groups with access to decision-making, through the development of a constituency relationship between the elected and the electorate. Furthermore, as will be discussed below, the lack of confidence in political parties is particularly important in understanding the increasing role that NGOs play in various areas – particularly in the case of HIV/AIDS.

With regards to 'camarillismo,' which is a central feature for the analysis of policymaking and the process of Mexico's transition to democracy, it has been argued (See Camp 1999b) that even though traditionally defined camarillas are not likely to disappear, they have been going through some important transformations. Moreover, scholars have suggested that during the transition years the cohesive nature of camarillas began to break down (See Camp 1990; 2000; 2003; Ronfeldt 1989). Originally, for example, a more limited personal profile regarding family relations, public career, and education background was the most important determinant for the recruitment of camarillas' members. In recent years, however, among other changes, there has been an elevation of private over public university education among the political leadership. Additionally, the traditional distinction between social and educational backgrounds of political and business leaders (See Camp 1980; Smith 1979) is becoming increasingly blurred, especially with Vicente Fox himself and some of his closest collaborators having a strong entrepreneurial background (See Camp 1999b; 2002; 2003; D'Artigues 2002).

The increasing presence of a technocratic elite has also been a relatively recent trait of camarillas' composition, and as such it has been fully documented (See Camp 1980; 1990; Smith 1986; Teichman 1988; 2001; 2004), particularly in relation to the process of economic reforms. In this regard, it is important to underline the fact that according to Camp, "the assertion by some scholars that technocrats lack political skills is incorrect and misleading...[t]he political-technocrat, a more apt label, is primarily distinguished from the politician of the 1960s or 1970s by lack of party experience, by the fact that he or she has never held elective office, and by specialized education abroad" (Camp 1999b, p. 121).

As will be shown in the following chapter, this trend towards the increasing presence of technocratic members in the political elite plays a central role in the analysis of the constraints imposed on health sector reforms. Furthermore, it is precisely with the intention of shedding light on the transformation of camarillas, and their impact on policy formulation and implementation, that we adopt the concept of policy networks for the analysis of health and HIV/AIDS). As argued before, the examination of the formation of these networks will also allow us to look at the institutionalization of power relations both within the network and the broader socio-economic and political context. It will further allow us to move beyond considering state-society relations in Mexico through the prism of pluralism or corporatism.

It is necessary to emphasize that although some characteristics of the Mexican political system are in fact changing, with their subsequent impact on policymaking, significant inertial forces remain in place. As expected, whenever there is a transition process, such as the Mexican process of democratization, with new spaces for participation in decision-making opening up, this generates some tension and disagreements between political and social actors. Juan Linz (1973) called these political situations poorly institutionalized. It is also expected that after a long past of a traditionally closed and rigid system, a transition government would inherit institutional structures that are not designed to be permeable. Under these circumstances, often, the agenda-setting process continues to be endogenous; social problems continue to be perceived and translated by different groups of specialists in each area, with discussions and negotiations taking place at the level of Secretariats and camarillas. In fact, in most cases, and the health sector is certainly not an exception to this, since the cabinet Secretary[61] continues to be the key figure in initiating policy proposals. However, as will be argued below, policy networks have become increasingly influential in the definition of public policymaking.

At the risk of stating the obvious, it is necessary to underline the fact that even though electoral competition is necessary, it is not sufficient for a successful transition to democracy. As Jonathan Fox (1994) points out, "increasingly, political scientists are stressing the Tocquevillian idea that democratic governance depends on the density of associational life in civil society" (p. 152). In other words, changes in electoral rules, while potentially a hugely important step, do not by themselves suffice for the transition to democracy. In the case of Mexico, and in spite of the significant changes discussed above, Baer (1999, p. 91) underlined the fact that "the cultural values needed to underpin democratic governance – tolerance, compromise, and civic participation – remain weak," all of which are necessary elements for the consolidation of democracy. Thus, the need to look at the participation of civil society beyond electoral reforms.

The Role of Civil Society and Sexual Minorities

Some groups within civil society deserve a significant share of the credit for the changes made to the electoral system, since more often than not, PRI's electoral defeats were conceded in response to mass civic antifraud protests rather than as spontaneous and actual respect for ballot results.[62] In general, Mexicanist scholars agree that there has been a proliferation of popular movements and NGOs in the last few decades (See Chalmers and Piester 1996; Foweraker and Craig 1990; Camp 2003). However, it is true that not all popular movements evolve into formal NGOs (See Haynes 1997). Yet in the case of sexual minorities and HIV/AIDS activism in

---

[61] It is important to make explicit the rationale behind the use of Secretary/Secretariat as opposed to Minister/Ministry in the Mexican context. The fact of the matter is that Mexican politics is defined by a presidential system, in which cabinet members are not elected representatives – as is the case in a parliamentary system (ministers) – but are employees appointed by the executive with no need for ratification by the legislative power. This has a great significance in reminding us of the highly personalistic tradition of the concentration of power in the executive branch of the government.

[62] Levy and Bruhn (2001) provide one of the best overviews of the process of civil society activism before and during the transition period.

Mexico, those groups fully engaged in the promotion of a more democratic process of public policymaking, which are referred to as action groups by Haynes (1997, p. 15-16), and have been clearly identified as formal NGOs. Furthermore, as will be argued in chapter four, some HIV/AIDS NGOs have gained influential power and become much more than simple service providers.

But going back to what could be called the general awakening of several civil society groups in the course of the last few decades, this phenomenon can be seen as the consequence of six different historical moments. First, many groups with different political, economic, and social interests grew out of the general malaise that resulted from the 1968 student massacre. Secondly, some of these groups were given an additional boost and others emerged as a response to the 1985 earthquake that greatly affected Mexico City. Thirdly, civic mobilization right after the highly contested 1988 presidential elections, and the discontent with the political and economic (globalist) changes introduced thereafter, contributed to the increasing growth and strength of NGOs. In 1988, after a polemical electoral process, in which fraud allegations were widespread and the government was accused of robbing the PRD candidate Cuauhtémoc Cárdenas of the victory, Carlos Salinas de Gortari was declared elected president. At that point in time, the growth of opposition was faced with what has been argued to be the last extremely authoritarian exercise of power (Salinas' presidency). Under Salinas, various civil society groups were mostly ignored and manipulated, and opposition groups and individuals (particularly PRD members) were repressed (See Bruhn 1997; Sánchez 1999). Fourthly, if one considers the January 1994 Zapatista uprising, and now more than two-decade old movement, in a separate category (given its more radical character), one can also see that it has encouraged civil society groups (particularly indigenous groups) in their efforts to have a significant political influence. The fifth moment is the organization of civil society groups during the 1994 general elections, under the co-ordination of umbrella NGO 'Alianza Cívica' (Civic Alliance). In the months leading to the elections, Mexican NGOs banded together on a scale never seen before, with some 400 human rights and other civil society groups marshalling 20,000 volunteers to scrutinize the votes and carry out a series of crucial checks on the election process (Camp 2003, p. 154). Their efforts stimulated a civic ground swell that brought out an even larger number of observers belonging to labour unions, business organizations, and youth groups. Lastly, the sixth defining moment for the thrust of civil society mobilization was the 2000 elections, with the victory of PAN, which not only put an end to more than 70 years of PRI rule but also gave various groups within civil society new hopes for participation and effecting political change.[63]

---

[63] There are two more recent movements that have been considered by some as part of this trend. Although their impact on the electoral process or the transformation of the political system is not evident, or perhaps it is too early to tell; these are 1) the university students movement *#YoSoy132*, which got mobilized in 2006 against the PRI candidate (Peña Nieto) and the biased support he received from the private media, and 2) the *Movement for Peace with Justice and Dignity*, which was a reaction against the increasing daily violence and civilian killings that have accompanied the so-called "War on Drugs" started by Felipe Calderón (See Bizberg 2015).

Equally significant, for the emphasis on civil society's participation in the process of democratization, are some findings regarding the public perceptions about NGOs vis-à-vis public institutions. According to polls by *Este País*,[64] back in 2003, only 20 percent of the Mexican population believed in their government institutions, in contrast to the increasingly effective and visible NGOs which garnered a credibility rate of 80 percent (Camp 2003, p. 154). In this regard, Camp (1999b) points out that in Mexico, in general, "NGOs and [civil society] groups are characterized by their lack of partisan political attachments" (p. 149). In some cases, they took significant steps in lobbying the Congress, independently, for their respective causes (See Chalmers and Piester 1996). Therefore, in the context of some gains made on the electoral terrain and the previously mentioned lack of confidence in political parties, other kinds of formal and informal channels of civil society political participation have increased in importance.

Interestingly, and a key factor for the current analysis of the impact of globalization at the domestic level, often Mexican NGOs have more contact with their foreign counterparts than with their domestic colleagues,[65] establishing South-South and North-South partnerships. And although it is not the case in all issue areas, as we will see below, HIV/AIDS NGOs do belong to this group of interconnected organizations, which have also been quite active in establishing linkages at the local level. This has also contributed to an expansion of international influences in Mexico through NGOs' links to international actors. Camp (1999b) questioned, however, whether these civil society groups and non-violent popular movements can "go beyond making social demands to serving as a direct bridge to political change, establishing organizational and policy alternatives" (p. 152). This reality clearly speaks to the present analysis of HIV/AIDS and the ways in which, through its involvement in the formation of a policy network, civil society has been participating, with varying degrees of success in the formulation of HIV/AIDS and health-related policies.

As a matter of fact, the participation of NGOs is central to the analysis of the formation of policy networks and their role in the process of policymaking. The increasing importance of this sector is not exclusive to the case of HIV/AIDS or Mexico, but as argued by Duquette (1999), non-partisan civil society groups and NGOs have been thriving for years all over Latin America. Therefore, the efforts of HIV/AIDS and sexual minorities' activism must be put in context within the broader phenomenon of civil society mobilization in Latin America and Mexico. By way of consistently issuing demands, which are more or less formally met, some civil society groups have been able to expand "the realm of the politically possible" (Duquette 1999, p. 228). Mexico has been part of this trend, with the growth of political opposition and civil society mobilization weakening the state-dominated corporatism.

---

[64] The first political magazine in Mexico dedicated to surveys, whose editor, Federico Reyes Heroles, is a well-known intellectual.
[65] See David C. Scott, "NGOs achieve credibility in Mexico: http://www.oneworld.org/crosslines/xlines2_mexico.html.

Although, most Mexicans belong to no NGO (Camp 2003, p. 63), by 2003 there were more than 5,000 NGOs serving different communities throughout Mexico (Camp 2003, p. 154; See also Townsend 2001). Mexican NGOs are working in various aspects of development and differ in size, missions, capabilities, and in their political and cultural outlooks. Some provide technical and financial support for community initiatives, while others assist in Mexico's transition to a more open and accountable government. Some others, although possessing local knowledge and some organizational capabilities, lack the necessary funds, or the necessary technical knowledge (i.e., expertise on legislation and regulations, or scientific procedures) to attain a strong bargaining position before the Mexican government (See Townsend 2001). Hence, external support from more resourceful Northern NGOs and International Governmental Organizations is essential for them to succeed in their efforts. In some cases, though, a report culture, language and buzzwords, performance indicators, outputs, and over-reliance on paperwork rather than visits to the field, as well as complicated funding applications, prevent some local NGOs from getting into the loop of funding institutions. Additionally, and similar to HIV/AIDS NGOs, human rights and environmental NGOs have provided protection and support to otherwise voiceless groups.[66] It is interesting to note also that although, as pointed out by Castells (2996 and 2010), the use of new communication technologies has contributed to the strengthening of civil society movements and organizations, face-to-face encounters at international meetings tend to be the real spark-points of communication and partnerships (Interviews with representatives of various NGOs in Rio de Janeiro (2000), Havana (2003), Mexico City (2008); See also Townsend 2001, p. 15).

In our analysis of civil society groups and the process of democratization, we must also look at the role of sexual minorities. As stated in the first chapter, and without denying the importance and urgency of looking at women and the way they have been affected by the pandemic, the focus on sexual minorities responds to a long-overdue need to examine the links between health and sexual-minorities' politics as integral elements of the processes of development and democratization in Mexico. It is also necessary to underline the limited number of critical analyses of the politics of sexual minorities in Mexico (See De la Dehesa, 2010; Díez 2015). Sadly, many of the original participants in the movement have been victims of the pandemic and are not alive to tell their part of the story. So that the combination of these factors, as pointed out by Laguarda (2001), represents an obstacle to put together a complete picture of the movement's history.

The tension between globalization and globalism also becomes evident in the analysis of HIV/AIDS and sexual minorities. Here, it is important to draw from Dennis Altman's (2001) analysis of sex and globalization, and argue that globalism has contributed to the transformation of sexuality into a commodity. This has impacted on the national realities of many countries, resulting in the further social and economic marginalization of women and sex workers (male and female), worsening

---

[66] See David Winder's piece on Mexican philanthropy: http://www.fas.harvard.edu/~drclas/publications/revista/mexico/Winder.html

or reducing the possibilities of obtaining and processing the necessary information for sex negotiation and health protection. Moreover, insecurity and precariousness (vulnerability) reduce the motivation for postponing the satisfaction of basic needs (such as sexual intercourse) and increase the likelihood of future negative consequences (such as illness as a result of disease transmission).

Additionally, although a thorough analysis of tolerance falls beyond the scope of the present analysis, it is important to underline its centrality in the context of development, HIV/AIDS, and globalization. As such, tolerance is regarded as a virtue that is widely recognized as one of the core values and practices in democratic societies. In this sense, it has been argued that as a result of globalization and Mexico's integration through NAFTA with its North-American neighbours (namely Canada and the U.S.), the Mexican society is part of a world-wide cultural shift (See Inglehart, Nevitte, and Basáñez 1994). Yet according to the *World Values Survey* (Camp 2003, p. 75-97), back in 2002 less than 40 per cent of Mexican families taught their children the importance of tolerance. In fact, human rights abuses related to HIV/AIDS and sexual orientation have been widely documented for more than a couple of decades now (See Reding 1995; Cleary 1995; Various Human Rights Watch Americas reports). The latest survey on tolerance, conducted by the National Council Against Discrimination (CONAPRED) in 2010, showed that about 44% of the people would not like to live in the same household with a lesbian or a homosexual (with important differences according to age group).[67] At the individual level, tolerance within the family unit may depend on the contribution of members of this minority to their family income, leading sometimes to a kind of 'modus vivendi' of 'todo hecho, nada dicho' (everything permitted, nothing said) (Lumsden 1991, p. 45). At the same time, others argue that the reality of the HIV/AIDS pandemic has triggered a breakaway from some of the long-held sexual inhibitions in Mexican society (Interview with the late Carlos Monsiváis, a well-known writer and gay Mexican intellectual, Mexico City, August 13, 2002).

In the analysis of democratization in Mexico, it is crucial to recognize that the struggle of sexual minorities for recognition has been an integral element and should be acknowledged as central to this process. In other words, organized LGBT groups efforts and their activism have been central to the democratization process, and not just a "side effect." In fact, the formation of some gay organizations coincided with the electoral reforms introduced by López Portillo in 1977, with significant linkages between them and the political Left. For instance, the 'National Front Against Repression'[68] was the first organization that embraced the Mexican Left, while 'Lamda' (another gay organization) was also responsible for introducing gay rights into the platform of the Left (Interview with Juan Jacobo Hernández, Mexico City, November 6, 2001; Interview with José María Covarrubias, Mexico City, October 20, 2001).[69] These groups developed ties with the Trotskyist 'Worker's Revolutionary

---

[67] For some updates see http://www.conapred.org.mx/userfiles/files/Enadis

[68] Frente Nacional contra la Represión.

[69] For a more detailed account of who these activists are and their organization see chapter four, section 4.3 and Appendix 4.2.

Party' (PRT[70]) (Lumsden 1991, p. 62). However, as pointed out by Lumsden, the marriage of convenience between the PRT and the movement could not last. Even though most of the early activists were nominally socialist, the explicit identification of socialism with homosexual liberation tended to alienate the majority of gay organizations' immediate supporters, for they were mostly middle-class and did not share their leftist political views. On the other hand, some members of the political Left were also afraid of alienating potential supporters for their association with sexual minorities' organizations. The late leftist politician Heberto Castillo represented one of the few most prominent cases of association between the Left and the gay movement. In 1988, Castillo was the presidential candidate for the Marxist Mexican Socialist Party (PMS[71]), and later withdrew from the race in favour of the candidacy of Cuauhtémoc Cárdenas (PRD). Heberto Castillo once publicly declared that "homosexuality is not only as normal as heterosexuality, but also revolutionary in the sense that regardless of the politics of individual homosexuals their demands imply a fundamental change in society because they open new spaces for creativity" (Lumsden 1991, p. 73).

It was the dismissal of a Sears department store employee in 1971, on account of his allegedly homosexual demeanor, which became the catalyst that brought together the first organized group of Mexican gays and lesbians in the country's history (Confidential interviews with gay activists, Mexico City, 2001/2002; See also Lumsden 1991). For the first time, they would publicly question and challenge society for their stigmatization and social oppression. Several consciousness-raising and political study groups emerged in the following years, aided and abetted by prominent intellectuals such as Nancy Cárdenas[72] and Carlos Monsiváis,[73] who had ties with gay activists in the U.S. and Britain (See Lumsden 1991).[74] Some leading gay activists, such as Juan Jacobo Hernández - who founded and currently directs HIV/AIDS NGO 'Colectivo Sol' - had lived in the U.S. and were much influenced by their exposure to the explosive assertion of gay rights that had taken place in the neighbouring country (Interview with Juan Jacobo Hernández, Mexico City, November 6, 2001).

By the early 1980s, the gay movement in Mexico, like in many other parts of the world, adopted the rainbow flag as the sexual diversity banner.[75] At the beginning though, some groups, like the 'Homosexual Front for Revolutionary Action,'[76] saw

---

[70] Partido Revolucionario de los Trabajadores.

[71] Partido Mexicano Socialista.

[72] Theatre professor at UNAM and respected intellectual, she was also host of various Radio and TV shows. In 1968, Cárdenas Martínez actively participated in the formation of 'Alianza de Intelectuales, Escritores y Artistas en apoyo al Movimiento Estudiantil' (Alliance of Intellectuals, Writers and Artists in Support of the Student Movement). She died of cancer in March of 1994.

[73] Considered one of the best contemporary Mexican writers and an influential intellectual. Monsiváis supported the fight against the pandemic and openly denounced discrimination against sexual minorities.

[74] In August of 1975 Nancy Cárdenas, Carlos Monsiváis and Luis González de Alba published 'El Primer Manifiesto en Defensa de los Homosexuales en México: Contra la práctica del ciudadano como botín policiaco' (The First Manifest in Defence of Homosexuals in Mexico) in the midst of the emerging homosexual movement.

[75] Designed by Gilbert Baker in 1978 for the gay pride march in San Francisco, California.

[76] Frente Homosexual de Acción Revolucionaria.

the term gay as a cultural imposition, yet it was later preferred for its neutrality (Laguarda 2001, p. 38; See also Lumsden 1991). Interestingly, and in contrast to the case of the U.S. or Canada, and in spite of the influence of the U.S. on Mexico's gay culture, for many years, there were no real gay ghettos as such in Mexico City, which is the most liberal and open city in the country. Furthermore, it has been argued that sexual identities in Mexico seem to be much more fluid and not nearly dichotomized into gay and straight "cultures" as in the rest of North America (See González Pérez 2001; Hernández Cabrera 2001; Núñez Noriega 2001). In one of the few detailed studies of Mexican men's sexual behaviours, by Joseph Carrier, for instance, it is estimated that 30 per cent of Mexican males between the age of 15 and 25 are bisexual to different degrees (Lumsden 1992, p. 46). In fact, the increasing number of women infected with HIV by their male partners might confirm Carrier's findings.

The history of the lesbian and gay movement is also reflective of the economic crises experienced in the last decades, which will be discussed in the following section. In 1982, the year of that the debt crisis publicly began and a significant peso devaluation, the organized movement (which was mostly based in Mexico City) entered a period of crisis of its own. By 1984, it had nearly collapsed, and by 1991 it had lost most of its political infrastructure. Not surprisingly, due to the 1982's economic crisis, gay and lesbians were much less willing to come out or to put their jobs in jeopardy as a result of their activism. Accordingly, for many years, the fragmentation of lesbian and gay organizations represented one of the greatest obstacles in the struggle for tolerance and the democratization of political life in Mexico. The energy, skills and experience of the movement's leaders became dissipated in personal recriminations. Such conflicts were major obstacles to the reformulation of the movement under difficult conditions, given the economic and social crises that by then had engulfed Mexico. A handful of strong organizations survived: 'Colectivo Sol,' 'Guerrilla Gay,' the 'Grupo Homosexual de Acción Revolucionaria,' and the 'Círculo Cultural Gay,' whose energies increasingly turned towards the fight against HIV/AIDS. Outside Mexico City, there were not any gay organizations of major significance in terms of their membership, public reach, and activism. One of the few examples is the 'Homosexual Pride and Liberation Group[77]' (GOHL), which was created in Guadalajara, Jalisco (Lumsden 1991, p.80-81), which to this day fights against discrimination and police repression, offering some psychological and legal counselling services and HIV/AIDS information, a gay hot-line and a growing library and archives.

Paradoxically, as argued by some gay activists, for many years, PRI's pragmatism represented an advantage in the sense that it did not exercise power in the name of an official exclusionary ideology (Interview with Juan Jacobo Hernández, Mexico City, November 6, 2001; Confidential interviews with gay activists, Mexico City, 2001-2015). In fact, and in spite of some other criticisms directed towards its more than 70 years of rule, PRI's pragmatic coalition of forces had presided over a process that brought about an increasingly diverse society and a secular government

---

[77] Grupo de Orgullo Homosexual de Liberación.

(70s and 80s). Historically, the separation between the Church and the State dates back to the 1857 Mexican Constitution and the Liberal Reform Laws of 1858, which sought to diminish the traditional power of the Catholic Church and the centrality of religion in public life in general. One must not overlook, however, the fact that a characteristic of the Mexican State is the discrepancy between legal rights and the way authority is exercised in the name of the State. There are, for example, some moments, well-remembered by the gay community, in which the PRI government showed open signs of discrimination against this group. In his fourth State of the Nation Address, President Luis Echeverría (1970-1976) declared that "amongst other things that characterized the background of the terrorists operating in Mexico was a high incidence of masculine and feminine homosexuality" (Lumsden 1991, p. 55).[78] In contrast, the last PRI presidents, Miguel de la Madrid Hurtado (1982-1988), Carlos Salinas de Gortari (1988-1994), and Ernesto Zedillo Ponce de León (1994-2000), and more recently Enrique Peña Nieto (2012-2018) proved to be more liberal on sexual and cultural issues, despite the economic crises and the adoption of anti-popular globalist economic policies.[79] At the national level, and against the demands of such homophobic groups such as PROVIDA[80] (antiabortion group) and the National Union of Parents[81] (UNPF[82]) (which have been supported by the Catholic Church and for whom HIV/AIDS is the consequence of "anti-natural" and "disordered" behaviour), these governments did not allow the epidemic to be a pretext for increased repression of homosexuals. At most, the religious groups associated with the Right were able to prevent the Mexican government from expanding its safe-sex public education at some points in time, particularly with respect to the use of condoms (See González Ruiz 2002).

Although systemic persecution of homosexuals may not be official public policy in most parts of Mexico, harassment and exploitation of street homosexuals, cross-dressers and prostitutes remains a common practice – including in some cases police officers (See *Notiese* 2000-2016). Among other factors, the lack of wide coverage in the press has been blamed for the low level of political awareness of most homosexuals regarding their rights and the extent of police and social repression (Confidential interview with human rights and HIV/AIDS activist, Mexico City, October 15, 2001; several other confidential interviews 2002-2015). There have been a few major newspapers such as 'La Jornada,' 'Unomásuno,' and 'El Nacional' that

---

[78] Echeverría used the term terrorists to refer to some of the groups that grew out of the 1968 movement and some guerrilla-like groups that were present in some parts of the country (particularly in the south-west) during the first half of the 1970s (See Schmidt 1991, pp. 82-87).

[79] Although highly speculative, it is argued here that an explanation for the progressive views of the last four PRI presidents might be rooted in their personal and educational backgrounds, as well as in the highly secular tradition that distinguished their party. The first three of them attended U.S. universities for their graduate studies and were therefore exposed to both neo-liberal economics and relatively progressive moral views regarding sexuality. Furthermore, the pragmatism that has characterized PRI in accommodating various groups with diverse social and political views within its ranks can help to explain their relative openness.

[80] PRO-LIFE in English.

[81] Two of the most conservative groups whose role will be discussed in the chapter four.

[82] Unión Nacional de Padres de Familia.

are gay-positive and pro-feminist, which have covered some of the news affecting the gay population and exposed abuses to their human rights. For the homosexual population in Mexico, similar to Pecheney's (2002) observations in his analysis of sexual orientation and HIV/AIDS in Argentina, "legal rights are difficult to exercise if such acts entail revealing a socially stigmatized trait of one's identity" (p. 254). In Mexico, as in many countries in Latin America, the epidemic is still generally associated with people who are not very well-regarded socially, it is seen as "a problem of 'Maricones' (faggots), 'Putas' (prostitutes), or of promiscuous and depraved people" (Confidential interviews with gay activists, Mexico City, 2001-2015). Under these circumstances, concealment becomes a protective recourse that many "stigmatizable" individuals can exploit; the problem, of course, is that this recourse becomes a liability for political participation and the consequent public exposure of human rights abusers. Concealment represents then a major challenge for gay politics and for the fight against HIV/AIDS, given that visibility is essential for their success.

Similar to sexual minorities' politics, issues of discrimination and class in Mexico are understudied, particularly in terms of their link to homophobic manifestations. In general, Mexican society denies the impact of race and class on social mobility. Admittedly, Mexican racism is less acute and more "complex" as a phenomenon than that of the U.S. for example, but it is present; to be called 'indio' (native) is equivalent to being called a 'negro' or worse in the U.S., and the term 'indígena' or 'indito' (indigenous or little 'indio') is applied to those who are patronized or pitied (Lumsden 1991, p.40). From the time of the Spanish conquest and the appropriation of Indian women by Spanish males, racism has been tied to machismo and therefore to homophobia. When it comes to class and sexual orientation, some argue that the freedom and gains for the gay movement will be there only for the elite: "If you are nice and pretty you will be accepted, but the poor and transvestite are not welcomed" (Confidential interview with a transvestite and gay activist, Mexico City, August 20, 2002). As evidence of these class divisions, Lumsden (1991, p. 36) refers to the high admission charges at gay bars and restaurants, which are acceptable to their class-conscious patrons since they ensure that the 'chusma' (rabble) will be kept out. For some activists the fight then is not only against HIV/AIDS and homophobia but against the stigma and discrimination based on "race" and class too. As noted by José Joaquín Blanco (In Lumsden 1991, p. 36), "those precious locals who against everybody and everything have resisted a limitless inferno which we can't begin to imagine, are who they are with courage, dignity, strength and a will to live, which I and probably the reader lack."

It is important to state that the generalized sentiment among sexual minorities in Mexico is that their organized presence and mobilization have had a significant impact upon the sexual discourse and cultural politics of the middle class in Mexico. As we will see in the following chapter, the organization around the struggle against HIV/AIDS has resulted in major gains, some of which go beyond those related to the pandemic itself. For instance, a very important victory took place in November 2006, when gay and lesbian activists, with the support of some politicians, succeeded in pushing for the adoption on a new Law on Domestic Partnerships (Ley de Sociedades de Convivencia) in Mexico City, which, though limited in its scope, allowed for legally recognized unions between same-sex partners (See *Notiese* 2006). A similar and more ambitious law was approved three months later by the legislature in the state of Coahuila (Del Collado 2007). Even more recently, the Federal District's local assembly voted 39–20 (on December 21, 2009) in favor of same-sex marriage, including the right to adopt, representing a major success for the advancement of equal rights for sexual minorities, which has been seen as part of a general trend in Latin America (See De la Dehesa 2010; Díez 2015; Pierceson, Piatta-Crocker, and Schulenberg 2013). Notwithstanding the significance of these gains, however, many gays and lesbians (particularly the poor) remained vulnerable at the individual level to state and societal oppression. This has become strikingly apparent with the discriminatory medical treatment in public hospitals against people with HIV/AIDS from lower socio-economic strata; showing the persistence of institutional homophobia.[83] Thus, the LGBTT community still defines any meaningful homosexual liberation in terms of democratizing society and the state as a whole, and emphasize the need to create new and strengthen old effective civil society organizations that are capable of asserting and defending their rights. Additionally, many among sexual minorities' activists believe that the most pressing task is to insert the debate about issues of machismo, social oppression of homosexuals, and class-based discrimination into the discourse of mainstream institutions such as the mass media, the school system, trade unions, and political parties. For them, the strengthening of democratic institutions vis-à-vis a traditionally authoritarian and corporatist state is the best guarantor of civil rights, and the only way to be able to transform society's machista/homophobic character over the long haul. For many years now, activists have argued that a pre-requisite for any meaningful homosexual liberation requires the government and political organizations, at the very least, to respect those rights that already exist in form, if not in practice (Lumsden 1991, p. 93).

MEXICAN GLOBALISM AND THE HEALTH SECTOR

The following sections will provide an overview of the main economic reforms that have accompanied the process of social and political change, as well as the organization and recent reforms of the health sector. First of all, the declared purpose behind most of the economic reforms introduced since the 1980s to date has been the transformation of the Mexican economy into an open and free-market oriented one. Thus, of great significance to the present analysis is the impact that these globalist reforms have had on the limitations and opportunities for the definition of developmental strategies and social participation. Special attention will be given to the identification of the main actors and institutions, as well as the historical trends

---

[83] In interviews with some health care providers and volunteers working with AIDS patients, the discrimination that many patients still suffer in public institutions was a common complaint. There are also some reports by MEXSIDA, a watchdog network, on patients' rights abuses (See *Notiese* 2000-2015).

that have determined the definition of HIV/AIDS policies in Mexico. Of central interest are those aspects of the structure of the health care system and social security that more directly determine access to treatment and the promotion of prevention campaigns. As already stated above, we contend that the analysis of social policies in general, and HIV/AIDS and health-related policies in particular, speaks loudly to several issues: those related to state competence and inclusiveness in policymaking; to the linkages between state institutions and civil society groups; to patterns of marginalization; and to the broader struggle for democratization and development. The goal is to identify those health sector reforms that define the response to the pandemic in Mexico, as well as the key actors that have traditionally defined the policymaking process. Consequently, special consideration will be given to the description and significance of health sector and economic political cliques, traditionally known as sectoral 'camarillas.'

The Mexican Globalist Agenda

For decades, Mexico experienced not only political stability, but also, a relatively long period of sustained economic growth and sound finances. However, the 1968 Tlatelolco student demonstrations and massacre, together with a major doctors' protest movement, rural unrest, guerrilla organizations, and mobilizations by the urban poor for basic services and housing affected all dimensions of the country's life (See Appendix 3.1, for an overview of economic reforms from 1970 to 1982). These events, combined with years of following an Import Substitution Industrialization (ISI) model, contributed to the politico-economic system beginning to show symptoms of exhaustion (See Lustig 1992; Teichman 1988). Since then, the country was faced with a series of economic crises, and economic policy was increasingly dominated by a globalist agenda. As a consequence of the cycle that began with the 1972 Organization of Petroleum Exporting Countries (OPEC) embargo, which together with other international economic and political variables led to the world drop in oil prices and the rise in international interest rates, in late 1982 Mexico faced one of its worst financial and economic crises.

After taking office, at the end of 1982, Miguel de la Madrid Hurtado introduced a National Development Plan comprising an immediate emergency program of crisis management and a longer-term strategy to induce structural changes within the economy (See Teichman 1988; Ward 1985). Subsequently, De la Madrid's administration marked the ascendance and dominance within the PRI government of the politico-technocratic globalist elite. Following the International Monetary Fund (IMF) and World Bank's recommendations, the Mexican government adopted the First Stage of a Structural Adjustment Program (SAP) reforms in order to overcome the economic and financial crisis, of which a central element was the launching of a major process of trade liberalization (See Lustig 1992; Teichman 1988; Ward 1985).

Following the contested presidential elections of 1988, with public accusations of electoral fraud leading to the "victory" of the PRI candidate, Carlos Salinas de Gortari (1988-1994, who became De la Madrid's successor) deepened the Structural

Adjustment reforms and continued the process of privatization of publicly managed companies (See Lustig 1992). He privatized telephones, banks, and communal lands, while at the same time, deregulated businesses and liberalized investments, opening even some areas of the oil industry to foreign capital, and pushing Mexico into the North American Free Trade Agreement (NAFTA) (Levy and Bruhn 2001, p.12). In addition, Salinas decided to pursue a policy of limiting the depreciation of the exchange rate in order to bring inflation down. As a result, and combined with an increasing deficit on the trade balance, Salinas' exchange rate policy and financial de-regulation triggered the next big crisis faced by the following administration of Ernesto Zedillo (1994-2000).

As a consequence, between the end of 1994 and the first months of 1995, the Mexican economy experienced its worst economic and financial crisis ever, with a tremendous impact on income distribution and increased poverty. According to Pastor and Wise (2003, p. 183), Zedillo himself had unsuccessfully pressed for a devaluation in late 1994, before taking office. So that almost immediately after becoming president, his administration had to devalue the peso, which led to its free fall. These events marked in a significant way the rest of his administration, and uncovered some of the fundamental flaws of the liberalization and privatization processes (what we call the Mexican version of the globalist agenda). In particular, the re-privatization of the banking system proved to be plagued with irregularities and was followed by a series of bad loans by the new owners, which forced the government to step in and purchase those loans from them (Pastor and Wise 2003, p. 184). By February 1995, the risk of an international financial crisis of greater proportions forced the U.S. government of Bill Clinton to guarantee a $50 billion multilateral bailout package. To the surprise of many, the 1995 adjustment program was successful and, although slowly, and limited to the macro-economic indicators, the economy started to recover, significantly aided by an export boom (See Pastor and Wise 2003).

Zedillo's banking system bailout clearly put the interests of the financial sector first, and increased the burden on the tax- payers. The government has been paying the costs of this bail out since then, which as many private-sector analysts predicted would exceed 10 per cent of GDP over several years (See Fidler 1996). In contrast to the government's response to the problems faced by the big financial conglomerates, individuals and small businesses were left to their own misfortunes. Additionally, in the early 1990s, there was a rapid growth of consumer and mortgage credit, which meant that many more individuals suffered from higher interest rates than had been the case during previous economic setbacks. The lack of support from the government led to the emergence of a vociferous lobby group called *El Barzón* (the Yoke), which engaged in regular street protests aimed at encouraging the government to ease the debt burden of the middle classes (See Fidler 1996). Although El Barzón turned out to be an isolated case of relative success, the general trend showed that the weakened but still functioning corporatist and clientelistic arrangements helped contain dissent during the market reform process (Teichman 2001, p. 36).

In general, the government of Ernesto Zedillo was characterized by the continuation of the same globalist economic policies of his predecessors. As part of these policies, in 1997, his administration introduced a reform of the National Social Security Institute (IMSS[84]). According to the government and supporters of the reform - particularly with regards to its pension system -, this was necessary to help raise Mexico's inadequate savings rate. Yet it cost the budget 1.5 to 2 per cent of GDP in its first year (Fidler 1996, p. 716). These two factors (savings rate and the cost of the reform), combined with the broader economic crisis, seem to have left very little scope for the public sector to aid economic expansion and strengthen social welfare development. While the Mexican economy rebounded over the next several years, mostly due to a more competitive exchange rate, wages and employment lagged behind. Yet neither the level of GDP growth nor its pattern was sufficient to alter severe inequalities, or to reduce the number of people living in poverty (See IDB 1997). In a chilling understatement, the Inter-American Development Bank (IDB) conceded that "the relatively well-off groups of Latin American society appear to have benefited from the recovery of the 1990s somewhat more than the poorest classes" (IDB 1997, p. 18).

Zedillo's term in office coincided with the introduction of what has been identified as the Second Stage of Structural Adjustment (Cook et al. 1994; See also Naim 1994). This second stage was defined as a time for consolidation (See Box 3.1, next page).[85] An important feature of the implementation of these second stage reforms is the fact that, as pointed out by Naim (1994), the costs of institutional changes are likely to be borne by more specific groups, in comparison to the widely dispersed – socially and politically speaking - segments of society that bore the initial burden of macroeconomic adjustment. In turn, and given the similarly targeted impact of these reforms, one would expect to see more political organization and civil mobilization as a response. Indeed, as will be argued in chapter four, this has been the case for the organized HIV/AIDS activism and their opposition to further reforms to social security that threatened access to treatment and medication.

The next two presidential administrations under PAN's Vicente Fox (2000-2006) and Felipe Calderón (2006-2012), as well as the first half of the current administration of Enrique Peña Nieto (PRI), strongly favoured the continuation of a globalist agenda and, similar to their predecessors, rejected the consideration of taxes on capital flows, or other explicitly interventionist strategies. Among their proposals to deepen the

---

[84] Instituto Mexicano del Seguro Social (IMSS). IMSS's reform represents a central part of the transformation of the Mexican Health Care System, and will be discussed below in more detail.

[85] A significant change in Zedillo's administration was his departure from the strict hands-off market strategy, putting forward the new Program for Industrial and Foreign Trade Policy (PROPICE). This program offered information services for the production and marketing of exports; general assistance for exporters; and consultation on industrial policy needs from the numerous chambers of business and commerce (Pastor and Wise 2003, p. 192). The relevance of this attempt at introducing a timid kind of industrial policy is quite significant for the analysis of the globalist agenda and its influence in the case of Mexico, given that it represented a shift from the statement made by Salinas' Secretary of Commerce, Jaime Serra Puche, who declared that "the best industrial policy is no industrial policy" (Pastor and Wise 2003, p. 192). Zedillo's PROPICE, however, was also primarily led by market forces.

process of Structural Adjustment, labour reform - towards a more "flexible" market[86] – was a core initiative, which was eventually passed under the return of PRI with Enrique Peña Nieto (2012-2018). This trend also encourages export-oriented corporations in the maquiladora sector to hire subcontractors and to replace full-time employees with part-time workers. The consequences of these policies have had a severe impact on the financial solidity of the Social Security Institute (IMSS), given that it depends on the generation of full-time jobs in the formal economy. Furthermore, as will be shown below in our discussion of the development of the social security system, the weakening of IMSS has important implications for the current analysis, since it threatens the access to treatment for HIV/AIDS patients that has so far been guaranteed for social security affiliates.

Box 3.1: Main Features of Structural Adjustment's Second Generation Reforms.

Pastor and Wise (1999, p. 35) identified three different types of second-generation reforms: (1) market-completing measures designed to bring liberalization initiatives started under the first reform phase to fuller fruition; (2) equity oriented programs designed to ameliorate the region's widening distributional gap; and (3) institution-building initiatives aimed at 'good governance' and citizen input into the policy-making process. As underscored in their analysis, second-generation reforms pull policy makers in at least three potentially conflicting directions – market completion, distributional amelioration, and 'good governance.' Much of the debate over second-phase strategies has concentrated on the creation of more professional civil service, the 'modernization' of state governments, judicial reform, and much broader property-rights guarantees. It has also been argued that in order to sustain and deepen the changes brought about by the turn to the market and to address poverty alleviation, states would have to increase their technical and managerial capacities (See Naim 1994).

In sum, a major consequence of the series of economic crises for the formulation of public policy was the strengthening of the position and influence of the Secretariat of Finance and the Central Bank (Banco de México) during the last three PRI administrations of the twentieth century.[87] From the 1980s on, the Secretariat of Finance, the Secretariat of Programming and Budgeting, and the Bank of Mexico

---

[86] In practice, this means cracking down on unions, dismantling wage and benefit protections, and also loosening the rules for hiring and firing – changes that strengthen the hand of managers over workers (See Bayon, Roberts and Rojas 2002).

[87] It must be said, however, that the influence of the Secretariat of Finance is not new. It goes back to President Cárdenas' (1936-40) decision to enhance both the Secretariat's authority and its leader. Cárdenas allowed the Secretary to act as an arbiter in the allocation of funds to other agencies and to state governors in connection with the federal revenue-sharing program (Camp 2003, p. 170; See also Carrillo Flores 1977). Since then, other than the president, the Secretary of Finance – often a key member of the President's camarilla - became the central figure in distributing economic resources, as well as in determining financial policies.

became the driving forces of economic reforms. Out of these three agencies, the most politically influential, during its short life (1977-1992), was the Secretariat of Programming and Budgeting, which produced three consecutive presidents: Miguel de la Madrid Hurtado, Carlos Salinas de Gortari, and Ernesto Zedillo Ponce de León (Camp 2003, p. 170). More importantly, it produced a cadre of key politico-technocrats who dominated the Salinas-Zedillo camarillas, their political generation, and economic decision-making. Their power and influence is evident by the fact that even after the defeat of PRI in 2000 some key members of these camarillas—although in most cases not the entire camarilla —joined Vicente Fox's and Felipe Calderón's administrations. For instance, as will be further discussed below, Francisco Gil Díaz became Fox's Secretary of Finance, while Santiago Levy was appointed director of IMSS. Additionally, the globalist agenda has had a major and often negative impact on social policies in general, explaining in part the mobilization of some civil society groups to resist it. Thus, as part of the struggle against HIV/AIDS, pressure on state authorities for their responsibility in guaranteeing access to treatment and health-care services in general became one of the driving forces for activists and NGOs.

General Trends in Social Policies

A country like Mexico trails far behind other middle-income Latin American countries on human and social development (e.g., Costa Rica, Argentina, Uruguay, Chile, and Cuba) and finds itself in place 74th of the world ranking of the (UNDP 2015).[88] And although in the last 20 years social spending has doubled from 6.7% of the GDP in 1991 to 11.3% in 2010, it is quite low compared to Argentina (27.8%), Brazil (26.4%), and Chile (15.2%).[89] In fact, poverty and inequality are very much rooted in Mexico, as in other parts of Latin America, and it has been argued that there is a link between this and globalization (See Cordera and Boltvinik 1984; Korzeniewicz, Patricio and Smith 2000). As Bonfil Batalla (1987) argued three decades ago, in his seminal work on Mexican culture and civilization, there are at least two Mexicos - culturally, economically, and socially; a "modern," industrialized, urbanized and financially resourceful one, and an indigenous, marginalized, mostly rural and dis-empowered one. As evidence of this, in 2012, the wealthiest 10 per cent of families received 39.2 per cent of the national income, while the poorest two fifths received about 4.3 per cent; peasants, who represent one third of the total population, received less than 10 per cent of GDP.[90] Similarly, as Levy and Bruhn (2001) point out, one Mexico has access to modern health care facilities, while the other depends on folk cures and herbs, and bears the brunt of underweight births and deaths from curable diseases. These same inequalities in the access to health-care services are explained by the absence of a strong and territorially homogeneous health care infrastructure. As such, Mexico lacks a universal health-care system, and as will be

---

[88] See http://hdr.undp.org/en/countries/profiles/MEX
[89] See CEPAL, Panorama social de America Latina, 2012, at http//www.eclac.org/publicaciones/xml/5/48455/PanoramaSocial12012DocI-Rev.pdf
[90] See https://www.worldeconomicsassociation.org/newsletterarticles/inequality-in-mexico/

shown below, the very same structure of public health institutions reflects the highly unequal character of the Mexican society (See Flamand and Moreno-Jaimes 2015)

The central purpose of the following paragraphs is to show the impact that some of the historical and current political and economic factors have had on some key areas of social policy in general and the public side of health-care in particular. As stated at the very outset of this chapter, the focus is on those aspects of the structure of the health-care system and social security that more directly determine access to HIV/AIDS treatment and the promotion of prevention campaigns. With regards to treatment, access to medication, and equal treatment for HIV/AIDS patients are often treated as human rights issues. Yet the emphasis here is on a more holistic view that links equal access to health as an integral part of the expansion of citizenship and the process of democratization. This is particularly important in the case of Mexico, where HIV/AIDS continues to predominantly affect sexual minorities, a traditionally marginalized group. For its part, the analysis of the promotion of prevention campaigns will be dealt with in the following chapter.

In analyzing HIV/AIDS and health-related policymaking in Mexico, we must pay attention to the ways in which patterns of socio-economic change and a traditionally corporatist state have played a role in defining this process, and the extent to which access to social programs has been conditioned by political subordination. In doing so, special attention must be paid to the role of dominant groups in determining development strategies and programs, since a more structured and transparent policymaking process represents a threat to traditional forms of political mediation, which are often possible through patron-clientelism. In this context, although public health policy in general has been increasingly constrained by a series of globalist macro-economic policies, there have also been some openings in the process of decision making for the case of HIV/AIDS.

In his analysis of welfare politics in Mexico, Poitras (1973) argued that an institutional perspective – one that focuses on the internal dynamics, pressures, and complex patterns of interaction that characterize bureaucracies and their relations with trade unions – helps to explain welfare policy development on social security under PRI's corporatist tradition.[91] For his part, Mesa-Lago (1978) also argued that this approach helps to explain the highly stratified and unequal social security systems that exist in the Latin American region.[92] Additionally, in the last few decades, social policies in Mexico have gone through an initial cutback, followed by stagnation, and some more recent limited growth (See Brachet-Márquez and Sherraden 1994; Flamand and Moreno-Jaimes 2015). The concentration of decision-making in certain areas of the state bureaucracy has also gone through a series of transformations. Since 1986, these variations and transformations are partly explained, as pointed out by Jonathan Fox (1994), by the ascendancy of Mexican technocrats (who viewed the old-

---

[91] Similarly, for Latin America at large, and in spite of its limitations and the fact that this approach has been subjected to considerable criticism, Eckstein (1960) used this framework for his analysis of medical care policy.

[92] These ideas will be revisited below, when looking at past trends of the formation of health care institutions and social security.

fashioned brokers as both expensive and politically ineffective) and their decision to move social policy away from reliance on traditional patronage and generalized subsidies towards measures that ostensibly targeted the poor directly. The National Solidarity Program (PRONASOL [93]) is a prime example of this new strategy. PRONASOL was Salinas' master program, and the core of his strategy was to target the poor with electoral purposes. In his analysis of PRONASOL, which had a significant health content, Fox (1994) concludes that policy implementation responded to a combination of clientelist, semi-clientelist, and pluralistic patterns. [94]

PRONASOL was explicitly designed to make social spending compatible with neo-liberal structural adjustment strategies and to target social programs directly at those most in need. It was also a community-oriented program designed to involve community-generated projects. It bypassed traditional central corporatist and clientelist institutions and strengthened the control and power of the President (See Kurtz 1999). The basic mode of operation was through the local solidarity committees, of which 250,000 were operational during the six-year life of the program (Kurtz 1999, p. 25). It was part of a political strategy, in which resources were to be targeted not simply by degree of poverty, but also to areas of political opposition's strength, seeking to re-legitimate the government and turn back the challenging threat (See Horcasitas and Weldon 1994). It also helped to maintain discretionary control over funding, and it complicated the ability of local bosses to gain control of the spending (Bailey 1994, p. 116-117).

In general, apart from PRONASOL, other social policies suffered neglect after Salinas. The immediate consequence of the peso crisis of 1994, right after Zedillo took office, was the 12.7 percent decline in the social development budget and a 16 percent decline in funding for programs to combat extreme poverty (García-Junco Machado 1997, p. 22). Although resource limitations have definitely had a pronounced impact on welfare development in Mexico, and they clearly play an important role in the structuring of policy options, this factor alone does not explain the government's actions. Some critics (See Boltvinik 2001; Leal F. 2002) argue that the introduction of programs such as PRONASOL, which was later transformed into the more targeted and technocratic PROGRESA under Zedillo (the Program of Education, Health, and Nutrition[95]), Presidents Fox's and Calderón's 'Oportunidades,' and Peña Nieto's "Prospera" have responded to a lack of genuine political commitment to improve the welfare of the poor. [96] Instead, it is argued that the introduction of such programs is the outcome of a technocratic commitment to macroeconomic stability and economic growth, and the consequent need for

---

[93] Programa Nacional de Solidaridad.
[94] Fox focuses on PRONASOL, and the National Plan for Depressed Zones and Marginal Groups (COPLAMAR). In Fox's analysis, the first two rural development reform cycles are reviewed briefly to show how mobilization from below interacted with openings from above. PRONASOL officially targeted the urban poor, peasants, and indigenous peoples, with various programs for sewage and potable water, health, education, food distribution, electrification, street paving, housing, and soft loans for low-income rural producers.
[95] Programa de Educación, Salud y Alimentación.
[96] PRONASOL became PROGRESA, then 'Opportunities,' and more recently 'Prospera.'

"efficient" management (See Appendix 3.2, for an overview of the program's transformations, which became a poster child for Conditional Cash Transfer programs worldwide).

Health Care and Social Security

Although our focus of attention is the analysis of HIV/AIDS policies, it is necessary to look at some of the health-related policies that integrally define the government's response to the pandemic. Of particular significance are those policies that determine access to treatment, both in terms of medication and health-care facilities. As such, it is important to highlight that based on the Mexican Constitution (Articles 4 and 73) health-care is a central component of the infrastructure for which the state is considered responsible, regardless of whether the government or a private agent is the actual provider. However, as is the case with most other Latin American countries, even though the responsibility is clearly established in the Constitution, Mexico has never been able to consolidate a welfare state or a national public health-care system.

At the federal level, health policy in Mexico depends on the Secretariat of Finance for budgeting and the Secretariat of Health for planning and admistration. As part of the structure of the federal government, and as a reflection of the political system as a whole, the public health sector has been characterized by its centralism, which has led to an inefficient and unequal distribution of resources, as well as a lack of clear allocation and transfer of these resources to the state level. Similar to other areas of the Mexican bureaucracy, the health sector presents a collage of separate institutions, whose fortunes have fluctuated with administrations (See Torres-Ruiz 1997; Flamand and Moreno-Jaimes 2015). As such, the health sector is integrated by three types of institutions: 1) Secretariats of Health, both at the federal and state levels, which aim to provide primary health care services to the open or uninsured population (which by 2003, before the creation of a new program called 'Seguro Popular,' represented about 50 million people); 2) Social Security Services, with full benefits coverage for about 54-59 per cent of the population; and, 2) Private providers, which cover about 6 per cent (See Flamand and Moreno-Jaimes 2015; Ortiz 2006). Yet, due to the lack of actual access, it has been estimated that in reality at least 8 and 10 per cent of the national population was not covered by any formal health care services between 1995 and 2004 (Secretariat of Health/Pan-American Health Organization 1995, p. 15; See also Secretaría de Salud 2004). Of those who have access to primary care public services, it has been widely recognized that in spite of its ongoing problems, such as long waiting lists and deteriorating infrastructure, social security institutions provide a higher level of health care than the services offered by the Health Secretariats (See Frenk 1995; 1997; Laurell 1997).

The history of today's health care institutions goes back to the 1930s and 1940s, when there was a proliferation of social security policies in Latin American countries (See Spalding 1980), and an increasing association of these policies with progressive governments. Additionally, the ability of the International Labour Organization's (ILO) officials to supply technical assistance and encouragement allowed diffusion influences to play an important role in the design of the health sector (Spalding 1980, p. 427). And in the context of external influences, the continued lack of a social security program became a source of some embarrassment to Mexican leaders (See Cruz-Saco and Mesa-Lago 1998). This led to the creation of the Mexican Institute for Social Security (IMSS), in 1942, which provides full benefits coverage for workers in the private sector of the formal economy.[97] Some problems arose later on in the process of trying to incorporate new groups into the same scheme, and in the face of mounting opposition to the government's policies in this area, the regime adopted several strategies to dissipate conflict. For instance, railroad (FERRONALES[98]) and petroleum workers (PEMEX[99]) were allowed to keep their own social security plans. Also, in 1960 a similar institution for government workers was created – the Institute of Security and Social Services for State Workers (ISSSTE[100]), of which, almost all affiliates are urban and a high proportion of them lives in the Metropolitan Area of Mexico City (See Ward 1986). As pointed out above, altogether, those covered by social security represent 59 per cent of the total population (this includes workers and their families). The establishment and transformation of the social security system is particularly relevant for the current analysis, given that, until recently, access to treatment for HIV/AIDS had been predominantly determined by people's affiliation to one of the aforementioned social security institutions. Only recently, and as will be discussed in the following chapter, the Secretariat of Health at the federal level committed itself to full coverage of access to treatment for the open population.

Historically, with the highly unequal social security structure in place, those who wanted health care benefits offered through it were aware that to have access to them they had to secure a job in the formal economy, either in the public (ISSSTE) or the private sector (IMSS), where it is provided automatically. These circumstances contributed to the perception that the lack of coverage is the fault of the individual for not having the right job, as opposed to that of the state for failing to provide a universal service (See Ward 1986). In fact, corporatism and political power were the variables that exerted the major influence on the extension of coverage. Moreover, these two variables contributed to the highly unequal distribution of social security benefits among the Mexican population, given that in terms of political payoffs, a coverage policy that reflected political power seems to have been clearly preferable in the eyes of the political elite. As such, the state used its power in this area to reinforce sectoral stratification instead of challenging it (Spalding 1980, p. 431-432).[101]

In addition to the social security system, in 1974 under the administration of Luis Echeverría Alvarez, there was an unsuccessful plan to establish something closer to a

---

[97] It is estimated that the informal economy in Mexico represents about 50 per cent of the national economic activity (See Canada's International Development Research Centre document "Women and Men in the Informal Economy, at http://web.idrc.ca/es/ev-83644-201-1-DO-TOPIC.html).

[98] Ferrocarriles Nacionales.

[99] Petróleos Mexicanos.

[100] Instituto de Seguridad y Servicios Sociales para los Trabajadores del Estado.

[101] It is worth noting that in Spalding's (1980) examination of the expansion of social security protection, there is little evidence of a significant relationship between this and independent unionization, which suggests that a pluralist interpretation of program expansion could not be supported.

national and universal health-care system. A National Health Plan emerged following a Pan-American Conference on Health, and although it was originally designed to be implemented in two stages, it ended up being immediately scrapped in 1977 for lack of resources and unrealistic aims (Ward 1986, p. 117). The following administration of José López Portillo (1976-1982) selected only 2 out of the 57 programs contained within Echeverría's National Health Plan for their implementation: these were a program of community health centres and one for family care (Ward 1986, p. 118). By the end of the 1970s, the total share of resources allocated to social development declined relative to other sectors of federal expenditure. For instance, the proportion spent by health and social security institutions declined from 56 per cent of the social budget in the early 1970s to around one-half of that at the end of the decade (Ward 1986, p. 114). As it turned out, the government's priority for health and social security throughout this period was one of maintenance rather than development and expansion.

In recent years, a decentralization strategy and the reform of the social security system became the central features of the different governments' health policies. Unfortunately, the decentralization program has not been very successful and, in fact, its effects have evidenced the weak and unequal character of health infrastructure at the national level (See Appendix 3.3, on the decentralization strategy in health). The reality is that in spite of significant efforts in that direction, the sector remains highly centralized, with health policies – including HIV/AIDS – being predominantly defined at the federal level. Notwithstanding its shortcomings, throughout the early process of decentralization parastatal health agencies at the state level were created, with some autonomy provided in the management of financial resources and the administration of services. The long-term declared objectives of this reform were to expand coverage of health and social security benefits, to facilitate the affiliation of the informal sector, and to provide access to the urban and rural marginalized areas.

As part of the explanations for the relative failure of the decentralization strategy, there was a strong opposition from IMSS to it; a central reason for its resistance has been the interest in keeping a program called IMSS-Solidarity[102] under its own control (for budgetary and political reasons). Another factor contributing to the lack of success in health decentralization was the deepening of the 1994-1995 economic crisis, which hindered the allocation of the necessary resources for its successful implementation. Additionally, in their analysis of this process, Gonzalez-Block et al. (1989) point to two other important obstacles: First, the Health Secretariat and the Social Security Institute's authorities confronted a strong and resistant corporatist trade union structure, which opposed the weakening effects that the de-concentration of personnel would have on the IMSS' trade union power and control; Secondly, due to the uneven character of state level health infrastructure, the first stage of the

---

[102] IMSS-Solidaridad begun in 1973, with the intention of extending social security health coverage to segments of the population that were unable to pay into the social security system. As of 1996, the program served about 10 million people in 225 municipalities, and it had built 3,540 clinics and 67 hospitals in marginalized areas (See Giugale et al. 2001, p. 85-96). It later became a key element of Salinas's PRONASOL, and as such, it was closely tied to its electoral strategy.

process is considered to have had a negative impact on the equal access to quality health-care services for most of the population, resulting in further resistance. On top of these factors, as underlined by Cabrero Mendoza (1999), in a poorly democratized context real decentralization was highly problematic, given the traditionally patrimonial and clientelistic character of local governments.

In President Zedillo's National Development Plan ('Plan Nacional de Desarrollo 1995-2000'), of May 31 1995, the process of decentralization of primary and secondary health care was re-established. And on March 6, 1996 the public 'Health Sector Reform Program 1995-2000' was introduced. According to this reform, the federal Secretariat of Health was expected to be responsible for the regulation (normative side) of the public health-care system, while the provision of services (the operative side) pertained to the state level and federal providers of services. Of much more significance for the current analysis of HIV/AIDS policies in Mexico and their more inclusive character is the establishment of the National Health Council (CNS[103]), on August 20 of 1996, which officially launched the National Accord for the Decentralization of Health-Care Services. [104] The National Health Council is integrated by the President, his Secretary of Health and all the Sub-Secretaries, as well as the heads of health programs at the state level, including the HIV/AIDS program (See Secretaría de Salud 2004).

The 1994 General Health Law[105] officially created what was called the National Health System. Once again, the new reform program aimed at distributing resources to local governments responding to a formula based on mortality and poverty indicators, and at universal coverage and full integration of the different public health subsystems. The new distribution formula was supposed to take into account per capita spending recommended by the World Bank, the state's child mortality rate, and the marginalization index of the Population National Council (CONAPO[106]) to allocate the budget (See González-Block et al. 1989). However, wage commitments to unionized health-care employees and operative expenses hindered the distribution of resources according to this formula. All in all, efforts at the universalization of coverage and the full integration of the different subsystems have not been successful either. Both institutionally and organizationally, local governments are weak and often unable to fulfil their new responsibilities (See Cabrero Mendoza 1999; Cardozo 1995; Torres-Ruiz 1997; Flamand and Moreno-Jaimes 2014). As fundamental obstacles for the full integration of the health sector and a successful decentralization program, we can point to the unequal availability and distribution of resources, the weak health infrastructure, and the overall highly heterogeneous and segmented nature of the national health care system (See Box 3.2, below).

---

[103] Consejo Nacional de Salud.
[104] Acuerdo Nacional para la Descentralización de los Servicios de Salud.
[105] Ley General de Salud.
[106] Consejo Nacional de Población.

Box 3.2 - A Highly Heterogeneous and Segmented National Health System.

> The Federal District or Mexico City is approximately three times better off than the national average. Additionally, the lack of coverage for primary and secondary health care affects primarily those who have no social security. This is particularly the case for those living in the 9 states considered at the bottom in terms of public health levels and financial resources: Chiapas, Guanajuato, Guerrero, Hidalgo, Michoacán, Oaxaca, Puebla, Veracruz and Zacatecas.
>
> For the integration of the different public subsystems into a National System, one would need to assess the viability of this effort and its potential consequences. As suggested by Laurell (1997) if one adds the resources of the two major public subsystems (IMSS and the Secretariat of Health) one can distinguish three groups of states, with the states in of each of these groups being characterized by having the same need for resources. The first group, which includes 17 states, has enough public resources in order to cover the demand for primary and secondary levels of health care. Most of these states could be self-sufficient, due to the existence of two complementary subsystems that would facilitate their integration with favourable results. Therefore, in this category it would make sense to merge them towards universalization. The second group includes 6 states – Jalisco, San Luis Potosi, Sinaloa, Tlaxcala, Durango and Morelos, characterized by some need for extra resources and low complementarity between their respective subsystems. In these states there is a need to strengthen both subsystems before they can be integrated and full universalization can be achieved. The third group consists of the 9 states listed in the previous paragraph, which need a great amount of additional resources and where complementarity is basically non-existent between the two public subsystems. The integration in these states would cause serious problems in terms of institutional overload, adding scarcities as opposed to sharing and optimizing resources (Laurell 1997, p. 111-113).

In general, decentralization produced a decrease in resources for health. This situation worsened by the introduction of reforms to IMSS. In 1995, the first year of Zedillo's term, which was key for the introduction of controversial globalist policies, and following the World Bank's advice (See Giugale et al. 2001), the government introduced a major reform to the Social Security Law, which became functional in 1997. The central point of this reform was the privatization of the pension funds (See Bayon, Roberts and Rojas 2002). These changes in the administration of the pension funds represented a major reduction in the availability of financial resources for the maintenance and expansion of IMSS's health-care infrastructure (Se Laurell 1997; Leal 2000). In addition to the pensions reform, it included administrative de-concentration, budgetary autonomy of health zones, reductions in employer contributions, some services sub-contracting and the privatization of others. All these reforms led to fewer resources available for the services provided by IMSS. The successful passing of the IMSS reform was possible due to the fact that in 1995 the National Congress was still dominated by a PRI majority, and that the government obtained the support of most PAN members. During Zedillo's administration, it became clear that health and social security policies followed the World Bank's globalist agenda.

The so-called translator of the globalist agenda into concrete policies was Luis Téllez, who was the co-ordinator of Zedillo's advisers[107] (Leal 2001, p. 63). Téllez

---

[107] Luis Téllez then joined Desk group, a powerful financial consortium.

was in charge of imposing those guidelines on the then Secretary of Health Juan Ramón de la Fuente. Another facilitator of Zedillo's health agenda was Genaro Borrego - from PRI – who was appointed as the director of IMSS (Leal 2001, p. 68). And although Zedillo's intention was to proceed with similar reforms to the state worker's social security system (ISSSTE), this was not possible, given that as seen before, by 1997, the PRI had lost the majority in Congress and was facing increasing difficulties in passing legislative initiatives by the Executive.

The fact is that health and social security confront significant challenges in the pursuit of any real universalization, due to the lack of public spending in these areas and the segmentation of coverage. The loss of pension funds to the private sector added to the lack of increases in health expenditures as a proportion of the GDP throughout the 1990s, and it contributed to the continuing deficiencies in health infrastructure (González-Block and Gutiérriez 1998, p. 7). Although the discussion of whether or not privatization is a good alternative for the improvement of the health-care system in Mexico falls beyond the scope of the current analysis, it is important to underline that these reforms were conducted in a highly undemocratic manner, with little discussion, and almost no room for incorporating alternative views. Far more important for our analysis is the way in which the segmentation of social security, according to people's affiliation to different institutions, determined unequal access to health-care services and HIV/AIDS treatment up until 2003, when, as we will see in the following chapter, universal access to treatment was put in place by the federal government. If we consider that in 2001 the national census registered a total population of close to 100 million people, it is necessary to underline that, as pointed out before, only approximately 59 million (See Table 3.1, below, second line, membership total) of the population was covered by some form of social security (once again, this includes affiliates and their families). Of a total of close to 40 million workers in the formal sector, around 65 per cent of them were men, with 36 per cent covered by social security benefits. For their part, of the female population in the formal sector, which represented the other 35 per cent of the total, 43 per cent of them enjoyed social security benefits.[108] If we look at the population covered by the state level in 2001 (Table 3.1, bottom line), it is worth noticing that in spite of the persisting implementation of decentralization policies, this level of government covered no more than one and a half million people. Another interesting finding is that the IMSS's and ISSSTE's numbers of affiliates have steadily increased since 1995, which needs to be carefully considered in light of the current debate on the privatization of these two public institutions. Finally, it is also worth noting that the only reduction in affiliation seen between 1991 and 2001 was in the State-owned oil-company (PEMEX).

---

[108] These figures are based on the Mexican National Institute of Statistics, Geography and Information Technology (Instituto Nacional de Estadística, Geografía, e Informática, INEGI) (See http://www.inegi.gob.mx).

Table 3.1 - Population covered by Social Security Services per Institution 1991-2001.

Year	1991	1993	1995	1997	1999	2001
Membership	48 716 530	48 134 828	45 723 840	51 433 645	57 033 072	58 929 440
IMSS	38 953 374	36 737 601	34 323 844	39 461 964	44 557 157	45 872 403
ISSSTE	8 506 748	8 919 041	9 246 265	9 472 042	9 896 695	10 236 523
PEMEX	776 494	792 724	518 552	597 078	603 879	664 938
SDN	326 968	618 110	315 550	456 683	489 477	510 784
SM	152 946	143 855	216 310	183 972	232 528	213 275
State Services	N.A.	923 497	1 103 319	1 261 906	1 253 336	1 431 517

Source: Mexican Ministry of Health (Secretaría de Salud), Statistical Information Bulletins, numbers 11, 13, 15, 17, 19, 21.

During Fox's term in office (2000-2006), a new General Law for Social Development was issued (Ley General de Desarrollo Social 2003), which established a yearly increase in social spending, or at least proportionately with inflation, as well as the National Council for the Evaluation of Social Policy (Consejo Nacional de Evaluación de la Política Social). It is relevant to mention this law here, given that its most important result was the launching of the 'Seguro Popular' ('Insurance for the Poor'), which official name is Sistema de Protección Social en Salud con el Seguro Popular or SPSS). The new law and program were the foundation of a rights-based approach. Interestingly, the new 'Seguro Popular' or SPSS program was developed by FUNSALUD, a private foundation dominated by one of the strongest health groups or "camarillas" led by Guillermo Soberón, the former Secretary of Health under president Miguel de la Madrid (1982-1988).

SPSS has three sources of funding: federal government, state level governments, and individual contributions.[109] It promotes a culture of anticipated payments, with individuals' fees determined according to income level. However, up until 2015, only 0.5% of those covered by it paid some fees at all. The program is administered by the states according to an agreement signed by all in 2006, and by 2012 SPSS became the main provider of social security, covering about 38.5% of the total population (See Gutiérrez and Hernández-Ávila 2013). Although resources for SPSS have increased constantly since its creation in 2003 (it was 0.1% of total social spending in 2003, and 3% in 2010, closer to the aforementioned 'Oportunidades' program of 3.5%), the emphasis and actions during the two PAN administrations changed (Flamand and Moreno-Jaimes 2015, p. 221-222). With Felipe Calderón there was an expansion of

---

[109] See Ley General de Salud 2009.

the program with the 'Seguro Médico Nueva Generación y Embarazo Saludable' (Medical insurance for pregnant women), and under his administration SPSS operated also the health components of 'Oportunidades,' reaching a coverage of about 15.3 million people under that program in 2012. That same year, which was his last as president, Calderón proclaimed that total coverage had been reached, with 52.6 million people being insured under SPSS. Yet according to other sources, such as the Consejo Nacional de Población[110] and Coneval,[111] about 26.2 and 35.8 million, respectively, were still not covered in 2010, which makes it hard to believe the government's assertion and figures. In fact, according to Flamand and Moreno-Jaimes (2015, p. 233), and based on the numbers presented by the 2010 Encuesta Nacional de Salud y Nutrición (National Census on Health and Nutrition), coverage had reached 44.3 million, with 39.5% of the total population and 22.3% of the poorest without any social security at all. Additionally, and in spite of the increase in total federal expenditure in health from 3.3% in 2000, to 4.4% in 2010, according to the World Bank (2014) the out-of-pocket expenditure as percentage of household health costs is still quite high, representing 44% for Mexico, compared to 32% for Chile, 31% for Brazil, 20% for Argentina, and 14.8% for Colombia. Another serious challenge is the lack of sufficient investment in human resources and infrastructure, resulting in long waiting times and low quality services, with a very fragmented health system (See Lawson 2006). It is also a system that will suffer more and more from an aging population and the potential pension deficit.

It is too soon to assess the type of results that the ongoing policies implemented by Peña Nieto will have. However, and considering the fact that his first Secretary of Health, Dr. Mercedes Juan López (December 2012 to February 2016) has been part of one of the most powerful PRI health camarillas (See discussion of Guillermo Soberón's camarilla in section 3.3 below), and who headed a public health research group in FUNSALUD (which produced a study on the Universality of Health Services in Mexico) before joining again the federal government, it is relatively safe to say that there will be some continuity with the past policies initiated by Frenk under Fox. Similarly, Peña Nieto's most recent choice in appointing Juan López's successor, Dr. José Narro Robles, has also been well-positioned within the PRI camarillas. Yet again, as argued by Flamand and Moreno-Jaimes (2015, p. 254), the high level of inequality in the system makes it very challenging to unify the three systems (SPSS: 38.5%, IMSS: 32.2%, and ISSSTE: 6%), especially without paying any serious attention to the state level disparities.

On the other hand, and as argued before, the mobilization of civil society actors against further reforms to social security has increased in visibility and, as we will see in the following chapter, in cases such as the HIV/AIDS activism, their participation has been determinant in the definition of access to treatment policies and health-care for all. As previously stated too, the issue here is not so much an ideological position

---

[110] National Population Council.
[111] Consejo Nacional de Evaluación de la Política de Desarrollo Social/ National Council for the Evaluation of Social Development Policies.

with respect to the privatization of the whole or parts of the health-care system, but the way in which limitations have been imposed by the neo-liberal economic and hegemonic discourse as opposed to having an open and democratic debate on the matter.

In general, as a consequence of the implementation of the globalist agenda in Mexico, the rules of the game have often hurt domestic delivery of health-care, particularly for poor or marginalized populations (See Laurell 1997; Leal 1997). And the globalist agenda has been translated into various trade agreements' rules as well. In fact, there is an increasing importance of trade regimes for the analysis of health interventions and service provision. Similarly, the role of TNCs, especially big pharmaceutical and insurance companies, as well as private health care providers, has increased in the last few decades. Thus, in the case of Mexico, some attention must be directed to the roles of the WTO and NAFTA, as well as of TNCs themselves, all of which limit the policy options available to the government around health. Therefore, under today's world reality, the analysis of the Mexican governments' responses to the HIV/AIDS pandemic cannot be divorced from the challenges that accompany the phenomenon of economic globalization and trade liberalization.

For a country like Mexico, being a neighbour to the United States represents an additional and undeniable challenge, especially when it comes to the limiting of social policy alternatives (See Grinspun and Cameron 1993; Clarkson 2003; 2004). In recent decades we have witnessed the U.S. disenchantment, first with the General Agreement on Tariffs and Trade (GATT), and now with the WTO, which led to North American trade regionalism promotion, symbolizing a significant shift from multilateralism to regionalism (See De Gaay Fortman 2011; Manokha 2008), leading to the NAFTA's birth in the 1990s.[112] In this context, we must consider that of the three partners in NAFTA (Canada included), the United States, up until "Obamacare" (which as we know has faced a very strong opposition by the Republican Party in Congress), have had the least egalitarian health insurance plans administered by private firms (See Andrain 1998).[113] This represents an additional source of pressure on the Mexican health sector for further privatization under NAFTA's regulations. More concretely, there is a significant potential impact on public policy-making through compensation rules under Chapter 11, which sets the rules for the protection of foreign investment.[114] Furthermore, in July 1992 and as part of NAFTA's negotiations, the Mexican legislature had to elaborate a new health regulatory framework.[115] All the governmental regulatory health norms where expected to expire

---

[112] In the case of the U.S., NAFTA prevailed over domestic political opposition largely because of the well-concerted lobbying activities of large U.S.-based Corporations (Gray 1998, p. 70).

[113] For an interesting analysis of "Obamacare" or the *Patient Protection and Affordable Care Act* (PPACA), which was signed into law to reform the health care industry by President Barack Obama on March 23, 2010 and upheld by the Supreme Court on June 28, 2012, see: http://www.huffingtonpost.com/news/obamacare/

[114] As put by Clarkson (2003), in his analysis of the North American Continent "NAFTA established some very important rules that restricted Canada's and Mexico's capacity to maintain certain policies that differed from or were disapproved of by the United States" (p. 2).

[115] The new "Ley de Metrología y Normalización."

at the end of 1993, allowing for the elaboration of the new official norms that were supposed to describe the types of administrative and technical procedures that state institutions were to follow. These norms had to be adapted to the regulations of the other partners in NAFTA (Bronfman et al. 2000, p. VII-IX). Thus, among other things, under NAFTA regulations Mexico committed to fully opening the insurance sector by January 2000 to U.S. and Canadian companies, and to reforming its respective laws[116] in order to regulate its expansion (Leal 2001b, p. 107).[117]

Mexico is also part of the WTO, which as of November 2015 had 162 Member States.[118] The legal ground rules that guide the WTO are covered in multilateral agreements (along with annexes and schedules), four of which are particularly relevant to global health and HIV/AIDS; the aforementioned TRIPS, the Agreement on Technical Barriers to Trade (TBT), the Agreement on the Application of Sanitary and Phytosanitary Measures (SPS), and the General Agreement on Trade in Services (GATS).[119] The TRIPS agreement, for example, seeks to harmonize national regulations pertaining to intellectual property and broadens the scope and length of patents,[120] extending them for some drugs to 20 years (which varied from 0-17 years before TRIPS) (Kickbusch and Buse, in Buse et al. 2002, p. 713). In this regard, Sell (in Kaul et al. 1999, p. 171) provides a comprehensive account of the machinations of the Intellectual Property Committee, whose membership of twelve chief executive officers of U.S.-based TNCs succeeded in getting most of what they wanted from an intellectual property agreement, which now has the status of public international law. For its part, the concept of trade in services behind GATS is relatively new, and responds to the growing trade in services in different areas. In the case of health, it includes the following: the movement of consumers and providers across borders to receive and supply health-care; foreign direct investment in health; and the emerging area of electronic commerce and telemedicine (Ranson et al., in Merson et al. 2001, p. 27). Increase in health services can have benefits such as the needed technology, but it can also deepen inequalities in access and promote the migration of skilled health professionals from already under-serviced areas (Ranson et al., in Merson et al. 2001, p. 32). In fact, foreign commercial presence is typically restricted to foreign investment in some domestic health activities, such as hospital management and health insurance. Under these circumstances, often, joint ventures with local health

---

[116] The "Ley de Instituciones Mutualistas y de Seguros."

[117] In December of 1999, the Mexican Senate approved the reforms to the General Law for Insurance Companies, anticipating the establishment of 24 institutions specialized in health services, for a market of at least 5 million well-off families (representing not more than 1.5 per cent of the national market) (See Leal 2001b). In 2000, U.S. based New York Life bought one of the largest Mexican insurance companies 'Seguros y Fianzas Monterrey,' expecting healthy profits, according to its CEO (*La Jornada,* Feb 15, 2000).

[118] Over three-quarters of its members are LMICs, which forces the recognition of differences and the granting of some preferential treatment for some of them.

[119] In terms of controlling trade-restrictive measures, Fidler (2000) argues that the SPS Agreement (primarily) and the TBT Agreement (secondarily) are now of more importance from a disputes perspective than GATT Article XX.

[120] This includes—among other things—human and animal cell lines, genes, and umbilical cord cells, and it also extends the scope of patents to the products obtained by a patented process.

service providers have been encouraged by increased privatization in health-care provision in LMICs, promoted by the World Bank.

To be fair, it must also be recognized that just like any other trade agreement, NAFTA and the WTO included some exceptions and reservations. Under NAFTA, for instance, although a bit vague in its scope, "social services established or maintained for a public purpose" were exempted from the terms of the agreement (Romanow 2003, p. 235). Furthermore, a requirement of the agreement was that all provinces and states in Canada, Mexico and the United States list every program or service that they wanted exempt from NAFTA by December 31, 1995. The potential consequences, however, have remained long submerged due to its sheer technical complexity (the agreement has over 1000 pages and some of the wording is deliberately ambiguous) (See Gray 1996). The risk here is that once there is any significant foreign investment engaged in for-profit delivery of health-care services, any attempt to restrict its access to the market in the future could result in relatively high compensation claims (again, according to NAFTA's Chapter 11). On the other hand, at the global level, many of Mexico's obligations under WTO's GATS apply only to those services or sectors that are explicitly made subject to the agreement.[121] The problem is that, just like in the case of NAFTA, free-trade laws make reduction of the public component of the health system a one-way street. Once private firms acquire economic interests due to deregulation, the return to the status quo ante is possible only upon payment of compensation. In this context, international agreements represent an additional factor determining the room for maneuver that domestic actors have in the process of policymaking in health.

SECTORAL HEALTH "CAMARILLAS" AND ECONOMIC CLIQUES

For a better understanding of health sector, it is necessary to identify the groups that are at the core of the public policymaking process. As discussed above, the Mexican political system has long been defined by the central role of political cliques called 'camarillas,' which have been directly linked to the presidential system and the control over the public policy agenda. Thus, the composition of health 'camarillas' deserves special attention, whose members have had a great advantage in terms of available resources and power to shape policies and determine outcomes.

It has been argued that the system of political cliques is being altered by some of the structural changes forced by the PRI defeats at the state and federal levels (See

---

[121] In comparing the two, we can see that WTO's features are stronger than NAFTA's, due in an important way to the existence of the supranational Secretariat. Obligations under WTO are both more comprehensive and powerful, and "the disputes handled through the WTO's dispute body are more expeditiously resolved and more authoritatively applied than under NAFTA" (Clarkson 2003, p. 248). Furthermore, TNCs such as Pharmaceuticals exert greater influence in the formulation of policies that are instituted at the global level (i.e. TRIPS), forcing governments in North America and elsewhere to conform to their demands. As will be discussed in the following chapter, in this context, as a net importer of prescription drugs, Mexico is highly reliant on drugs developed and manufactured abroad.

Camp 2002). However, similar to some of the other traditional features of the Mexican political system, it is unlikely to see the complete disappearance of 'camarillas' in the near future. As argued by Douglas North (1990), in any political system, there are some inertial forces that explain certain path dependencies. In the case of camarillas, there have been two major reasons for their survival and some degree of continuity in their central role. On the one hand, there were serious compromises and strong alliances made with some of the traditional political cliques, made by the PAN administrations of Fox and Calderón. On the other, the return of the PRI under Peña Nieto represented a comeback of some of those same PRI groups to office. It is also true that other characteristics, some of which are associated with the definition of policy networks, seem to be gaining significance and as such contribute to transform the way political cliques function and policies are made. Furthermore, in the following paragraphs and the next chapter, it will argued that even though some camarillas have survived and remained influential (even after the 2000 PRI's defeat), arrangements like sectoral policy networks are gaining importance, while other factors are moderating their influence.

Although politico-technocrats have come to dominate some camarillas, they have also showed varying degrees of political skills. As economists, however, most of them identify themselves more with an international profession based in the U.S. and in some International Financial Institutions (e.g. IMF, World Bank) (See Camp 2002; Teichman 2001). Additionally, politico-technocrats, like former Presidents Carlos Salinas de Gortari and Ernesto Zedillo Ponce de León, had smaller camarillas due in part to their scarce political experience associated with their relative youth (Camp 2003, p. 124). Interestingly, to reiterate a point made earlier, today, in spite of the fact that the PAN victory in the 2000 presidential elections represented a decline of technocratic control over national political institutions, some key members of Zedillo's and Salinas' cliques were kept as part of Fox's and Calderón's economic teams.

Particularly interesting for the analysis of health camarillas, and their transformation or incorporation into a policy network, is the fact that a very common informal process such as networking remains central. Although, what has been occurring is that the network has expanded, from being mostly personal and party-based to a more professional and permeable one. Similarly, Mexico's political leaders continue to have extensive ties with prominent figures from other leadership groups (particularly the big-business community) -established through educational experiences, family, and career. [122] Yet, changes in the composition of the new political elites, such as the predominance of private schools versus public ones, were accentuated starting with Fox's team (See Camp 2002; D'Artigues 2002; Confidential and non-confidential interviews with several members of the network, Mexico City, 2001-2015). In the case of the health sector there is a set of clearly identifiable groups of people who have both professional and personal links. Although professional links

---

[122] Some examples of these close connections between public sector officials and the private sector will be shown in the next chapter.

might be thought of as especially important in the health sector, which to some extent requires an important degree of medical specialization, health camarillas had shown some of the same features of those in other sectors of the public administration. The interest in identifying the main health camarillas lies in the fact that some key members of these joined PAN administrations, and thus became key members of the new policy network being formed.

There are at least three clearly defined groups, with each of them led by a central figure and a close circle of collaborators who at different times have been well-positioned in the Secretariat of Health's structure. During the PRI years, and to different extents, these health camarillas and their respective leaders were directly connected to the President, and they functioned as the mechanism through which the Executive exercised its power in the health sector, imposing its views on them. This left little room for any single camarilla to define health policies according to its members' own views or much independent ideological or technical/professional positions.[123] First of all, there is the group formed around the late Dr. Ramón de la Fuente, a psychiatrist and founder of the National Institute of Psychiatry, whose son, Dr. Juan Ramón de la Fuente, a close friend of Ernesto Zedillo's (Confidential interview with Senior Official, Health Secretariat, Mexico City, October 25, 2001), became Secretary of Health under his government (1994-1999). Juan Ramón de la Fuente was then appointed, during the last year of Zedillo's administration, as the President ('Rector') of the National University (UNAM[124]). Although this group lost some influence in the health sector, from his position at UNAM, Juan Ramón de la Fuente became a visible political figure and was, for a time, identified as a potential candidate for the presidential election of 2006 (See Alvarez Béjar 2003).

Second, there is also the camarilla formed around the late neurosurgeon Dr. Manuel Velasco Suárez, who died in 2001, which is seen by some as in tension and competing for power with De la Fuente's camarilla (Confidential interviews with two health officials, Mexico City, November 14, 2001). President Echeverría supported Velasco Suárez as the PRI candidate for the state of Chiapas, and he became governor during Echeverría's presidency (1970-1976). Velasco Suárez was also the founder of the National Institute of Neurology and Neurosurgery (INNN). More recently, he was well-positioned not only in the health sector, but also within the governing elite during Salinas's presidency. One of his daughters – who died of cancer a few years ago- married Manuel Camacho Solís, who was then Salinas's close friend and collaborator. Under Salinas's government (1988-1994), Camacho Solís was Mayor of Mexico City, Secretary of Foreign Affairs, and Special Commissioner for Chiapas. After his death, Velasco Suárez's camarilla has lost influence, and currently none of its members hold any high-level position in the public administration.

The third camarilla, and some would say the most powerful and long-lasting, is that of Dr. Guillermo Soberón's. Soberón is the former Secretary of Health under

---

[123] As pointed out in the introductory chapter, no work has been previously done on the portrayal and analysis of health camarillas. Thus, the depiction of camarillas in this sector is based on a series of interviews—most of them confidential—with various participants in the health care sector in Mexico.

[124] Universidad Nacional Autónoma de México.

Miguel de la Madrid Hurtado (1982-1988), and has been the Executive President of the National Foundation for Health (FUNSALUD[125]) since 1988. Soberón was quite successful in positioning some members of his camarilla in Vicente Fox's government. From 1988 to 2000, however, Soberón himself did not play a central role. During Salinas' presidency, Dr. Jesús Kumate - a member of Soberón's group - was appointed Secretary of Health, but Kumate was known for being more independent from the camarilla leader and for having his own views on health reform. However, Kumate too was constrained by the priority Salinas gave to PRONASOL (Leal 2001, p. 105). Additionally, during Salinas' term, two health camarillas were well positioned and in tension for the President's attention: that of Soberón's and Velasco Suárez's.

It is important to underline that under Zedillo's administration, Soberón's camarilla was excluded from the close circle of power in the Secretariat, by the appointment of Juan Ramón de la Fuente. De la Fuente was the head of this sector until the last year of Zedillo's term, when José Antonio Fernández González replaced him.[126] In 2000, however, Soberón's group made a successful come back, when Fox appointed Dr. Julio Frenk Mora as Secretary of Health - who is one of Soberón's most successful disciples. To some, the appointment of Frenk as Secretary of Health came as a surprise, given that Dr. Carlos Tena Tamayo, who was Fox's Secretary of Health during his tenure as Governor of the State of Guanajuato, was supported by a significant portion of the medical community. According to some, although Tena Tamayo was part of Fox's transition team, as well as Frenk, the fact that he was a doctor from IMSS created some worries in the Secretariat (See Scherer 2000). As an additional explanation to Frenk's appointment, it is necessary to mention that during the 2000 campaign, Soberón provided financial support for Fox, although he also helped fund the PRI's presidential candidate, Francisco Labastida Ochoa (Interview with Gustavo Leal, Mexico City, July 13, 2002).[127]

Julio Frenk is a PRI member since 1985 (*El Universal*, February 13th, 2001, insert UCA p. 8), and was the first director of the National Institute of Public Health (INSP[128]) in the city of Cuernavaca, which was founded by the then Secretary Soberón. Frenk was also director of the Centre of Economics and Health at the National Foundation for Health (FUNSALUD) (1995-1998), and from 1998 to 2000, he worked for the WHO in Geneva as Executive Director of Research and Information for Public Policies. Previously, Frenk had worked for the Secretariat of Programming and Budgeting during Lopez-Portillo's presidential term, and under Soberón's guidance at the Secretariat of Health from 1982-1988 (See Scherer 2000).

---

[125] Fundación Mexicana para la Salud.

[126] At the end of his administration, Ernesto Zedillo's appointment of Fernández González was seen as an unprecedented move, given that he was not a medical doctor, and for the first and only time so far, someone outside the profession and with no affiliation to any health 'camarilla' was appointed Secretary of Health.

[127] See also Leal (2001, p. 67), where he documents the source of this support: 50 million dollars of a contribution from Nestlé to the National Foundation for Health, an organization head up by Soberón, went into Fox's campaign.

[128] Instituto Nacional de Salud Pública.

It was during Calderón's government (2006-2012) that we saw a temporary and limited interruption of the continuity of PRI-linked health camarillas at the federal level, with his appointment of PAN member from Guanajuato Dr. José Ángel Córdova Villalobos as Secretary of Health, for most of his administration.[129] With PRI's comeback to the presidency, however, and the appointment of long-time PRIístas Dr. Mercedes Juan López and Dr. José Narro Robles, under Peña Nieto, we have witnessed the strengthening of Guillermo Soberón's camarilla again, and very likely some continuity with the past policies initiated by Frenk under Fox.

As discussed before, just like in other areas of the Mexican government, it is not surprising that after a 70-year PRI rule, camarillas remain central in the recruitment process of the Secretariat of Health. And although until very recently this remained a key variable in determining who went to the top of the political ladder, in the context of the transition to democracy and globalization, other factors are gaining importance and tend to moderate camarillas' influence. Furthermore, and as will become clearer in the two following chapter, Frenk's appointment represented the strengthening of the links between the domestic and international HIV/AIDS policy networks. As Secretary, Frenk showed independence with respect to Soberón's group and incorporated a more diverse set of actors into his team. Although the discussion of the formation of the policy network will take place in the following chapter, here it is important to emphasize that as such, the domestic HIV/AIDS policy network began its formation even before Frenk became Secretary of Health.

But before turning our attention to the ways in which members of these health camarillas have shaped HIV/AIDS and other health-related policies, it is important to address the influence of the Secretariat of Finance and the survival of its entrenched economic camarillas. And although the Secretariat of Health is responsible for health, the Secretary of Finance has a great discretionary power in terms of the budget, the distribution of resources and their allocation to all sectors, including health. As Secretary of Finance, Fox appointed Francisco Gil Díaz, who has been part of the market reform policy networks, and who kept many of his collaborators in the Secretariat. Apart from Gil Díaz, of particular significance for the analysis of economic camarillas during Fox's administration are the appointments of Santiago Levy (Director of IMSS) and Benjamín González Roaro (Director of ISSSTE) as key players in the reform of social security. In particular, Levy was not only a close collaborator of Zedillo's but also the author of the then government's anti-poverty program: PROGRESA (Teichman 2001, p. 155). He had been the co-ordinator of advisors of Jaime Serra Puche[130] in the Secretariat of Commerce and Industrial Development (SECOFI[131]) under Salinas' presidency. Levy was later appointed as Sub-secretary of Public Expenditure of the Federation (in the Secretariat of Finance)

---

[129] In fact, Córdova Villalobos as Federal Deputy and head of the health commission approved the budget for civil society organization's with work on HIV/AIDS under Fox.

[130] Dr. Serra Puche led the negotiation and implementation of NAFTA as Secretary of Commerce and Industrial Development under Salinas de Gortari's administration.

[131] Secretaría de Comercio y Fomento Industrial.

under Zedillo. He is also known for being behind the 'Puebla-Panama Plan' and as an economist who represents a very neo-liberal (globalist) orthodoxy (See Boltvinik 2001; Leal 2002).

As director of IMSS, in an official speech on the 28th of July 2002, Levy presented an apocalyptic view of the future of social security, in which he portrayed it as tragically ill, and according to Leal (2002, p. 96) presented and manipulated OECD's data to try to solidify his viewpoint, arguing that without further reform there would be no social security in the future. As some of the reasons put forward for the further reformation of IMSS (See IMSS 2004), the Fox administration argued that 20 per cent of its resources went to cover the needs of less than 2 per cent of its affiliates' needs (e.g., treatments for HIV/AIDS, diabetes, and neuro-pathologies). Furthermore, it was argued that by December 31st, 2001, of each 100 pesos required to pay for pensions, IMSS had only 6.7, and that in the following 4 years the payroll for retirees would increase in 9 billion pesos. It was estimated that by the end of the decade there was going to be 1 pensioner for each 2 workers (the ratio then was 1 to 3.5) (See IMSS 2004). Yet the negative effect of the privatization of the pension funds was not and has not been recognized as an explaining factor for the weakened financial status of IMSS. In addition to Levy's appointment, Fox also left ISSSTE in the hands of Benjamín González Roaro - a loyal follower of Elba Ester Gordillo. Gordillo is a long-time PRI member and close collaborator of Salinas de Gortari, and she became a close friend of Fox's and a political ally of his and Calderón's. In the case of ISSSTE, the reform agenda moved more slowly, given the internal opposition and the obstacles faced by Levy himself in the pursuit of IMSS's further reforms.

Apart from the inertial forces behind the continuing role of camarillas in different sectors, according to Leal (2002), Fox's decision to place members of the PRI-era camarillas, such as Gíl Díaz as Secretary of Finance and Santiago Levy as director of IMSS, was an expression of gratitude towards Zedillo, who sympathized with the 'Alliance for Change' [132] of Fox's electoral campaign. Zedillo facilitated the alternation of power and some of his collaborators were allowed to continue serving as strong globalists in Fox's cabinet. In the case of the Secretary of Health, as pointed out above, the appointment of Frenk is partly explained by Soberón's support during Fox's electoral campaign. Yet, as will be discussed in the following chapter, Frenk's appointment was also explained by the domestic and international support within the health community that Frenk himself was able to attract.

RECENT HEALTH SECTOR REFORMS

In looking at the current health-sector reforms relevant to the analysis of HIV/AIDS policies, it is necessary to focus on two opposing trends; the remaining exclusionary practices in the process of public policymaking, and the opening up and incorporation of new actors in some policy areas.

---

[132] Alianza por el Cambio.

As we have seen so far, some members of the traditional camarillas have remained influential in the process of public policymaking in the health sector, even after the defeat of PRI in 2000 and the incorporation of new actors into the federal administration. In the health sector, the designation of Julio Frenk as Secretary of Health was regarded as key for the positioning of Soberón's camarilla under Fox's government. Yet it is necessary to emphasize that although Frenk's appointment showed the strength of long-existing political cliques, it will be argued that it also represented a shift in terms of their composition, their functioning, and their influence. It must also be underlined that Frenk had no formal camarilla of his own, which contributed to explaining why he allowed a more diverse set of collaborators into some policy areas, such as the national HIV/AIDS program.

There are of course some criticisms raised against the lack of change in the way public policies have been made. As an example, Frenk's health program has been criticized for its lack of responsiveness to some of the concerns expressed to Fox by the population in his electoral campaign (See Boltvinik 2000; Leal 2002). Among others, throughout Fox's electoral tour of the country, people expressed their increasing preoccupation with access to more and better medicines, the improvement of the existing health-care services, and the completion of ongoing projects to strengthen ISSSTE, IMSS, and the Secretariat of Health, especially the improvement of their facilities (*Reforma*, October 8th, 2001; See also Leal 2001; 2002). The point here is that although Frenk's team claimed that the National Health Plan 2001-2006 represented a response to a series of citizen consultations, the veracity and significance of this consultation have been questioned in terms of its actual responsiveness to people's demands. According to Carmen Soler (head of Mexico City's HIV/AIDS program until 2007) (Interview, Mexico City, September 13, 2002), for example, "the National Health Plan did not incorporate even one bit from the suggestions coming from the states' governments and NGOs." Furthermore, according to Gustavo Leal (Interview, Mexico City, July 13, 2002) - one of the National Health Plan's harshest critics - although "they talk a lot about equity and universal coverage, it is not clear how they plan to achieve this, given the complaints concerning the services provided by IMSS, and the undergoing efforts to privatize it." In Leal's view, the official health plan was nothing else but the third volume of FUNSALUD's series on health (See Frenk 1995; 1997), while the so-called 'three pillars' of health reform (financial protection, quality, and equity) were of their own creation, and not - as they claimed - the result of consultation. The issue of financial protection, for instance, Leal and Martínez (2001) argue, was proposed only in two of the discussion tables of the consultations, and in one of them it was Julio Frenk himself who put it forward. In fact, they concluded, the idea of financial protection came from Frenk's World Health Report of 2000 for the WHO.

The fact is that since the year 2000 the federal government has sent contradictory signals to those concerned with public health and universal access to health-care services and medicines. On the one hand, Fox and his Secretary of Health publicly declared their commitment to universal access to health-care and to treatment for HIV/AIDS patients. At the same time, from the beginning, Fox's Secretary of Finance

- Francisco Gil Díaz[133] – pushed for the application of the value-added tax (IVA[134]) to medicines, books and food, as part of the fiscal reform promoted by the federal government (*Proceso*, December 3, 2000, pp. 46-51, No. 257). This gave rise to strong opposition and demonstrations against the fiscal reform (both from the public at large and in the National Congress), and polarized the debate over health reforms and access to medications (*La Jornada*, May 27, 2001). On the other hand, Frenk's central health policy involved the creation of the previously discussed 'Insurance of the People'[135] or SPSS program, which in theory would give access to limited social security to all – particularly the poor and marginalized- and would reduce the impact of the so-called catastrophic health expenses ('gastos catastróficos') (See Secretaría de Salud 2004).

Additionally, the Fox administration proposed a further reform for IMSS and a similar one for ISSSTE, with a new model of integral service provision. On October 3, 2001, Fox sent to the Congress the proposal for a new IMSS reform, of which fraction IV clearly opened the possibility for referral to private institutions for the provision of health-care services. Fox's proposals responded to a similar rationale as Zedillo's reforms and can be seen as the result of the incorporation of key Zedillo's collaborators in the new government, namely Santiago Levy (IMSS) and Benjamín González Roaro (ISSSTE). The same globalist economic/financial logic that led to the privatization of the pension system was behind the lack of overall government support for IMSS and ISSSTE. While the introduction of private health insurance in large institutions such as the National University (UNAM) and the Metropolitan University in Mexico City (UAM) further weakened IMSS' financial situation (Interview with Carolina Tetelboin, Mexico City, July 31, 2002). Additionally, the lack of formal employment generation has contributed enormously to the deterioration of the employment-based social security system. Moreover, as part of both the austerity plan and an internal campaign to undermine the financial position of the institution, there has been a policy of not filling up the low-level positions left vacant at IMSS and the reduction of the real salaries of its employees (Confidential interviews with IMSS's high-level officials, Mexico City, 2001-2006). One of the main problems with the reforms to social security lies in the way they have been carried out, which consists of lack of willingness to engage in an open debate and to consider other alternatives to the globalist interpretation of the issues and solutions.

For his part, in 2001, Julio Frenk presented the 'National Health Program 2001-2006'. [136] This was followed by the launching of the new federal 'Law for Transparency and Public Access to Governmental Information,' [137] which was promulgated on June 10, 2002, and led the government to organize the

---

[133] As discussed above, Gil Díaz himself belongs to one of the economic 'camarillas' associated with Zedillo and Salinas' governments.

[134] Impuesto al Valor Agregado.

[135] Seguro Popular.

[136] Entitled, 'La democratización de la Salud en México; hacia un sistema universal de salud' (The Democratization of Health in Mexico: towards a universal health care system).

[137] Ley de transparencia y acceso a la información pública gubernamental.

aforementioned series of public 'Citizens Forums on Health'[138] (See Secretaría de Salud 2001). The official position has been that of consultation in the process of setting the priorities for the health ministry. Yet there has been a tendency to push for the continuation of the privatization of insurance and social security services. Under the 'Seguro Popular' or SPSS program, for example, the idea has been to give the poor the "choice" of health-care provider, with their payments for insurance varying according to income level (See Secretaría de Salud 2004). According to some critics though, the government's hope is that most people will opt out for private insurance, which would further weaken the social security system (Leal 2002, p. 96; Interview with Carolina Tetelboin, Mexico City, July 31, 2002). Another criticism directed towards this scheme is that according to its operation rules, services must be provided by the state-level health institutions, with a special clause, according to which state governments must agree to take full responsibility for the coverage in the event that unexpected budgeting problems force the federal government to withdraw (*Diario Oficial de la Federación*, May 15, 2003).[139] In general, Fox was criticized for adopting a social policy inspired by the notion of philanthropy, whose sole purpose was to provide the minimum to maintain the legitimacy of his government in order to avoid social explosions (See Semo 2000). The real challenge has been, critics argue, to put in place an economic policy with social responsibility in order to respond to the urgency of addressing poverty and disease (See Castro 2000; Cordera 1997; 2000).

With regards to HIV/AIDS, federal public policies have reflected different visions and varying responses to the pressures from several civil society groups. As a response to the pressures from NGOs and to their active participation in the formation of an inclusive HIV/AIDS policy network, the federal government in general, and the health authorities in particular, have committed themselves to further inclusion of civil society groups and individuals in policy formulation and implementation. As mentioned above, public authorities also committed themselves to universal coverage of Anti-Retro-Virals (ARVs) and against discrimination based on sexual orientation.[140] Furthermore, as will also be shown in the following chapter, some changes introduced in 2003, such as the re-structuring of the federal body in charge of the national program for the prevention and control of HIV/AIDS (CONASIDA[141]), represented key signs in terms of the inclusion of other actors in the process of decision-making.

---

[138] Foros Ciudadanos de la Salud.

[139] Changes to the General Health Law, Title number Third-b, of the section on the social protection of health, Chapters I to V, and Chapter VI, of the Fund for the Protection against catastrophic health expenses.

[140] As publicly expressed by Julio Frenk in his presentation of the 'Action Program for the Prevention and Control of Sexually Transmitted Diseases and HIV/AIDS 2001-2006,' at the III Symposium on HIV/AIDS of the Mexican Association of Clinical Infectiology and Microbiology, August 21 2001, Mexico City.

[141] Consejo Nacional para la Prevención y el Control del SIDA.

CONCLUDING REMARKS

In spite of its shortcomings, if we define political democracy in classic procedural terms, namely free and fair electoral contestation for governing offices based on universal suffrage, guaranteed freedoms of association and expression, accountability through the rule of law, and civilian control of the military, then one can argue that Mexico has made important progress in the last four decades. The transition to democracy, however, has been characterized by both significant changes in some aspects of the Mexican political system and the persistence of some other features. On the one hand, the Executive powers have been lessened, with greater autonomy for a multiparty-controlled National Congress. These changes have led to the reduction of - and less centralized – Executive control over the public policymaking process. Additionally, as will be discussed in the following chapter, as a consequence of more transparent elections and greater pluralism resulting from the slow breakdown of corporatism, some civil society groups have gained confidence in their capacity to effectively participate and influence public policy in some issue areas. On the other hand, some major obstacles remain on the road to "full democracy." For instance, there are still some remnants of clientelism, as well as the persistent presence of some authoritarian redoubts. Similarly, some old style political cliques or camarillas remain influential, with some of their members being well-positioned within the government structures. Also, and in spite of the major steps forward in the transparency of the electoral process, civil society in general shows a persistent lack of credibility in political parties. In contrast, NGOs' credibility is much higher.

It is particularly significant to note that the unfolding of the transition to democracy has been determined, and shaped, by the ways in which more and less authoritarian factions within the state react to growing civic pressure from below. As such, some civil society groups have been part of the driving force for the democratic gains and the inroads made in terms of increasing participation of a wider segment of the population in politics. Furthermore, the activism of some civil society groups, such as those engaged in the struggle for the recognition of sexual minorities' rights, has been able to open up the debate of formerly taboo issues that are central to public policymaking discussions. In fact, there is a strong link between the fight for the recognition of sexual minorities' rights and the process of democratization.

As will also be shown in the following chapter, beyond electoral participation, the politics of social policymaking can tell us much more about the non-electoral dimensions of democratization. Indeed, perhaps the most obvious weakness in measuring Mexico's democratic achievements might be in the economic policy arena, since, as we have seen above, in recent years, presidents narrowed the range of acceptable policy alternatives in the economic realm - with a globalist agenda dominating the debate. When it comes to its health-care system, historically, Mexico has been characterized by its lack of equality, both in terms of access as well as the quality of the services provided by its different institutions (i.e., IMSS or ISSSTE versus Health Secretariats). It also suffers from a long history of centralization and unequal distribution of resources among different jurisdictions. Furthermore, attempts aiming at the universalization of coverage have failed, and as such, it remains highly heterogenous and segmented. Once again, since 1982, and as a response to the various economic crises, policy in Mexico has been increasingly determined by the globalist agenda. As a consequence, the neo-liberal economic model has limited the options for social policies, which a has determined as well the state's capacity to respond to the HIV/AIDS epidemic. To different degrees, globalist policies have shaped the reforms introduced to the health sector in the last six federal governments, of both PRI and PAN, and as such, the long-term implications of these reforms are not very encouraging for sustainable human development, given the pre-existing lack of both a strong health-care infrastructure and a clear commitment to create it.

Additionally, the continuing presence of some members of the long PRI-era camarillas, as part of the federal economic team and the social security bureaucracy, represents a further obstacle for an open debate on a wider variety of alternatives for the future of health care. Thus, it is in the context of the previous analysis of some of the main features of the political system and the health-care sector, that chapter four will offer a closer look at the formation and operation of domestic and international HIV/AIDS policy networks. The central aim will be to determine the degree to which the various responses to the pandemic and the interaction between domestic and external actors represent catalyzing forces for the democratization of the public policymaking process in Mexico, and whether they provide some hope for the future of health, democracy, and development.

In sum, the overall aim of this chapter was to argue that the political and economic reforms of the last few decades have redefined the socio-political context within which domestic individual actors and institutions participate in the formulation and implementation of HIV/AIDS and health-related policies. Furthermore, it provided some evidence of the ways in which significant changes are taking place in the health sector, explained by the broader process of democratization, and in spite of the fact that some features of the long-lived one-dominant-party regime still survive. Based on these findings, the following chapter's analysis will show that even though public health policy in general has been significantly influenced by a series of globalist macro-economic policies, there have also been some openings in the process of decision making, in particular for the case of HIV/AIDS policies.

CHAPTER 4

HIV/AIDS and Sexual Minorities in Mexico

The domestic and external factors determining the formation of the HIV/AIDS policy network are strongly intertwined. Even though this chapter will mainly focus on the domestic side of the analysis, it will be argued that the participation of some civil society actors in the formation of a new and relatively inclusive domestic HIV/AIDS policy network has been strengthened by their strong connections with their external counterparts. As a consequence, their role in the process of policymaking, both in terms of access and influence has also gained in strength. In other words, although significant limitations remain – imposed by some of the features of the Mexican political system and the impact that the globalist agenda has had at the national level – the formation of an HIV/AIDS policy network has resulted in the inclusion of formerly marginalized groups. These groups have been successful in translating their inclusion in the policy network into influence on policy outcomes.

In fact, what we are witnessing in the case of HIV/AIDS represents the emergence of a new type of policy network. This is a type of network that, contrary to those already in place in other issue areas (i.e., market reform or health care financing), is relatively more inclusive and institutionalized. And its emergence has led to significant changes in the attitudes and actions of public health authorities towards the pandemic. These changes have been reflected in their assessment of the pandemic as a public health priority and in their recognition of the need to address some of the broader concerns of gay men and other sexual minorities. Furthermore, the increased funding, both domestic (from public sources) and external (i.e., World Bank loans and from UNAIDS), for treatment and prevention has been a direct result of the HIV/AIDS policy network's success in exercising domestic and global influence and in obtaining concrete results.

This chapter is divided into three sections. The first one provides an overview of HIV/AIDS in Mexico, as well as of the main policies implemented by the different governments to confront the pandemic in the last few decades. In it, it will be contended that some of the most recent changes are the result of the formation of a clearly identifiable HIV/AIDS policy network at the domestic level. The second and central section will outline the composition and operation of the network; identifying those actors or stakeholders, who are part of the policy community at large and those who are members of the actual network, to show how they participate in and influence the formulation and implementation of policy. Additionally, section two provides a brief discussion of the role that traditional camarillas still play in the process of policymaking and their place within the newly formed policy network. It provides a description of the emergence of the policy network and the role of some civil society groups, namely HIV/AIDS and sexual-minorities' activists, in the significant reorientation of public policies. The emphasis is placed on their preoccupations with epidemiological and marginalization issues, as well as on their general lack of actual affiliation to political parties. And special attention is paid to the links between the domestic network and its international counterpart, drawing from chapter two's discussion on the emergence and operation of the international HIV/AIDS policy network.

Lastly, the third section provides a brief account of some of the remaining challenges in the fight against the pandemic, including a discussion of the role of socially conservative groups and the Catholic Church, and their positions regarding prevention campaigns and discrimination based on sexual orientation. Special interest is directed to uncover the ways in which powerful and influential entrepreneurs have joined efforts with some socially conservative groups to influence public policies, in their attempts to undermine the gains made regarding the control and prevention of the pandemic. The focus is on their successes, or lack thereof, in advancing their economic and religious/moral agendas. Of special significance is the fact that some civil society organizations (members of the HIV/AIDS policy network) have gained power and been able to thwart the wishes of some conservative groups against the violation of human rights. As a result, issues such as the need to fight discrimination against sexual minorities and prevention campaigns among MSM have entered the political agenda and have been translated into concrete public policies.

At the outset, it must also be underlined that, for reasons that have become evident in the previous chapters, most of the attention is devoted to the national vis-à-vis the state or municipal levels. As will become clearer in the discussion below, the centralization and concentration of power that are characteristic of the Mexican political system and the public sector are also reflected in the organization and functioning of civil society groups in general, and HIV/AIDS NGOs in particular. However, among sub-national entities, the State of Jalisco and Mexico City deserve special attention and will be briefly discussed.

In sum, the central aim of this chapter is to show the extent to which the activism of civil society groups, the sense of urgency in the response to the HIV/AIDS pandemic, and the broader process of transformation of the Mexican political system have all contributed to the formation of a more inclusive and influential HIV/AIDS policy network. Thus, the following pages provide the domestic side of the supporting evidence for the central argument, which complements the analysis presented above on the international level. The overall argument is that some of these domestic forces and changes have been significantly galvanized by external influences. Thus, despite the continuity of some entrenched practices and exclusionary features of the Mexican political system, and the constraints imposed by the globalist agenda and its supporters, significant democratic openings have occurred in the case of HIV/AIDS policies.

MEXICO'S RESPONSE TO HIV/AIDS

The first case of HIV/AIDS in Mexico was registered in 1983. As in other countries, at the beginning of the pandemic, the government engaged in an attempt to deny or conceal its existence with very concrete negative consequences. For example, during the 1980s, the refusal of Mexican health authorities to recognize the presence of the epidemic within the national borders, and their negligence in the implementation of the necessary preventive measures resulted in a major scandal of tainted blood (See Liguori and González-Block 1992; Galván et al. 1991).

Today, the estimated rate of people living with HIV is less than two per 1,000 inhabitants (approximately 190,000 people) of which 103,726 have access to anti-retroviral treatment. Of all accumulated cases, 80.2 percent correspond to men and 19.8 to women, which represents a proportion of 4 to 1, with MSM, Male Sex Workers, and Transsexual Women representing almost 70% of the total (See table 4.1, below). By age, the prevalence is as follows; 2.1% under 15 years old, 34% between 15 – 29, 63.4% 30 and older; and 0.5 unknown. In 2015, of the total new registered cases 98% were sexually transmitted, 1% from mother to child, and another 1% through intravenous drug use, with no cases of blood contamination.[1]. Since the 1980s, there has been a trend defined by a growing rate of infection in rural areas, with a significant increase also in the proportion of women (Cáceres 1999, p. 232; See also Secretaría de Salud 2015). This is closely related to the growing rate of infection among legal and illegal migrants and residents of Mexican origin in the U.S., who often go back to their communities and infect their female partners (See González-Block and Liguori 1992; Brofman et al. 2002a; 2002b). In 2000, the rate among Hispanic immigrants in the U.S. was 22.5 per 100 thousand people - more than three times the rate for the white population of European origin (6.6) (See report by U.S. HIV/AIDS Prevention Centre, October 2001; *La Jornada*, July 17, 2002). And as showed in Truby's (2014) analysis of the Northern and Southern Mexican borders, there are special patterns associated with migration trends and marginalization that help explain the persisting higher rates of infections among migrant workers.

Without any intention of underestimating the importance of looking at other population groups, and due to the fact that the HIV/AIDS pandemic has had a major impact on the visibility and activism of sexual minorities in Mexico – which is also the group most affected by the pandemic to this day - the present analysis focuses on gay men and MSM. Not only is information scarce with respect to women and how they have been affected by HIV/AIDS, but there has also been comparatively less women's activism in this issue area vis-à-vis MSM's (See Appendix 4.1, on women and HIV/AIDS in Mexico). Interestingly, and contrary to other cases (e.g. China and Russia) (See Whiteside and Barnett 2002), in which there has been an alarming increase in the rate of infection among drug users, in Mexico this population represents only 2.5 per cent of those infected. Furthermore, and as clearly stated at the very outset, our analysis focuses on and responds to a long-overdue need to examine the links between health and the politics of sexual minorities or the LGBT community in the context of democratization – two aspects of the Mexican reality that have been

---

[1] The number of cases is registered and regularly updated by the Secretariat of Health on its website. However, the figures provided by the Mexican government must be taken with some caution, since critics argue that one of the major problems is the under-registration of cases, and that the government has privileged the registration of AIDS over HIV infections.

largely neglected in political economy, as well as in globalization and developmental studies.

Table 4.1 - Estimated prevalence of HIV/AIDS cases per population group. *

Group	Percentage
Men who have Sex with Men	17.3-25
Male Sex Workers	24.1
Transsexual Women	15.5-20
Intravenous Drug Users	2.5
Female Sex Workers	0.7
Others	27.7

Elaborated by the author, based on data from the Secretariat of Health: http://www.gob.mx/salud

The emergence of the pandemic in Mexico coincided with various other circumstances – some of which were discussed in the previous chapter – such as recurrent economic crises and the processes of political and social transformations that characterized the 1980s. In a way, the advent of HIV/AIDS contributed to the unveiling of the façade of national "progress" that characterized the previous decades. In fact, in the analysis of the Mexican context, the epidemic has been portrayed as a ghost that became visible on the horizon of the celebrated "subterranean" city life of large metropolitan centres (e.g. Guadalajara, Mexico City, and Monterrey) (See Sefcovich 1987). At first, according to Sefcovich's (1987) analysis, the economic and political crises "practically extinguished the middle classes along with their hopes for the tolerant, if not supportive, coexistence of all of [society's] members" (p. 227) - including and especially sexual minorities. Both old and new right-wing conservatives lashed out against homosexuals who ostensibly threatened the progress of the "West" with their 'fiebre rosa' or pink fever, as HIV/AIDS was initially referred to in the press (See Rubio Carriquiriborde 1994). As put by Rubio Carriquiriborde, "un virus logró catalizar rencores y enfrentar en un nuevo terreno a viejos enemigos" [A virus managed to catalyze animosities and brought old enemies face to face on new grounds[2]] (p. 53). Immediately after the first official case of AIDS in 1983, a wave of persecution against homosexuals swept through Mexico again, and was stopped (at least temporarily) only by the devastating earthquake of September of 1985 (Schaefer 1996, p. 135). Yet, in recent years, socially conservative groups and the Catholic

---

[2] Translation is the author's.

Church have increased their efforts and exercised some influence in order to counterbalance the influence and gains made by sexual minorities to combat discrimination and marginalization.

As a consequence of the different historical moments behind the mobilization of some civil society groups and as part of the process of democratization, we have witnessed the increasing significance of what Camp (2003, p.54) calls a "political culture of participation." This has been a reaction to the demands for entrance into the political system by large groups of people who have been at the margins of politics. Sexual minorities have not been an exception and, as victims of the disease and as active participants in the fight against the epidemic, they have made their voices heard. Moreover, they have made relatively small but visible steps to enter mainstream politics in Mexico (See Lumsden 1991; Shaefer 1996; De la Dehesa 2010; Díez 2015). Some gay activists and people living with HIV/AIDS have joined and formed organizations involved in different ways in the fight against the disease (See García Murcia et al. 2010; and Appendix 4.2, for an overview of various HIV/AIDS organizations, some of which will be mentioned in sections 4.2.2 and 4.2.3 below), and have established strong and helpful links with international organizations, both non-governmental and governmental (the focus of chapter two). These civil society organizations have also established partnerships with some sectors of the government, resulting in what could be seen as a type of relationship that – although perfectible - could be a model for civil society-state engagements.

In addition to the increasing involvement of civil society groups in the fight against HIV/AIDS, the private sector has become more active as well in some health-related areas. The globalist agenda (i.e., free trade and social security privatization), together with the new circumstances defined by the HIV/AIDS pandemic (e.g., costly treatment and strained public budgets) have generated new expectations and opportunities for the private sector to participate in different health-related activities. These have been translated into the private sector's increasing presence in areas such as financing (i.e., private insurance), infrastructure (e.g., clinics and hospitals), and treatment (i.e., the pharmaceutical industry).

In this context, the study of the response to the HIV/AIDS epidemic allows us to explore the various ways in which a diverse set of actors is increasingly participating in public policy formulation and in shaping the process of democratization in the health sector. And as will be further discussed in the rest of the chapter, in the last couple of decades, the HIV/AIDS policy network has been successful in influencing and shaping HIV/AIDS public policies. Amongst the most significant and concrete gains, members of the network participated in the negotiation and drafting of a major World Bank loan, which provides funds for prevention among MSM and HIV/AIDS treatment. They worked intensely and successfully to extend treatment coverage for IMSS affiliates and to reduce the price of ARVs drugs. The network has also succeeded in its efforts to press the government to legislate against discrimination based on health status and sexual orientation. And more recently, after the creation of the NGO department within the national HIV/AIDS program, the HIV/AIDS policy network was effective in its battle to guarantee universal access to drugs for AIDS treatment. But before moving on to the more detailed discussion of the formation, operation, and influence of the HIV/AIDS policy network, the remaining paragraphs of this section will present some important facts regarding the development and implementation of HIV/AIDS policies in Mexico in the course of the last thirty years.

In February of 1986, under Soberón's supervision (De la Madrid's Secretary of Health[3]), the Mexican government created the National Committee for the Prevention of AIDS (CONASIDA[4]), which represented the first official effort to respond to the epidemic at the national level. In its early years, the Committee did not incorporate or consult any civil society actors and thus was not very responsive to the actual needs of those affected by the disease. In 1988, before leaving office, De la Madrid decreed (See presidential decree in *Diario Oficial de la Federación*, August 24, 1988) a new and higher status for the Committee, transforming it into the National Board for the Prevention and Control of AIDS (it kept the same acronym: CONASIDA). Under Salinas' administration (1988-1994), although as a result of its new status CONASIDA was given some more federal resources, most of its operations continued to be carried out with international financing - mainly funds from the then Global Program on AIDS of the WHO (See Saavedra et al. 1999). In 1997, Zedillo's government decided to consolidate CONASIDA as a deconcentrated body of the Secretariat of Health. Later on, and as part of the decentralization reforms in the health sector, councils at the state level were also created (COESIDAS). Yet again, as we will see below, until the last couple of years of Zedillo's term, no official civil society participation was considered in the process of HIV/AIDS policymaking (See Córdova Villalobos et al. 2008; Torres-Ruiz 2006; 2011; 2013).

In contrast, more recent reforms to the HIV/AIDS program have increasingly been the reflection of the emergence of the policy network. For instance, between 1999 and 2000, for example, a major World Bank loan – with a substantial HIV/AIDS component - was negotiated with the involvement of civil society organizations. Also, in July 2003, CONASIDA became the collegiate body of co-ordination,[5] which is formed by the Secretaries of Health and Education, the Directors of the two main social security institutions (IMSS and ISSSTE) and the National Institute for Nutrition and Medical Sciences (INN[6]). Its new mandate was to strengthen cooperation and coordination among public entities for the prevention and control of HIV/AIDS and other sexually transmitted diseases (*Diario Oficial de la Federación*, July 5, 2001). According to these reforms, the functions previously assigned to CONASIDA are now the responsibility of the Centre for the Prevention and Control of HIV/AIDS (CENSIDA[7]). Thus, CENSIDA not only continues to perform the same functions assigned to CONASIDA before, but its Director General also functions as the Technical Secretary of CONASIDA, as established in the decree for the reform of CONASIDA (article 46) (*Diario Oficial de la Federación*, May 15, 2003). More

---

[3] See discussion of health camarillas in chapter three, section 3.3.
[4] Consejo Nacional para la Prevención y el Control del SIDA.
[5] Órgano Colegiado de Coordinación.
[6] Instituto Nacional de la Nutrición.
[7] Centro Nacional para la Prevención y Control del VIH/SIDA.

significantly, for the purposes of the present analysis, is the fact that as part of CENSIDA's restructuring and as a result of the pressure exercised by the NGO community, some civil society groups have been incorporated as members of its Department of Civil Society Organizations, whose role has been determinant in the definition and implementation of recent policies in this area.

With regards to the resources devoted to the fight against the pandemic, it is necessary to underline that even though there has been a significant increase in the total amount, most of these are dedicated to treatment, with much less left for prevention campaigns.[8] In 2002, for example, the Congress approved a budget of $11,062,637.00 pesos for prevention and $39,098,047.00 pesos for treatment, while the approved amounts for 2003 were $9,914, 456.00 and $372,435, 237.00 pesos respectively (*Letra S*, in *La Jornada*, October 7, 2004). The major increase in the budget for treatment in 2003 was a reflection of the policy network's pressure to secure the commitment of the Secretariat of Health to universal treatment coverage for all HIV/AIDS patients by the year 2006 (*Letra S*, in *La Jornada*, October 7, 2004). Unexpectedly, by the end of 2003, the goal was reached – in terms of resources available for the implementation of such program – three years earlier than planned. This was possible through the creation of the Fund for Catastrophic Health Expenses (which was part of the corresponding reforms to the General Health Law) (*Diario Oficial de la Federación*, May15[th], 2003).[9] This is not to say that all patients in need of treatment immediately had access to it. As recently as 2015, due to problems regarding the lack of proper health infrastructure and accessibility (See table 4.2, below), of the 190,000 registered cases only 103,726 have access to treatment with ARVs. It must also be underlined that even in the case of IMSS and ISSSTE, which are committed to providing treatment to all of their respective affiliates, there have

---

[8] It is difficult to know for certain how much is being spent by the various government agencies working on HIV/AIDS. Some budgeting problems are associated with the lack of proper accounting systems for the resources dedicated to HIV/AIDS. Although the UNAIDS initiative for Latin America and the Caribbean (SIDALAC) has supported efforts to account for these resources, significant problems remain regarding this matter region-wide. In the case of Mexico, which also presents several problems, CONASIDA's is the only budget that is accounted for methodologically. This becomes even more of a serious issue if one considers that in spite of being the central agency in this issue area, CONASIDA represents only 5 percent of all the estimated expenses on HIV/AIDS, and for many years it has been the only public institution that had a special budget for prevention and education (See SIDALAC 2004). For the rest of the public institutions working on HIV/AIDS, SIDALAC has come up with some estimates, taking into account all related expenses by institutions, public and private, domestic and external. Some of the problems with the collection of this information arise from the fact that some people think that they cannot give out information without the consent of their superiors. Additionally, PEMEX, the Army, and the Navy, as well as state level ISSSTE, all of which also provide services for HIV/AIDS patients, have differing accounting systems. In those cases, the budgets they present to the Secretariat of Finance and the Congress are used by SIDALAC as its main source of information.

[9] Through the creation of the Fund for Catastrophic Health Expenses, the government guaranteed the provision of ARVs to all Mexican Citizens in need of treatment (See Notiese 2003). For many years, however, it had been unsuccessfully pointed out that the provision of ARVs with public resources for those who have already developed AIDS would represent an affordable budget effort; for Argentina, Brazil, Colombia Chile, Costa Rica, Ecuador, Mexico, Panama, Paraguay, Peru, Venezuela and Uruguay, it would not represent more than 0.06% of their respective GDP. It would actually represent only 1 percent of public central spending, and a small fraction of the current budget for health and defense (Saavedra 1999, p. 160).

been reports of lack of availability of ARVs and other drugs needed for the treatment of HIV/AIDS patients at some of their clinics (Various Confidential Interviews with activists and people living with HIV/AIDS, Mexico City, 2001-2015). And until the creation of the *Seguro Popular* (Insurance for the Poor, see sections 3.2 to 3.4 of last chapter), both people under this new scheme and those completely uninsured patients with HIV/AIDS were referred to units of second and third level of the Secretariat of Health, to health care centres of CONASIDA, or to private physicians.

Table 4.2 - Registered HIV Cases and People Receiving Treatment*

PEOPLE LIVING WITH HIV	190,000
PEOPLE WITH ACCESS TO TREATMENT WITH ARVs	103,726
NEW CASES PER YEAR	4,800
DEATHS DUE TO AIDS PER YEAR	4,720

*Elaborated based on data from the Secretariat of Health:
http://www.gob.mx/salud*

Prior to the aforementioned changes in accessibility, in the event that drugs were prescribed patients were expected to pay from their own pockets (Confidential interviews with CONASIDA officials and members of HIV/AIDS NGOs, Mexico City, 2001-2002). In contrast, today the public funds to pay for the treatment are available, and the aim is to reach all those who need and want to be treated. The reduction in prices of the ARVs – with Merck Sharp & Dohme, for example, reducing the price of its AIDS drugs by 82 per cent - has also contributed to the availability of publicly funded treatment (*Notiese*, Jun 25, 2004-2015).

Before moving on to a more detailed analysis of the composition and functioning of the HIV/AIDS policy network at the national level, it is necessary to highlight some efforts made at the state level. In some cases, the differences between the state and federal responses manifest themselves not only in the different approaches in dealing with HIV/AIDS, but also with respect to a broader conception of the role of the government in health care and the provision of social security. Here, it must be underlined that in spite of the persisting limitations, the democratization process and the reforms introduced in the health sector have contributed to the dialogue and debate between the different levels of government. Of special importance are the regular meetings of the National Health Council,[10] in which the heads of all the state health programs participate and important decisions are made on a wide range of issues affecting health policies nationally.[11]

Unfortunately, and despite the aforementioned creation of AIDS Committees (COESIDAS) in all 31 states, only a few of them have actually committed sufficient resources and engaged in successful efforts in this area: the state of Jalisco and the Federal District (D.F.) (or officially now Mexico City) being the most noteworthy

---

[10] See discussion on the composition and functions of the Council in chapter three, section 3.4.
[11] See on-line documentation of the meetings of the National Health Council, which provides dates and abstracts of all meetings and discussions: http://www.gob.mx/salud

cases. In the case of Jalisco, the main area of activity and relative success has been a significant effort in prevention campaigns (See Romero Keith 2002). This has been facilitated and reinforced by the earlier process of municipal decentralization under Zedillo's government (See Torres-Ruiz 1997), with the creation of Municipal Committees for AIDS Prevention (COMUSIDAS [12]). The formation of these committees started in 1997, and it included 36 different rural municipalities, characterized by an important proportion of migrant populations. Due in part to funding from the World AIDS Foundation and an increase of more than 1,000 per cent in the state budget for HIV/AIDS, by the year 2000, the program had been expanded to 30 per cent of all of Jalisco state municipalities. This allowed the provision of some basic resources in the amount of US$3,000.00 for each community, and the training of close to 1,200 volunteers (Romero Keith 2002, pp. 54-60). Among other things, this program has improved people's knowledge and attitudes towards the understanding of HIV transmission and the proper and regular use of condoms.[13]

In contrast to other states, it is important to briefly discuss the case of the Mexico City government. As such, it has been regarded as an alternative model vis-à-vis the federal level, in terms of the role of the state in the health sector (Interview with Gustavo Leal, Mexico City, July 13, 2002; Interview with Carolina Tetelboin, Mexico City, July 31, 2002).[14] Under the direction of then PRD's member Andrés Manuel López Obrador (Governor from 2000 to 2006) and Cristina Laurell (his Secretary of Health), the government of Mexico City committed significant resources to health and HIV/AIDS, which were increased through the freezing of and reductions to civil servants' salaries, the reallocation of financial resources, and the combating of corruption.[15] Since its inception, the local program on HIV/AIDS has been committed to fighting the stigma attached to the epidemic, engaging in prevention campaigns, and providing treatment for those already infected and the sick (Soler 2002, pp. 119-126). It can be argued that the actions taken against discrimination are the result of the strong links between the Mexico City program and the HIV/AIDS policy network. Although López Obrador was criticized for some homophobic attitudes (Various interviews with gay and HIV/AIDS activists, and owners of gay bars in Mexico City, 2001/2002/2005; See also *Notiese* 2002), the positioning of various influential policy

---

[12] Comités Municipales para la Prevención del SIDA.

[13] Various studies, looking at the knowledge and sexual practices among the sexually active population in Mexico, show high levels of ignorance about the disease and lack of regular use of and access to condoms. In the northern city of Monterrey, for example, similar results were obtained for both heterosexuals and MSM (presentation by Juan Alfonso Torres Sánchez and Victor Ricardo Rosales García, representatives of the NGO "Identidad Saludable, A.C., at the Regional HIV/AIDS Conference in Rio de Janeiro 2000). An abstract of the presentation is available in the annals of the conference (Fórum 2000, p. 949).

[14] This is also the perception expressed by Inter-American Development Bank officials in confidential interviews at the regional conferences on HIV/AIDS of Rio (2000), Havana (2003), and Mexico City (2008).

[15] From 2000 to 2003 there was an increase of more than 70 per cent in the budget for health, representing close to 13 per cent of the planned spending of the local government. Close to 2 billion pesos of the new monies were obtained through salaries' reductions and targeting corruption (See Laurell 2002). Compared to its state-level counterparts, the Mexico City government has implemented a wider range of policies to combat and control the epidemic.

network actors within his government contributes to explain the strong program against the pandemic and discrimination based on sexual identity at this level of government. Two of these individuals were Dr. Jorge Saavedra and Dr. Carmen Soler. During the previous, and first democratically elected Mexico City's administration of Cuauhtémoc Cárdenas (also a founder and former PRD member), a specialized HIV/AIDS clinic ('Clínica Condesa') opened its doors in February of 2000, under the direction of Jorge Saavedra.[16] As an openly gay academic and public official, Saavedra has long worked on issues related to MSM and between 1997 and 2000 worked as an adviser to the Mexico City government.

For her part, Carmen Soler – who has also been involved in different ways in the fight against the epidemic since 1987 - became the new head of both the clinic and Mexico City's HIV/AIDS program from 2001 to 2007. During her tenure 'Clínica Condesa' provided treatment to about half of the registered cases in Mexico City, while the other half was covered by IMSS (Soler 2002, p. 119). As part of this program, 20 Centres of Counselling and Free-Diagnosis[17] were created, of which probably only 5 are fully functional due to the lack of appropriate personnel and infrastructure in the other 15 (Interview with Carmen Soler, Mexico City, September 5, 2002). Today, Clinic *Condesa* has about 11,000 registered patients, and a second one has opened in Iztapalapa, with about 500 patients. The gap in number of patients between the two clinics is due in part to lack of awareness and organizational capacity to publicize the opening and availability of the second one (Interview with Miguel García Murcia, Mexico City, April 23, 2015). Similarly, there is a preoccupation with the lack of clear and formal institutionalization of procedures that would give continuity to the program and the services it provides. However, and notwithstanding their shortcomings, both Mexico City and the State of Jalisco are the only two examples of significant progress at the state level in the fight against HIV/AIDS. And the greater success in the case of Mexico City is very much explained by the strong links that have been established between some members of the HIV/AIDS policy network at the local and national level. As an example of this, in 1999, national and local activist, the late Arturo Díaz Betancourt, started a group called "Grupo de Jóvenes Gays y Familias por una Comunicación Asertiva" (Gay Youth and Families for an Assertive Communication), which is still running today under its new name, "Cuenta Conmigo, diversidad incluyente," (Count on Me, Inclusive Diversity), and providing counselling to parents and children with support from the Mexico City government.

HIV/AIDS AND HEALTH POLICY NETWORKS

Before fully engaging in the depiction of the HIV/AIDS policy network at work in Mexico, it is important to refer again to the definition of policy networks introduced in chapter one. In it, and based on the analysis of the Mexican case, a policy network

---

[16] And, as will be discussed below, Jorge Saavedra was later appointed as the head of CENSIDA.
[17] Centros de Consejería y Diagnóstico Voluntario y Gratuito.

was defined as a permeable cluster of interdependent organizations and individual actors (public and private), with frequent interactions and a common interest, connected to each other by resource dependencies, with a core and a periphery, whose members participate in the formulation and implementation of a set of policies. It is important to remember also that, as in Marsh and Smith's (2000) analysis of policy networks, often the formal and informal or the institutional and the interpersonal linkages among its members are not so clearly distinguishable in the composition and dynamics of this type of networks. Yet, in the case of the HIV/AIDS policy network in Mexico, interpersonal linkages among the network's members have been significantly institutionalized based on three key variables. First, there is the shared knowledge or expertise in a policy domain among the network's members. Second, there are strong resource dependencies among various public and civil society actors. And third, the presence of public officials provides the network with the institutional base, which also translates into the ability to have a real impact on the public policy process. As a matter of fact, the institutionalization of the links among its membership, through the incorporation of NGOs into the national program (CENSIDA) and their resource interdependency, represents one of the characteristics that distinguishes the HIV/AIDS policy network from other types of professional networks, coalitions, and epistemic communities. Once again, this does not mean that some kind of informal relationships do not persist, but most of these are established or strengthened based on the more formal or institutionalized ones.

In distinguishing between the HIV/AIDS policy network and the policy community at large (See definition and contrast of both concepts in chapter one, section 1.3), we need to point to the main variables that allow us to identify those actors who are part of the network and those who are left out. To begin with, some members of the policy community share the technical expertise and a set of common goals (e.g., prevention campaigns, universal access to treatment, and the fight against discrimination against sexual minorities), which allows them to establish and strengthen both professional and personal linkages. Their expertise and involvement in the fight against the pandemic facilitates access to the same sources of funding, which in turn creates resource interdependencies amongst them. In some cases, membership in a health camarilla represents an advantage in positioning certain individual members of the network as public officials, which serves to facilitate the transition from a closed public policymaking process to a more open and inclusive one. Furthermore, power relations within the policy community and in the broader socio-economic and political context determine network membership and influence. Also, and as discussed in chapter one, power is defined as a relational concept between individuals, groups or agencies, where one party in the relationship is able to get the other party to do something that the latter would not otherwise do, or to thwart the other party's wishes by preventing some issues from entering the political agenda. Thus, in the analysis of power relations both within and outside the policy network, one must look for manifestations of dominance, manipulation, or persuasion in the process of HIV/AIDS policymaking to further identify the various members of the network.

The structure and composition of the policy network reflects the broader process of political transition that has taken place in Mexico in the last few years. In particular, it has been the result of a series of fundamental changes that led to the end of the long period of sole PRI rule (the so-called transition to democracy). And as emphasized above, for many years, HIV/AIDS was a health policy area dominated almost exclusively by PRI camarillas. Yet more recently, this health policy area has increasingly been defined by the presence of a more inclusive policy network, which has been the result of broader changes experienced in the liberalization of the political system and the increasing pressure from civil society groups to be incorporated into the process of policymaking.

The selection of the aforementioned criteria for the identification of the network's members and their influence is based on the analysis of the Mexican reality. And although it could raise some criticisms about its limitations, it does allow us to emphasize the distinction between access to and influence on public policies. In other words, some actors within the broader policy community come to exercise more influence than others based on the distribution of power in the form of technical expertise, political connections, and financial resources.[18] In this context, however, it is important to recognize that in spite of the increasing inclusiveness that characterizes the HIV/AIDS policy network there are still some members of the policy community who face obstacles in having access to and becoming part of it. As put by some NGOs representatives in various confidential interviews, in some cases they do not always know how the political system functions and are not so familiar with its intricacies. In other cases, some civil society groups have been intentionally kept out of the policy network; particularly those organizations that have been reluctant to give up the function of providing treatment for patients – due in part to the fact that there has been much more money involved there than in prevention - even after public authorities have officially committed to universal access to treatment. Some other organizations simply lack the necessary expertise to be considered for funding and official programs. Admittedly, there are other variables such as the continuing stigma and discrimination based on "race" and class, as expressed by some activists. Although these variables do play a role in the inclusion or exclusion of some members of the HIV/AIDS policy community at large from the policy network, they fall beyond the scope of the present analysis and are hard to document.[19]

---

[18] When looking at power distribution, it is necessary to consider its various sources and the ways in which a network and members within it can resist change, influence it or challenge official authority.

[19] It is worth mentioning that in some of the author's interactions with various HIV/AIDS policy network members, in seminars and at the various interviews, it became clear that class and "race" determined the acceptance of some and the rejection of other members of the policy community.

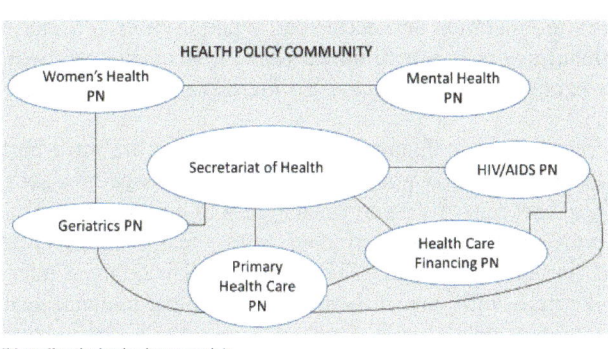

Figure 4.1 - Issue-Areas Health Policy Networks*

* Elaborated by author, based on the current analysis

Figure 4.1 (above) graphically represents the way in which the health policy community is formed by a diverse subset of actors; each one of them could potentially form distinct health policy networks, all of them linked to the Secretariat of Health, which would find itself at the centre of each network, given its decision-making and resource allocation powers. Some of these issue–area based networks might potentially establish contacts with others, and although there will be some overlaps, their interests and immediate concerns with certain policies would clearly distinguish them from one another.

In the discussion that follows, the attention will be directed to the actual findings for the case of HIV/AIDS, and the actors who are part of the HIV/AIDS policy community. Some of those actors have come to participate in the formation and functioning of the policy network, while others exert various degrees of influence on it. The aim is to illustrate the emergence of a more formalized and inclusive policy network vis-à-vis traditional political cliques or camarillas. Furthermore, the depiction of the HIV/AIDS policy network will contribute to contrast this new type of arrangements with other more exclusionary ones, such as those engaged in market reform.[20]

The Role of Traditional Camarillas vis-à-vis Policy Networks

Our more detailed analysis of the composition of the HIV/AIDS policy network begins by directing special attention to the ways in which health camarillas have been affected by exogenous changes and become integral parts of this network. Here, and in accordance with the earlier discussion on policy networks, major change in public policies is conceived as triggered by one or more of the following factors: economic

---

[20] As discussed before, Teichman's (2001) analysis of Mexico, Argentina and Chile, for example, has focused more on exclusionary market-reform policy networks.

(i.e., the various crises experienced in the last couple of decades) or political transformations (i.e., electoral democracy and alternation of the party in power at the federal level), variations in party or government ideology (i.e., the emergence and relevance of the globalist agenda), knowledge evolution (i.e., HIV/AIDS specific), the increasing mobilization and active participation of civil society, and the influence of international actors and institutions (the focus of chapter two). All of these factors together explain the emergence of an inclusive HIV/AIDS policy network and policy change.

As represented in figure 4.2 (next page), for the most part of the PRI rule, the health sector in Mexico was defined by the presence of a set of clearly identifiable camarillas. These groups determined access to public positions and the formulation of health policies, responding, of course, to the directives, interests, and conditions imposed by the presidential office and the PRI regime. Under the latter, camarillas would alternate, with one of them dominating the national health agenda for the six years of the presidential term. Once in power, the different camarillas would respond only marginally to the pressures of some civil society groups, who comprised the broader policy community. And for the most part, civil society groups were excluded from camarillas, which functioned as the vehicle through which the President would control the health sector and establish the policy guidelines during his term in office.

As previously stated, health camarillas have not disappeared, and at least some members of one of them, notably Secretary Frenk (during Fox's administration), and more recently Secretary Mercedes Juan López (under the current administration of Enrique Peña Nieto), have remained at the centre of the health sector in Mexico, exercising great influence over policy at the national level. Yet, in spite of the fact that Frenk – a member of Guillermo Soberón's camarilla (See discussion in section 3.3, previous chapter) – was appointed Secretary of Health in 2000, the camarilla itself was less dominant. In fact, most of its members became part of domestic and international health policy networks, of which the HIV/AIDS policy network is a prime example.

Similar to camarillas, the HIV/AIDS policy network is also defined by the presence of some individuals with strong personal qualities. These personalities are essential for the establishment and maintenance of strong links among the network's members. This is not to say, however, that there are not more formal or institutional linkages being defined, but the continuing significance of individuals explains the incorporation of old-style political cliques into the newer and more inclusive policy network. Moreover, based on the evidence, in contrast to the case of camarillas, to which entry depended on personal loyalties, more clearly defined common policy interests and expertise seem to increasingly secure entry into the HIV/AIDS policy network. Thus, the following section will provide an overview of the emergence and composition of the HIV/AIDS policy network and the ways in which different groups have positioned themselves within it. This will allow us to identify the roles that different actors have played in either exercising some influence or participating in the formulation of HIV/AIDS and health-related policies.

Figure 4.2 - The Traditional Influence of Camarillas and NGOs on the Secretariat of Health
(Most of PRI's regime since the appearance of HIV/AIDS, 1980s - 2000)*

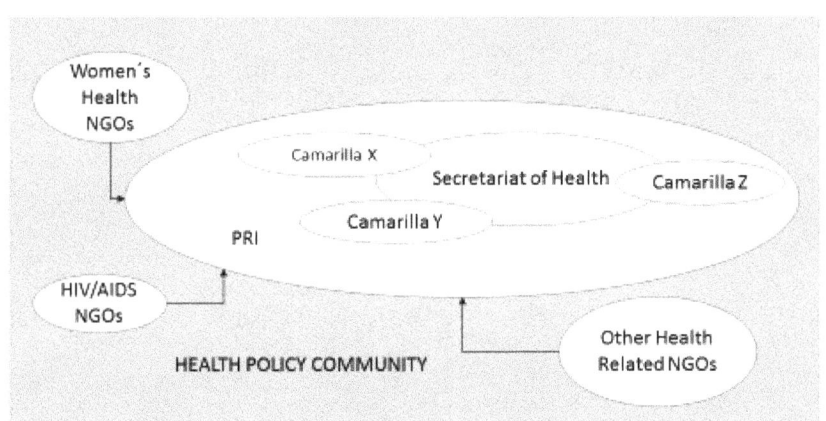

Elaborated by the author, based on extensive confidential interviews with health officials, members of health camarillas and the health community at large, as well as on the analysis of various related sources (periodicals, archives, etc.). Camarillas X, Y, and Z correspond to the three groups introduced in the previous chapter (section 3.3), namely those of Ramón de la Fuente, Velasco Suárez, and Guillermo Soberón.

The Emergence and Operation of the Domestic HIV/AIDS Policy Network

At the outset, it is necessary to emphasize that, as suggested by the evidence at hand, the formation of a policy network is more clearly observed at the sub-sectoral level (i.e., HIV/AIDS policy), which is partly due to the more narrowly defined goals and the mobilization of some civil society groups. It can also be argued that the emergence and nature of policy networks vary depending on policy issue-area, which becomes clearer in the Mexican case when looking at the differences between social security and HIV/AIDS.

As represented in Figure 4.3 (below), the HIV/AIDS policy network consists of a subset of the policy community and includes a cluster of interdependent organizations and individual actors (that is governmental and civil society ones) connected to one another by resource dependencies (i.e., common sources of funding). Clearly, not all members of the policy community are part of the policy network (See other NGOs, figure 4.3). The ones who are part of the network participate in the formulation and implementation of a specific set of HIV/AIDS and health-related policies, with frequent interactions and common interests, namely the fight against the pandemic and discrimination, and in favour of proper access to treatment (a list of the specific NGOs is provided in Table 4.3, below, p.
177). But before moving on to the analysis of each of these different sets of actors, we need to go over some of the other general characteristics of the policy network.

Figure 4.3 - HIV/AIDS Policy Community and Network under Fox's Administration (2000 - 2006)*

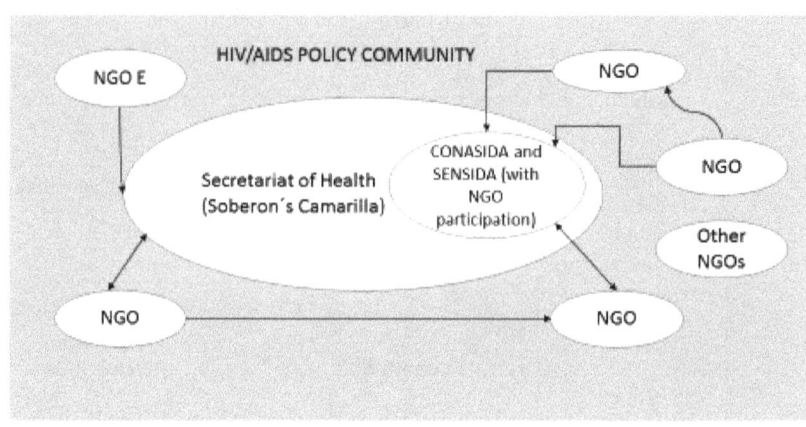

* *Elaborated based on the author's observations and analysis*

As mentioned, another central element of the definition of the HIV/AIDS policy network is the existence of resource dependencies among its members. In this case, these resource dependencies are represented by the common sources of funding for the implementation of a wide variety of HIV/AIDS and health-related projects and programs. In this case, the policy network mainly relies on the budget for health approved by the Secretariat of Finance and the National Congress (main beneficiaries: Secretariat of Health, CENSIDA and NGOs), on funds from the Secretariat of Social Development (main beneficiaries: NGOs), and on loans from the World Bank (benefiting all participants). Additionally, "public" and private external funding from UNAIDS, various foundations, and Pharmaceuticals represents alternative sources for some members of the policy network. Monies obtained from all these sources are essential not only for the functioning of the various NGOs but for CENSIDA and state-level programs as well. Interestingly, at the VIII Meeting of the Global Fund for the Fight Against HIV/AIDS, Malaria, and Tuberculosis (June 2003), and as a result of the active participation of some individuals with the support of NGOs, it was agreed that middle-income countries such as Mexico (despite its membership in the OECD) were also going to be eligible for funding from this source.[21]

For its part, the set of policies around which the policy network comes together is determined by the sharing of two basic common interests; namely the need to prevent and control the spread of the pandemic, and the provision of the appropriate attention to those living with HIV/AIDS, including and especially sexual minorities. This, in turn, forces one to direct the attention to the active participation of the different members of this policy network in those health-related policies, such as prevention, access to treatment, and against discrimination. In the analysis of the Mexican case,

---

[21] See http://www.salud.gob.mx/unidades/conasida/elegible.htm

this also forces one to consider the reforms to social security that directly impact the access to both the drugs for treatment and to the adequate public health infrastructure.

In addition to the shared expertise, common goals, and resource dependencies, frequent interactions and personal linkages among all members constitute key features of the HIV/AIDS policy network. At the national level, CENSIDA holds regular meetings[22] that allow all members of the network to participate with varying levels of influence in the discussion, formulation, and implementation of public policies. Meetings of the National Health Council[23] also represent an opportunity for some members of the network to discuss issues of common concern, particularly for the heads of the HIV/AIDS state level programs. Although, as expected in any transition process to a more open or democratic regime, there might be some limits to the full participation of all in decision making, there is also clear evidence of an ongoing dialogue and an open debate in these meetings.[24] Additionally, regular national and regional conferences and seminars represent other meeting venues for the HIV/AIDS policy network and the broader policy community to engage in the discussion of common concerns.

At the core of the structure of the policy network, there are governmental institutions such as the Secretariat of Health itself, CONASIDA, CENSIDA (including its Department of NGOs), and to a lesser extent the different HIV/AIDS-state programs (COESIDAS). Although the Secretariat of Finance plays a significant role in determining the federal budget for the health sector, as a matter of fact, it is not part of the network. As discussed before, it has lost influence on and participation in social policymaking, and it lacks the expertise, common concerns, and links with the network's members. However, it continues to represent an "external" factor capable of hindering or facilitating the network's efforts. For its part, the inclusion of some civil society groups in the structure of CENSIDA is fundamental for our definition of the HIV/AIDS policy network and the institutionalization of the linkages between civil society actors and governmental members of the network. As can be seen in table 4.3 (next page), some NGO members have found themselves at different points in time at the core of the network, while others have remained at the peripheral level from which they exercise various degrees of influence. And although they do not have direct access to decision-makers, in most cases they do feel that their interests are represented by those civil society groups that are at the core (Interviews with various HIV/AIDS and Gay activists, Mexico City, 2001-2015). At the level of the individuals, we will also identify some women and men who not only are key members of these organizations (both governmental and non-governmental), but who are also decision-makers. As represented in table 4.3 (below), and in figures 4.2 and 4.3 (above), what for many years was a health policy area dominated almost exclusively by PRI camarillas, has come to be defined by the presence of a more inclusive policy network.

---

[22] All CENSIDA members meet three to four times a year for three days each time.

[23] As mentioned in chapter two, the National Health Council is integrated by the President, his Secretary of Health and all the sub-secretaries, and the heads of health programs at the state level

[24] See minutes of all these meetings on the Secretariat of Health's website: http://www.gob.mx/salud

Table 4.3 - Actors involved in the HIV/AIDS Policymaking Process*
From Camarillas to Policy Networks

	1980 - 1997	1997 – 2015
CORE	*Secretariat of Health *CONASIDA	*Secretariat of Health *CONASIDA *CENSIDA (Including some NGOs: MEXSIDA, Colectivo Sol, FRENPA VIH, FUNSALUD, Letra S, Ave de México) *COESIDAS * Social Security Institutions
PERIPHERY	*COESIDAS * Social Security Institutions	* Other NGOs
OUTSIDE	* NGO Community at large * Socially Conservative Groups * Pharmaceuticals	* NGO community at large * Socially Conservative Groups * Pharmaceuticals

Elaborated by the author, based on the current analysis

This policy network has been part of the broader changes experienced in the democratization of the political system, and the result of the increasing pressure from civil society groups to be incorporated into the process of policymaking. In the following paragraphs, we will look at the ways in which different domestic actors and social groups (all members of the policy community) have participated in the formation and operation of this network, while others have been excluded from it (i.e., socially conservative groups). Interestingly, as we can also see from table 4.3 (above), while some actors have been able to move from the outside to the periphery (i.e., some NGOs), others, with the required expertise and personal and professional links have been successful in positioning themselves at the core (e.g., NGOs 'Ave de México,' MEXSIDA, FRENPAVIH, FUNSALUD, 'Letra S').[25] Some of the most recent changes to CENSIDA, in terms of the incorporation of NGOs at its core, strengthened the increasing responsiveness of policies to the actual concerns and demands of the periphery, and to a lesser extent to the entire policy community.

While the emergence of the HIV/AIDS policy network is directly related to the increasing organization of civil society groups working on HIV/AIDS and health-related issues, it is also explained by other domestic and international factors. And although the role of international influences has already been discussed in chapter two, it is important to underline here that domestic actors themselves point to the significant impact of the international dimension on the organization of domestic activism (Interviews with various HIV/AIDS activists, Mexico City/Rio de Janeiro/Havana, 2000-2015; Interviews at International AIDS Conferences in Rio de Janeiro 2000, Toronto 2006, and Mexico City 2008). In fact, without disregarding the significance of the first protest march in Mexico around HIV/AIDS that took place in 1987 and the efforts thereafter, most NGO representatives agree that a truly strong citizen participation in the fight against the pandemic in Mexico started only in 1996. Before then, there had been some limited engagements, but a more visible activism was triggered by an international event; namely the World Conference on AIDS, which took place in Vancouver in June of that same year. This conference represents a milestone at the world level, because in 1996 long-held ideas around the disease changed. Until then, in most cases, HIV/AIDS was regarded as a death sentence. At the World Conference, however, a series of new drugs were presented; the anti-retro-virals (ARVs), and more specifically the Proteasa inhibitors. This made it possible to think of AIDS not as a terminal disease anymore but as a chronic and treatable one. From that moment on, the fight for access to treatment for people living with HIV/AIDS world-wide, including those in LMICs, became the new challenge and a source of renewed hope and combativeness.

In essence, before 1996, people working on HIV/AIDS were more focused on dealing with the emotional impact that the disease had on its carriers' lives and their families. Yet after 1996 the mobilization of civil society groups and its influence on the elaboration of public policies became much more visible. In the words of a Mexican activist living with AIDS (Confidential interview, Mexico City, November 13, 2001), "then, us, the people who live with the virus, with renewed hope started to get organized." People living with HIV/AIDS started to create groups and networks of organizations working on advocacy. Various NGOs began lobbying for the promotion of universal access to integral health services – this included access to all the ARVs that were available, which would allow people to have a higher quality of life. The

---

[25] Some of these NGOs are introduced and their roles discussed in Box 4.1, below, and Appendix 4.2.

'Front of People Affected by HIV' (FRENPAVIH[26]) and other smaller groups organized protests to plea for treatment for HIV/AIDS patients and successfully demanded to be part of the Integral Attention Committee of the national HIV/AIDS program then called CONASIDA. Another central concern was access to the necessary laboratory tests for proper prescription of drugs and the monitoring of the health status of patients treated with them. Civil society groups also engaged in the fight for access to prophylactic drugs, which help people infected with HIV not to fall sick or to avoid getting opportunistic diseases. Increasingly, the NGO community's fight incorporated a concern with the need to improve the infrastructure of health services, including out-patient consultations and hospitalizations related to the attention of people living with HIV/AIDS and the population at large.

Not surprisingly, the emergence and functioning of NGOs have been reflective of the centralized nature of the Mexican political system and the country's highly urban character. More than half of the 5,000 of such groups - by the mid-1990s – were located in Mexico City, and around 25 percent of the total were found in four other major cities: Guadalajara (Jalisco), Tijuana (Baja California), Oaxaca (Oaxaca), and Saltillo (Coahuila) (Camp 2003, p. 154). Similar to the growth and mobilization of civil society groups in Mexico in general, discussed in chapter three, it has also been manifested in the response to the HIV/AIDS pandemic (See Box 4.1). Nation-wide, there are 112 different NGOs registered by CENSIDA working exclusively on HIV/AIDS. As it is the case with NGOs in general, more than half of these organizations is based in the Metropolitan Area of Mexico City, and they engage in a wide range of activities. Some of these HIV/AIDS NGOs provide services and information to the population at large, others focus on the more vulnerable groups, while, until recently, others provided medical care and administered drug banks, establishing strong links with external actors. Some NGOs have been central to the formation of the HIV/AIDS policy network, and one of them, with national reach and at the core of the policy network, is the aforementioned FRENPAVIH (See table 4.3, above). In 1996, FRENPAVIH's activism played a central part in the resignation of the then president of the national Red Cross, José Barroso Chávez.[27] Based on moralistic reasons, Barroso Chávez opposed the spending of any money on people with HIV/AIDS (Interview with Anuar I. Luna Cadena, Mexico City, December 12, 2001; González Ruiz 2002, p. 241), however, and as a result of the pressure from the NGO community, since then there has been a series of mixed public/private follow-up commissions, which have contributed to the improvement in the quality of medical attention by the Red Cross.

---

[26] Frente de Personas Afectadas por el VIH.
[27] A central figure, and to whom we will further refer below, as part of the analysis of conservative groups and the private sector.

Box 4.1 - An Overview of Early HIV/AIDS Organizations and their Activities.

There is a great degree of concentration of HIV/AIDS NGOs in Mexico City, which privileges its population, giving it access to a larger variety of services than their counterparts in other states. 'La Casa de la Sal, A.C.,' for example, was established in 1986 and provides medical attention to orphan children and adults. They also visit hospitalized AIDS patients, provide individual and couple psychological therapies, and administer a drug bank (Interview with Lic. Remedios Ramos Vargas, current director, in Mexico City, October 2002). Other similar programs, such as 'Alianza México,' have expanded across different states, and since 1998 they have new facilities in the states of Oaxaca, Yucatán, Puebla, Guerrero, Campeche and Quintana Roo. The population living in Mexico City and the Metropolitan area has access also to a hot phone line, 'Diversitel,' whose mission is to assist sexual minorities between 12 to 29 years of age. Another significant effort is the web-site Amigos contra el SIDA (Friends against AIDS: http://www.aids-sida.org/indice.html), which is not only a good source for general consultations regarding the efforts to combat the disease, but it also represents a valuable source of scientific information for other NGOs and people living with HIV/AIDS. There are other kinds of civil-society groups too, which through theatre performances raise awareness among the population at large regarding prevention and means of infection (See Tirso Clemades Pérez de Corcho, Brigada Callejera de Apoyo a la Mujer "Elisa Martínez, A.C.", Prevención del VIH/SIDA y de otras IT'S A través de la narración oral escénica en trabajadoras/es sexuales mexicanos/as, in Fórum 2000, p. 7630).

Some organizations have made significant efforts to extend their reach beyond the capital region. 'Colectivo Sol' represents a good example of a nation-wide effort in prevention campaigns. One of their programs involves a Condomóvil (a car called like this after a condom), in which they travel providing information on HIV/AIDS, STDs, and unwanted pregnancy, visiting towns and cities in other states (Fórum 2000, p. 794). For its part, the Mexican Network of People living with HIV/AIDS (MEXSIDA), which was founded in 1995 has a reach and a mission that extend beyond the capital region. Recently, they have put together a national campaign against the value-added tax (IVA) on medicines (The slogan for their campaign was 'IVA a medicinas igual a muerte y SIDA' [IVA to medicines equals death and AIDS]). As part of their work, they organize workshops for smaller NGOs from across the country, in Mexico City and Monterrey, in order to talk about empowerment, nutrition, home care, sexuality, and treatment adherence for those living with HIV/AIDS (Fórum 2000, p. 859). The organization 'Ave de México' has also played a central role, since its creation in 1988 by Francisco Estrada Valle – a prominent activist who was assassinated in 1992. Since 1992, Carlos García de León Moreno replaced Estrada as president of the organization and has actively participated in the fight against the pandemic, with much of their efforts focusing on MSM and the end of discrimination based on sexual orientation. Additionally, there are two major media organizations that collect and disseminate information on HIV/AIDS, health and sexuality; the news agency 'Notiese', and 'Letra S.' 'Letra S' is a monthly supplement of the national newspaper La Jornada, while 'Notiese' represents an important archival source that provides services to journalists and researchers. It reaches 45 local newspapers in 26 states, 20 national circulation media, 18 radio shows and the 4 main TV national stations (Fórum 2000, p. 797). Notiese also sends out its information material to 213 different NGOs in Mexico, Latin America, the US, and Europe (http://www.laneta.apc.org/mailman/listinfo/agencia_noticsc). Alejandro Brito and Arturo Díaz Betancourt are among the founders of Letra S and current leading figures within the HIV/AIDS policy network and community.

Another key actor in the formation of the policy network is the 'Mexican Foundation for Health' (FUNSALUD[28]). FUNSALUD is also part of the core of the network and was founded in 1985, with impresario Carlos Abedrop as the founding president of the directive council. Another 100 Mexican entrepreneurs have contributed to FUNSALUD, which first operated under the direction of Guillermo Soberón.[29] In 1995, the World Bank requested FUNSALUD to host the initiative for Latin America and the Caribbean for the control of AIDS and Sexually Transmitted Diseases (SIDALAC), designating José Antonio Izazola as its director. SIDALAC's goal was to trigger and strengthen national and international efforts to combat the epidemic in the region, and José Antonio Izazola's work significantly contributed to the government's recognition of HIV/AIDS as a public-health emergency, as well as the commitment to more public financial resources. During his appointment as head of SIDALAC, Izazola publicly and repeatedly stated that to succeed in the fight against the pandemic it was necessary to deal with one of the central problems of the Mexican reality, namely the persisting discrimination against homosexual men. In all interviews with members of the Mexican HIV/AIDS policy community, it became clear that as an openly gay man himself, and as an influential member of both Soberón's camarilla and a more broadly defined health policy community, Izazola contributed to the advancement of an agenda that addresses issues of discrimination and the transmission of the virus among MSM. Furthermore, his efforts were also translated into financial resources for HIV/AIDS prevention programs that did not exist before, some of which have been persistently opposed by powerful socially conservative groups.

For their part, NGOs 'Ave de México,' MEXSIDA, and 'Letra S' (See Box 4.1, above) also played central roles in the formation and functioning of the policy network. In the case of 'Letra S,' the late Arturo Díaz Betancourt was very active in the promotion of a human rights agenda to fight discrimination against sexual minorities. Since 1986, Díaz Betancourt put together workshops on safe sex, and in 1989, together with Francisco Galván (from 'Ave de México'),[30] organized the first national meeting of NGOs working on HIV/AIDS. After the assassination of Francisco Galván in 1992, Carlos García de León Moreno was appointed president of 'Ave de México,' and has been very active in the promotion of prevention campaigns for MSM. Furthermore, it is of special significance to point to García de León's role, for some years, as the Mexican liaison for the International Council of AIDS Service

---

[28] Fundación Mexicana para la Salud. In its first 10 years, FUNSALUD has administered close to 300 funds of a total of around US$40 million, of which 56.4 per cent have come from external sources. Nestlé, for example, finances its nutrition division, with a donation of more than half a million dollars for this area alone (See FUNSALUD's web site: http://www.funsalud.org.mx). Throughout the years, other donors have been big pharmaceutical companies, such as Merck Sharp & Dohme, which have provided smaller sums for health research and ill prevention (*Novedades*, February 23 2001, p. 12).

[29] As discussed earlier (chapter three, section 3.3), Soberón is the head of the most powerful health 'camarilla.'

[30] A leading gay and HIV/AIDS activist, who was killed in 1992 as the result of a homophobic crime.

Organizations (ICASO).[31] Both Díaz Betancourt and García de León worked with CENSIDA in the creation of the Department for NGOs, putting together for the first time a national database of all the civil society organizations working on this issue-area. Even more significantly, between 1999 and 2000, together with Silvia Panebianco (from MEXSIDA) and José Antonio Izazola (from SIDALAC), Díaz Betancourt worked on the elaboration of the proposal for the HIV/AIDS content of the major World Bank loan for health and HIV/AIDS mentioned above.

The World Bank loan has been the most important source of funding for HIV/AIDS. It was part of a larger loan of US$350 million for the Program for Quality, Equity and Development in Health (PROCEDES[32]), for the Secretariat of Health and CENSIDA (Secretaría de Salud 2004). The purpose of the HIV/AIDS content of the World Bank loan – which amounted to US$20 million - was to finance a five-year program, whose aim was to expand prevention campaigns through the strengthening of the NGO community (with a special emphasis on MSM). The negotiation of this loan is a prime example of the way in which the HIV/AIDS policy network worked together, allowing members of the NGO community full participation and influence in the formulation of the policies to be implemented with the Bank's funds. Key NGO members of the network (MEXSIDA and 'Letra S') worked together with the regional program (SIDALAC), and with the full of support of CENSIDA (especially the then director Patricia Uribe[33] and the one-year Secretary of Health José Antonio Fernández González),[34] in drafting and negotiating the conditions for the World Bank's loan during Zedillo's administration (Interview with José Antonio Izazola, Mexico City, November 27, 2001: Interview with Arturo Díaz Betancourt, Mexico City, September 10, 2002). MEXSIDA and 'Letra S,' both at the core of the policy network (See Table 4.3, and Box 4.1 above), put pressure on the government and worked shoulder to shoulder with other members of the HIV/AIDS policy network in order to secure the World Bank loan that specifically and openly addressed prevention among MSM (Interview with Silvia Panebianco, Rio de Janeiro, November 7, 2000). According to the parties involved in the negotiations, in the months between the 2000 elections and the transfer of power to the right-of-centre president elect, Vicente Fox, the strategy was to leave the 'hot potato' of prevention among MSM in the hands of the new conservative government.

The negotiations for that loan represented a major success for the emerging policy network, and their efforts then focused on making sure that those resources were going to be appropriately used. As mentioned above, out of the US$350 million, 20 million were allocated to HIV/AIDS programs in the course of 5 years. The original idea was to target 13 cities, with 60 per cent of the funds for the strengthening of local and regional NGOs, while 40 per cent was to be dedicated to the strengthening and monitoring of state programs (Interview with Díaz Betancourt,

---

[31] As has been pointed out before, ICASO has been part of the UNAIDS Programme Coordinating Board. Its role and links to the Mexican NGO community will be further discussed in the following chapter.
[32] Programa de Calidad, Equidad y Desarrollo en Salud.
[33] Dr. Patricia Uribe was appointed head of CENSIDA again by Peña Nieto, in 2013.
[34] Appointed Secretary of Health by president Zedillo.

Mexico City, September 10, 2002). As expected in a more inclusive process of decision making, there was some debate regarding the use of these funds within the network. In 2000, for instance, Jorge Saavedra, who was then the director of the 'Clínica Condesa'[35] and who in 2003 became the head of CENSIDA, pushed for the program to be expanded to include 40 cities, against the will of other members of the HIV/AIDS policy community at large. There was a heated debate on the issue, and in the end the program included 40 as opposed to the 13 cities originally contemplated, which represented a compromise between less resources for each and a broader geographical reach. The program had three components, each of them addressing three vulnerable populations; MSM, sex workers (male and female), and iv-drug users (See Secretaría de Salud 2004). The introduction of the issue of MSM into the National Program against HIV/AIDS has been a great success not only for the HIV/AIDS policy network but also for gay male activists and sex workers. As a result, gay activists have been working with the National Institute for Public Health (INSP[36]), offering a summer course focusing on health and sexuality with a special focus on MSM. Additionally, similar to the case of Brazil – which has received a series of equivalent World Bank loans -, they decided to work towards the creation of a special task force, with three components: raising awareness about MSM, getting more actors involved to stir support and resources, and creating an inventory of the programs in place nationally (Interview with Arturo Díaz Betancourt, Mexico City, September 10, 2002: Interview with Alejandro Brito, Mexico City, December 5, 2001).

The increased participation of the NGO community in the discussion of HIV/AIDS and health-related policies was accompanied by the emergence of common sources of funding for most NGOs and CONASIDA/CENSIDA, which further strengthened the aforementioned resource dependencies that define the policy network as such. Apart from the World bank loan, which represented the most important source of funding, the Secretariat of Social Development (SEDESOL) provided some funds in the amount of MEX$150 thousand for each project/organization (approximately US$13 thousand) (See SEDESOL 2004). Although this did not represent that much, together with funds provided by the Institute for Social Development (INDESOL) - which is part of the same Secretariat - these represent vital sources of funding and official recognition for NGOs. Some NGOs, however, have identified a few obstacles in accessing these resources. According to most applicants, in order to have access to these funds, people must demonstrate themselves to be experts in the field and have a lot of patience when it comes to the bureaucratic processing of their applications, being ready to compete with 5,000 other organizations (Interviews with various Mexican NGO representatives, Mexico City, 2001-2015). Additionally, for some years, external foundations, such as MacArthur and Ford, were important sources of funding for the

---

[35] The specialized clinic for HIV/AIDS of the government of Mexico City mentioned above.
[36] Instituto Nacional de Salud Pública.

work of many NGOs.[37] Since 1992, however, when as part of Salinas' globalist agenda Mexico joined the Organization for Economic Co-operation and Development (OECD), Mexican NGOs were no longer eligible for a significant number of sources on the basis of the country's new status as part of the wealthy countries' club.[38]

In December 2000, as another example of the positioning of the HIV/AIDS policy network, most members of its core (CENSIDA and NGO representatives) were one of the first groups to be received by the newly appointed Secretary of Health, Dr. Julio Frenk. This meeting allowed them to secure the commitment of the new Secretary to the allocation of funds from the World Bank loan in accordance to the terms defined by the previous government (although the loan was not confirmed until April of 2002) (Interview with José Antonio Izazola, Mexico City, November 27, 2001; Interview with Patricia Uribe, April 10, Havana, 2003; Interview with Artuto Diáz Betancourt, Mexico City, September 10, 2002). Their success in getting a renewed commitment with regards to the World Bank's loan by the new federal government was not considered enough, and the HIV/AIDS policy network demanded that the new Secretary of Health put more money into the fight against the pandemic and more pressure on the state level governments to contribute as well. These negotiations, which took place at the National Health Council,[39] were successful and in principle health authorities agreed and committed themselves to the allocation of more financial resources for HIV/AIDS and health in general (See Secretaría de Salud 2004). To the US$350 million from the World Bank, the federal government added US$231.2 million, for a total of US$581 million (*Notiese*, February 11, 2003). It was then publicly declared that a separate US$20 million program for HIV/AIDS would cover five big cities: Mexico City, Monterrey, Guadalajara, Durango, and Gómez Palacios. The goal of this second program was the implementation of prevention campaigns and diagnostic facilities, and the identification of NGO partners through competitions established by CONASIDA (*Novedades*, March 13, 2002). Given that organizations would have to compete for all these funds, the network made sure that each state would have a set of clear criteria and policy implementation rules, in order to make the allocation of resources the most transparent possible (Interviews with members of SIDALAC and MEXIDA, Mexico City, 2001-2002). Additionally, a Plural Advisory Commission was created in order to allow organizations to complain when they felt excluded.[40] Of greater concern was the need to ensure that local NGOs in the states had the required capabilities to perform effectively.[41] Hence, the NGO

---

[37] In particular, various projects of 'Colectivo Sol' (See Box 4.2) have been funded by external organizations (See presentations by Colectivo Sol in Foro 2003 and Fórum 2000).

[38] This was a constant complaint expressed by members of the NGO community interviewed in Mexico.

[39] See discussion of the creation and composition of the National Health Council, in chapter three.

[40] This came as a result to the complaints raised regarding a similar program in the case of Brazil. Originally, there were resources for two hundred organizations, then only twenty were considered, and in the end only twelve of them got it (Confidential interview with Brazilian program co-ordinator, Rio de Janeiro, November 8, 2000).

[41] This has become a particularly serious problem, given the availability of resources coming from the World Bank's loan, and the intention to work together with civil society organizations nation-wide. Therefore, in preparation for the World Bank's loan, in 2001, the Secretariat of Health and CONASIDA

'Colectivo Sol' implemented the so-called 'Alianza México' initiative, which consisted in the training for prevention campaigns of other smaller NGOs in different states (Interview with Hilda Pérez Vásquez, Mexico City, November 6, 2001). More recently, in 2011, civil society members of the network successfully lobbied to obtain a new 62 million pesos (about 5 million dollars) project for prevention for five years, financially supported by the UNAIDS Fund against AIDS, Malaria and TB (See UNAIDS 2015).

In August of 2001, key members of the policy network (NGOs representatives, CENSIDA officials, and the Secretary of Health) went to New York City to the UN General Assembly's special meeting on HIV/AIDS with a common agenda.[42] At that meeting, Secretary Frenk made a joint declaration with the rest of the network in order to make sure that the issue of prevention among MSM was at the forefront of the official delegation's position (*Notiese*, September 5, 2001). For some NGO members of the network, the government's declaration in New York City has been regarded as another example of the successes obtained by civil society groups as a result of a long and sustained battle since the beginning of the pandemic (Interview with Arturo Díaz Betancourt, Mexico City, September 10, 2002). For the longest time, not only civil society groups working on HIV/AIDS and in favour of sexual minorities' rights were excluded from any official act but government officials were very reluctant to recognize the urgency and importance of the problem. According to Díaz Betancourt, for example, the then Sub-Secretary for Health Prevention and Protection, Roberto Tapia Conyer, had long neglected and minimized the necessity of incorporating the MSM population into the planning for the pandemic. Yet today Dr. Tapia has become one of the main advocates for the promotion of prevention campaigns among the homosexual community.

Two subsequent changes in the national program can also be regarded as concrete successes of the HIV/AIDS policy network. First, as part of the restructuring of CONASIDA and the creation of the Centre for the Prevention and Control of HIV/AIDS (CENSIDA[43]), in July 2003, some civil society groups were incorporated

---

called for NGOs from all states to send their applications for funding for HIV/AIDS prevention campaigns among MSM. This was meant to be a trial program, in order to assess the actual numbers of existing NGOs with the necessary capabilities to undertake the responsibilities involved in the implementation of effective prevention campaigns. In June of 2002, out of only 12 applicants, 8 were selected, each of them receiving annual renewable funding in the amount of 125 thousand pesos (approximately US$12,000.00). The selecting criterion was based on objectives, viability, and the fulfilment of other stated requirements. The selection committee was integrated by the Secretariat of Health and CONASIDA officials, as well as members of FUNSALUD and the thematic group of UNAIDS. The recipients were eight different organizations. In the States: 'Asociación Queretana de la Educación para la Sexualidad, A.C.' (AQUESEX) (State of Querétaro), 'Juntos por Amor A.C.' (CD4) (State of Morelos), and 'Vihtalidad Vihsual e Identidad Saludable A.C.' (State of Hidalgo). In Mexico City: 'Compañeros en Ayuda Voluntaria de México' (AVE de México), 'Centro de Capacitación y Apoyo Sexual Humanista' (CECASH), 'Colectivo Sol', 'La Manta de México', and 'Centro de Atención Profesional para Personas con VIH/Sida' (CAPPSIDA).

[42] Representatives of NGOs 'Ave de México,' MEXSIDA and FRENPAVIH accompanied Secretary Frenk. Members of the Mexican Congress were also invited by Frenk to participate in the meeting (*Letra S, in La Jornada*, November 8, 2001).

[43] Centro Nacional para la Prevención y Control del VIH/SIDA.

as members of CENSIDA's Department of Civil Society Organizations. Second, of major significance was the appointment of Jorge Saavedra as CENSIDA's new director on September 2003, after a wide consultation process within the HIV/AIDS policy community. As an openly gay academic and public official, who has long worked on issues related to MSM, he had the legitimacy and support of most members of the policy community and the network. And between 1997 and 2000, Saavedra worked as adviser to the Mexico City government (from the left-of-centre party PRD), and was the first director of the 'Clínica Condesa.' Before assuming his new position (under the right-of-centre government of Vicente Fox), Saavedra was the adjunct general director of the World Bank-funded program PROCEDES at the Secretariat of Health.

In addition to the aforementioned commitment to universal treatment coverage, the various members of the policy network worked together to promote a reform to article 1st of the Constitution to prohibit all forms of discrimination. Their efforts resulted in the issuing of the Federal Law for the Prevention and Elimination of Discrimination,[44] which explicitly includes sexual orientation and health conditions (Secretariat of Health Press Release No. 209, September 23, 2003). Based on this new law, individuals cannot be tested for HIV for hiring purposes. As such, it can be argued that the renewed support of the right-of-centre government of Vicente Fox for treatment and against discrimination was the result of a series of positive developments in the fight against HIV/AIDS in the course of previous 20 years or so, and it reflected the active engagement of the policy network in policymaking and their impact on policy outcomes. Furthermore, as we know, a central component of an effective response to HIV/AIDS is the adoption of domestic legislative measures to guarantee individuals and communities access to effective judicial or other appropriate remedies in the face of human rights violations concerning their sexual health and/or sexuality. Yet, in Mexico, persistent problems in the administration of justice and the impunity of violators confirm the often-argued disconnect between the law and its observance (Panebianco 2000; Reding 1995). It must be acknowledged, however, that with increasing social pressure, some gains have been made in improving the country's legal framework for combating discrimination based on sexual orientation and HIV status, especially at the federal level and in Mexico City (formerly known as the Federal District). These include the aforementioned creation of the National Commission for Human Rights (CNDH) and the National Council to Prevent Discrimination (Consejo Nacional para Prevenir la Discriminación, or CONAPRED), on July 11, 2003, with the appointment of long-time activist and respected political figure Gilberto Rincón Gallardo as president until his recent death.[45] For its part, Mexico City's government introduced sexual orientation among the issues addressed in the July 2006 Law to Prevent and Eliminate Discrimination in the Federal District (Ley para Prevenir y Erradicar la Discriminación en el Distrito Federal), as well as the creation of the Council for the Prevention and Elimination of

---

[44] Ley Federal para Prevenir y Eliminar la Discriminación.

[45] It is important to remember that the late activist Arturo Díaz Betancourt, mentioned above, participated in the creation of CONAPRED and became one of its most engaged and active board members.

Discrimination in the Federal District (Consejo para Prevenir y Erradicar la Discriminación en el Distrito Federal) in October 2006. This council has a mandate and objectives similar to those of CONAPRED but with jurisdiction limited to Mexico City. Additionally, in 2010, the government of Mexico City, through its Ministry of Culture, launched the first publicly sponsored radio show with exclusive content on diversity called *Código Diverso,* its host, Gabriel Gutiérrez García worked diligently to make the voices of the LBGT community heard during his four years of broadcasting. Gutiérrez García was nominated and appointed as CONAPRED's Ambassador Against Discrimination in 2009, and has been the spokesperson for different initiatives on Human Rights and Sexual Diversity, participating in several legislative fora on LGBT issues at the local Assembly of Mexico City.[46]

Very importantly, and as part of CONAPRED's work and in coordination with the HIV/AIDS policy network, the right-of-center federal government of Vicente Fox launched a national radio campaign against homophobia in 2005. The campaign, which was very explicit and challenged traditional conceptions, was organized by CONAPRED and CONASIDA, with full support from the national Secretariat of Health and financial support from the Pan-American Health Organization (PAHO) and UNAIDS (La Jornada, March 23, 2005; for a transcript of the actual campaign (in Spanish), see also Saavedra 2007a, 2007b, and Appendix 4.3). The very launch of the campaign points to the surprising effectiveness of the policy network's work within a PAN administration, given that, in the case of Mexico, sexual minorities seem to have traditionally benefited from their alliance to and participation in a more progressive political front (De la Dehesa 2007). In a way, and paraphrasing Alejandro Brito, the construction of the policy network and collaboration with the government might be considered a sign of maturity and tolerance on all counts (See Frasca 2005).

When it comes to the relationship between the HIV/AIDS NGO community at large and the Security Institute (IMSS), overall, this had been of mutual understanding and co-operation. IMSS' authorities had shown a high degree of sensitivity towards HIV/AIDS patients until the appointment of firmly convinced globalist Santiago Levy as its director, in 2001. For instance, IMSS had provided treatment to the majority of AIDS patients in Mexico City, so that the activists' fight concentrated on those without social security. The position of the federal government and IMSS' authorities had reflected their conviction that Mexico could not stay behind other nations, and should provide treatment to all social security affiliates. Thus, during the years

---

[46] Gabriel Gutiérrez García has also been a presenter and facilitator on issues pertaining to culture, sexual health, and HIV/AIDS at workshops and seminars organized by many public and private institutions, such as the INAH, IPN, ITAM, UAM, UNAM, UCSJ, Sedesol-DF, CONALEP, etc. He actively participated in the lobbying for Same-Sex Marriage Legislation in Mexico City, for the change in a Federal Decree to declare the National Day Against Homophobia, and has worked as an academic research assistant. During a stay in Canada, he volunteered for the Centre for Spanish Speaking People, the 519 Community Center, and Amnesty International, and worked as an outreach worker with a focus on Hispanic communities on sexual diversity issues, as well as immigration, refugee claims and HIV/AIDS. He is a former fellow of the U.S. State Department, as an International Visitor Leadership Program (IVLP), and writes for various publications such as the weekly magazines *Tiempo Libre* and *La Guía de México.*

leading to the appointment of Levy, IMSS increased the number of treatments provided. In 2000, even before his appointment as director of IMSS, Santiago Levy had publicly positioned himself against the allocation of 10 per cent of the Institute's budget for the treatment of AIDS patients (at a time when he was still in the Secretariat of Finance, under president Zedillo). In 2002, then as the new head of the institute, Levy authorized the withdrawal of benefits to 1,119 IMSS subscribers who had lost their jobs and who were in need of treatment, causing a public outrage and a series of protests (*Notiese*, September 14, 2003). With a strong globalist agenda, Santiago Levy had been resistant to an open discussion. His decision to exclude those people who lost their jobs, and therefore IMSS affiliation, from being eligible for treatment showed Levy's and his advisors' stubbornness in pursuing their globalist agenda.

As a response to Levy's position and in line with the HIV/AIDS network, in appearances before Congress, Julio Frenk clearly stated the Secretariat of Health's arguments in favour of keeping IMSS' workers under treatment. From the beginning, the Secretary's proposals looked at two options. The first one would have involved the enrolment of these individuals in the voluntary social security scheme under IMSS. While the second one – and the one which was actually approved - would be to provide the necessary financial means for their treatment under the Fund for Catastrophic Health Expenses (conditioned to additional funds approved by Congress)(See Secretaría de Salud 2004). Since then, HIV/AIDS activists at large organized massive campaigns, and unsuccessfully demanded Levy's removal through a petition submitted to the federal government, with the signatures of 60 thousand people (*La Jornada*, May 9, 2002). In spite of the shift in IMSS's policies, and the disengagement of some civil society groups from any dialogue with the Institute's authorities, other groups such as FRENPAVIH and MEXSIDA – both at the core of the policy network - continued to work directly with it. They successfully demanded that IMSS cover all insured patients with the necessary treatments, including those who had lost their jobs. Eventually, the fight for access to treatment went beyond IMSS, and NGO members of the policy network persistently and successfully pressured Congress to authorize the budget for the provision of drugs for all HIV/AIDS patients in the amount of MEX$461 million (*Milenio*, November 27, 2001). Obviously, given the difficulty in assessing the reasons behind their success, the jury is still out regarding whether it was a product of old-fashioned lobbying or the increasing leverage that the existence of a policy network represents. The best one can do is to argue that both factors combined help to explain the outcome.

For his part, the then Secretary of Finance, Francisco Gíl Díaz (2000-2006), tried to exercise some political control over the aforementioned World Bank loan for health and HIV/AIDS (PROCEDES). Although the World Bank money was already in the Secretariat of Finance by July 2002 and was expected to be released by October of that same year, Gíl Díaz made its release conditional on political support in Congress for the approval of the fiscal reform proposed by the Executive (*La Jornada*, December 1, 2001). Yet due to pressure from the HIV/AIDS policy network, including the Secretary of Health himself, and in spite of the lack of congressional support for the Executive's proposal for fiscal reform, some of the funds were eventually released in June of 2003. Some members of the Legislative body were also critical of and opposed to the influence of Fox's Secretary of Finance in the area of health. For instance, Carlos Rojas Gutiérrez - a PRI senator – argued that in 2001 there were $1.3 billion pesos authorized and assigned for health by Congress that were not released by the Secretariat of Finance (*Notiese*, April 23, 2002). Interestingly, in spite of the Secretary of Finance's efforts to influence social policymaking, his actual power to formulate HIV/AIDS policies was close to non-existent, and the Secretariat's capacity to control access to public funds has declined and been restricted by Congress.

The appointments of Santiago Levy as the Director of IMSS and Gíl Díaz as Secretary of Finance represented prime examples of the persisting presence of some well-positioned market reform camarillas. Although significantly less powerful than in the past, these camarillas - with a strong globalist agenda – still constrained the capacity of maneuver of the Secretariat of Health. In fact, the differences between the Secretariat of Health and the other two institutions, that is IMSS and the Secretariat of Finance, showed the persisting tensions between the still strong and exclusive market reform camarillas on the one hand, and the more inclusive HIV/AIDS policy network on the other.

With regards to the role, or better perhaps, the non-role of the National Congress as an active participant in the fight against the pandemic, the NGO community has repeatedly expressed regret at the lack of interest from most representatives (Confidential interviews with various HIV/AIDS activists, Mexico City, 2001-2015). This lack of interest in Congress is a consequence of the fact that HIV/AIDS has not been a central concern for political parties (Interview with Hilda Pérez Vásquez, Mexico City, December 6, 2001).[47] Under these circumstances, HIV/AIDS NGOs have participated in the creation of the policy network, which allows them to work outside the party system, with further links to international actors (focus of chapter two). As in other issue areas, ranging from environmental to human rights allies (Camp 2003, p. 155; See also Keck and Sikkink 1998), many of these Mexican organizations either established or strengthened their links with peer groups in other countries.

---

[47] In more than one occasion, upon request, Congress has invited a group of organizations engaged in the struggle for access to drugs to working meetings with Congress Commissions in charge of the elaboration of the health budget. Civil society organizations saw these occasions as opportunities to lobby them to authorize the necessary resources for the provision of treatment for all people living with HIV/AIDS and without social insurance. Yet NGOs representatives complain that whenever they went to Congress, its members "listened" to them while at the same going through their mail, writing a memo, or checking their e-mails. Under those circumstances, activists argue, the fact that the Secretary of Health had publicly expressed his commitment to their cause was essential for them. As put by some of them, although Frenk was not in charge of the elaboration of the budget, the fact that he had declared HIV/AIDS as a priority did represent a strong argument for them to get Congress members' commitments. The problem then, in the opinion of most members of the policy community, was how to 'amarrar' (roughly translated as to moor, or to secure) the commitment of public officials and Congress members beyond promises, and make sure that those commitments were translated into concrete programs and budgets. As discussed before, for many years, the political system was hermetic, with hidden rules known only to PRI "ghettos."

Based on the above discussion, it becomes clear that some HIV/AIDS activists and members of the gay community in Mexico have positioned themselves at the core of the HIV/AIDS policy network. This is the result of sexual-minority groups having been organized to effect change through their engagement in the fight against the pandemic. And in spite of the many obstacles, since the early 1980s homosexuality began to emerge from its social invisibility. Triggered in an important way by the urgency of the HIV/AIDS epidemic, the increasing activism forced both the government and civil society at large to publicly discuss such topics as homosexuality and sexuality in general. In a way, as argued by Altman (2001), there has been a kind of legitimization through disaster. Although, it must be underlined that HIV/AIDS has helped to legitimate a sexual conduct and not so much the gay movement as a whole. In fact, the organization and participation of gay activists and HIV/AIDS NGOs in Mexico has not been easy; it has been part of the broader process of democratization and as such has been an exercise of trial and error. At the beginning, most people got organized to respond to the needs emerging from their most immediate and urgent circumstances, such as the need to provide care for the friend or relative who was dying from the disease. Slowly, they came to the realization that although the care and prevention work they were engaged in was essential, they were also faced with a broader political fight. As a result of this realization, there were a few individuals amongst the gay population and the HIV/AIDS policy community at large that successfully put their energies into the creation – perhaps unconsciously at the time – of the HIV/AIDS policy network.

Among some of the key individuals, who not only were full participants in the fight against HIV/AIDS but also openly gay men, one case is especially significant for the analysis of the HIV/AIDS policy network. Jorge Saavedra (the head of CENSIDA during Fox's and part of Calderón's administrations), as an openly gay man living with HIV, with a good record of activism and expertise, as well as the required political links with key individuals within the government and traditional camarillas has come to represent the success of a long fight for recognition by sexual minorities. This has given them decision-making power in public policies, and it explains their success in expanding the access to treatment and the attention to MSM in prevention campaigns. Additionally, the full support of an individual like the Secretary of Health, Julio Frenk, resulted in the strengthening of an HIV/AIDS policy network that was already in the making in the years leading to the 2000 election. Outside the network, there have been other allies, who have also contributed to the efforts to combat the pandemic. For instance, it has been widely recognized the significance of the remarks made by the then Mexican Secretary of Foreign Affairs, Jorge Castañeda (from 2000 to 2003), who in 2002 declared HIV/AIDS to be a national security issue (*Novedades*, June 4, 2002). His support helped to raise the profile of the Mexican government at the international level regarding its strong commitment to the fight against the disease and for human rights enforcement.

Ultimately, HIV/AIDS activism in Mexico has had concrete and positive effects on the visibility and empowerment of sexual minorities. In particular, through their NGOization and active participation in the creation of the HIV/AIDS policy network, activists have made specific gains in terms of public policy making and implementation, as well as in transforming and expanding the public sphere (See De la Dehesa 2010; Díez 2015). The increasing engagement of civil society actors in Mexico is also partly explained by the fact that, in the 1990s, major donors broadened their focus on NGOs and began funding a more diverse set of civil society groups. As a consequence, an important number of HIV/AIDS NGOs were created and received a steady stream of funding from international agencies. Yet this increasing interest in the promotion of NGO activities responded also to one of the central tenets of the globalist agenda: the insistence on less government and reduced public budgets.

Once again, observers of NGOization warned about the consequences this phenomenon can have on the weakening of social movements' autonomy and their causes (Álvarez, Dagnino, & Escobar, 1998). However, in spite of some of the risks associated with the close collaboration required between governmental and non-governmental actors around the pandemic, there have been some positive outcomes. In particular, we have witnessed successful initiatives around human rights issues being brought forward, some of which go well beyond the more narrowly defined goals of HIV/AIDS and health-related policies. In fact, some NGOs and individuals (part of the policy network) have been able to strategically engage with the state and mobilize resources, while prioritizing their own agendas and retaining their character. This has allowed them to advocate for the legal recognition and enforcement of more broadly defined sexual minorities' rights. The LGBT community elaborated a broader agenda based on the notion of sexual health as a basic human right and built on the idea of legal entitlements of individuals before the state, other individuals and institutions, which has been supported by the UN system. This discourse has been reinforced by the 2006 Yogyakarta[48] principles on the application of international human rights legislation around sexual orientation and gender identity issues. Furthermore, in the process of redefining the discursive field by adopting the human rights framework, civil society actors realized the need to establish direct relations with the official structures of the state, given that in the modern world, the enforcement of human rights (or Hannah Arendt's right to have rights) continues to rest on the state's commitment and ability to do so (See Parekh 2008). As such, the effectiveness of this strategy is also explained by the association of this discourse with the notion of modernity, which although often contested on the basis of having a 'western' bias, has led to many state governments doing whatever is necessary in order to appear as 'modern' in the eyes of the international community.

Finally, and as pointed out at the beginning of this chapter, in spite of the increasing inclusiveness that characterizes the HIV/AIDS policy network, it is important to recognize that there are still some members of the policy community who face obstacles in having access to and becoming part of it. In some cases, the exclusion of some NGOs might be due to lack of expertise and of the necessary personal and professional links, as well as lack of familiarity with the intricacies of

---

[48] See the 2006 Yogyakarta principles on the application of human rights to sexual orientation and sexual identity: http://www.yogyakartaprinciples.org/index.html

the political system, which prevents them from becoming part of the core or joining the network. Another plausible explanation for the exclusion of some groups - one that falls beyond the scope of the present analysis and which should be further investigated - is the role that issues like class and "race" seem to play, which has been intuitively suggested by the analysis of sexual minorities' activism (See discussion in chapter three). More problematic were the multiple complaints, during Calderón's term, about CENSIDA's director José Antonio Izazola, regarding accusations about corruption and misallocation of funds during his tenure.[49] According to some activists, there was some co-optation, and complicity among NGOs due to fear of losing their economic support, with little to no evaluation or auditing (Interview with Luis Adrián Quiroz, Mexico City, April 24, 2016; Interview with Miguel García Murcia, Mexico City, April 23, 2016.). Although some of those issues seemed to have been resolved under the new directorship of Dr. Patricia Uribe, lack of sufficient attention to transparency can potentially result in most NGOs losing some autonomy and taking unfair advantages from their own positioning. Thus, the need at the CENSIDA level to put in place mechanisms that could lead to greater transparency in the relations with the civil society side of the HIV/AIDS policy network, and some evaluation mechanisms for the performance of governmental actions. These improvements could help shed light on the processes of recognition or exclusion of concrete NGOs and other civil society groups. More importantly, according to some activists, as of today there is a lack of real commitment from president Peña Nieto, like the kind that was shown by Fox, who understood the need for leadership from the presidential office. In fact, the only meeting with the president took place with Fox, while Saavedra was at CENSIDA (Interview with Luis Adrián Quiroz, Mexico City, April 24, 2016). And since the radio and television campaign of 2005 (See Appendix 4.3), there has not been one of that scale.

Nevertheless, by way of participating in the formation of the HIV/AIDS policy network and positioning themselves at its core, some members of the NGO community succeeded in opening the process of policy formulation and implementation, from the closed camarilla-driven style to a more inclusive and participatory one. Furthermore, in this process, some spaces have also been opened for sexual minorities. The formation and makeup of the HIV/AIDS policy network has forced public authorities at the highest levels to listen to some civil society groups. Moreover, through the emergence of new institutionalized settings (i.e., CENSIDA's Department of NGOs), key members of the NGO community have actively participated in the definition of the official discourse in this area.

As expected in any network that aims to be more inclusive, there have been differences regarding some decisions and strategies among its members (i.e., scope of programs and allocation of funds). Yet, in general, these differences have been

---

[49] In 2012, the was a major scandal involving the "Circuito de la Diversidad Sexual "(Cidisex, Sexual Diversity Circuit), whose leadership was accused by fellow activists of misappropriation of public funds (See Notiese, July 25, 2012: http://www .notiese.org/notiese.php?ctn_id=5823). More recently, and under Izazola's directorship, there was a reality show on YuTube that costed 5 million pesos and nobody really saw.

resolved through dialogue and compromise. So far, the internal tensions have not been significant enough to impinge on the cohesiveness of the policy network or the capacity to present a common front in the fight against the pandemic. In fact, most of the differences, as identified by various members of the network in confidential interviews, tend to be of a personal nature and are kept private. Admittedly, some challenges persist in the fight against the pandemic. Thus, in the last section of this chapter, we will turn to the presence and power of several conservative groups, as well as economic interests that do not always go hand in hand with the goals pursued by the HIV/AIDS policy network. But before doing so, we will briefly look at some of the links between the domestic and international dimensions, drawing also from chapter two's analysis.

The Significance of Domestic and International Links

As a result of the efforts made by key individuals and organizations within the policy network and their supporters, Mexico has been more actively engaged in the struggle against the pandemic at the regional and global levels. For instance, Mexico joined other countries in the Latin America region, as part of an international initiative among public authorities in the creation and functioning of the Technical Co-operation Horizontal Group.[50] This group brings together all national HIV/AIDS programs, to co-ordinate their activities and to share their experiences. Furthermore, from 1998 to 2000, Mexico held the presidency of the governing council of UNAIDS (*Letra S*, in *La Jornada*, June 1, 2000). In 2003, at a regional meeting in Panama, and in recognition of some of Mexico's recent efforts and policies around the pandemic, the country's health authorities were elected as the representatives for Latin America in the Global Fund for Malaria, Tuberculosis, and HIV/AIDS, by 14 governments, and 6 NGO national and regional networks (See *Notiese* 2003).

The incorporation of members of the NGO community within the UNAIDS structure served as an example and as leverage for the efforts of domestic civil society groups, which resulted in the creation of the NGO Department within Mexico's HIV/AIDS program (CENSIDA). In contrast to the World Bank, the WHO and UNAIDS have not shared the former's view regarding the declining role of the state in the health sector, thus counterbalancing - at the core of the policy network - the Bank's privatizing proposals and their effects on the formulation of HIV/AIDS and health-related policies at the domestic level. It is possible then to establish significant parallels between the domestic and the international policy network, both in terms of the establishment and institutionalization of the linkages between civil society groups and governmental bodies. Moreover, the establishment of various links between local and international NGOs reinforces the idea of a domestic and an international HIV/AIDS policy network working together.

Among some of the specific links between members of Mexico's domestic network and their international counterparts, for instance, since the late 1990s the

---

[50] Grupo de Cooperación Técnica Horizontal (See SIDALAC's website: http://wwwsidalac.org.mx).

International HIV/AIDS Alliance (based in London, England) has worked together with local NGOs and served as an international liaison for some of them (e.g., Colectivo Sol, FRENPAVIH, and MEXSIDA) (Interview with Anuar I. Luna Cadena, Mexico City, December 12, 2001; Interview with Silvia Panebianco, Rio de Janeiro, November 7, 2000). The *International HIV/AIDS Alliance* continues to provide support for various communities in LMICs, both in HIV prevention campaigns as well as AIDS care for all people affected - with a special focus on children (See http://www.aidsalliance.org). It has also promoted the involvement of those most affected by HIV/AIDS to assess their own vulnerability, to initiate their own responses, and to make decisions about interventions which affect their lives, all of which have been shown to improve the effectiveness of HIV/AIDS programs.

Especially significant for the analysis of the Mexican case is the fact that at a meeting in Paris, in December 1989, the late activist Arturo Díaz Betancourt (From 'Letra S' and CONAPRED), together with other international activists, founded the International Council of AIDS Service Organizations (ICASO). Since its creation, ICASO has served as a co-ordinating body and as a permanent liaison for civil society groups that are part of the international HIV/AIDS policy network (Interview with Mary Ann Torres, Toronto, October 23, 2000). More importantly, for the analysis of the policy network, in 2003, ICASO had a seat on the UNAIDS PCB. Since its creation, the work of ICASO within UNAIDS resulted in the increased commitment of the international policy network to the expansion of prevention campaigns for MSM and access to treatment for all (Interview with Mary Ann Torres, Toronto, October 23, 2000; Confidential Interviews with UNAIDS official, Rio de Janeiro, November 2000, and Mexico City, August 2008).

As seen in chapter two, MSF actions at the international level also had major effects at the domestic level in many countries, Mexico included. For example, although CONASIDA had initially argued that ARVs were not essential and that the government did not have the resources to pay for them and provide access for all, pressure from within the policy network by MSF and other NGOs on UNAIDS and the World Bank led to the softening of the Mexican government's position. Additionally, civil society organizations had threatened to sue the Secretariat of Health and IMSS, following the example of activists in Costa Rica, Venezuela, and Brazil (See *Notiese* 2000). At that point in time, domestic and international health authorities saw a major problem looming, which forced UNAIDS and the World Bank to seriously look into the negotiation of the costs of medications with Pharmaceuticals. Thus, in the case of Mexico, the combined effect of the work of domestic NGOs and the external pressure resulted in the government's decision to provide full coverage of ARVs for all those in need of treatment.

Particularly interesting for our analysis, of the effects that globalization and globalism have had on Mexico's quest for democracy and development, is the agreement amongst most NGOs' representatives on the fact that Carlos Salinas de Gortari's presidency represented a big step backwards in terms of external funding from various public and private organizations. As part of his globalist agenda and his pursuit of the WTO presidency at the end of his administration, Salinas made sure to tell the world that Mexico was a wealthy country. Through his efforts and negotiations, Mexico joined the OECD in 1992, and was then officially regarded as the new member of the wealthy nations' club. At that point in time, the country stopped being considered a priority for international agencies, with international financial aid being cut down.[51] Two concrete examples of this were the MacArthur and Ford foundations, which withdrew from work on HIV/AIDS and cancelled all their ongoing projects (Interview with Hilda Pérez Vásquez, Mexico City, December 6, 2001).

PERSISTING DOMESTIC CHALLENGES IN THE FIGHT AGAINST HIV/AIDS

The analysis of HIV/AIDS in Mexico would be incomplete without looking at the efforts of some socially conservative groups to impose religious and moralistic principles on sexual conduct. As such, moralistic considerations in the formulation of sexual health policies can become obstacles for the provision of services for the sick and for the success of prevention campaigns. Moralistic attitudes imposed by religious institutions can further contribute to worsen problems related to public health, such as unwanted pregnancies in adolescents, and the spread of sexually transmitted diseases, in clear violation of the officially recognized human rights for all.

So far, socially conservative groups in Mexico have remained outside the HIV/AIDS policy network. Yet their influential power can still be exercised through other means, particularly given the strong links that some of them have with an influential institution such as the Catholic Church and various PAN members. Moreover, in a country like Mexico, where religion has traditionally played a very important role (privately and publicly), socially conservative groups must be carefully considered. In 1994, for example, three-quarters of all Mexicans described themselves as practicing Catholics (in 2000, the percentages by affiliation were as follows: 85 Catholics; 4 protestants; 4 other affiliations; 6 none) (Camp 2003, p. 85). However, the Catholic Church, together with the business sector and the military, is one of the groups that were traditionally excluded from the PRI party structure (Camp 2003, p. 158). Furthermore, for the most part of the PRI regime, the Church's role as an interest group was limited due to the antichurch rhetoric that was incorporated into the public education of each child in Mexico - the origins of which can be traced back to the Liberal Reform Laws of 1858. Yet in 1992 Salinas de Gortari – as a consequence of the contested federal elections and in need of support from powerful groups to legitimize his presidency - introduced constitutional reforms, which were also part of his globalist/modernization agenda, to make the Catholic Church a more active actor in the political system. Under Salinas' administration, constitutional amendments were meant to benefit the Church's political activism. Up until 1992 clergy of all faiths did not have a legal right to vote, although many actually did (Camp 2003, p. 138). Yet as put by Camp, as a result of the introduced changes "numerous bishops

---

[51] Apart from the World Bank and UNAIDS, among public agencies, the only one still present in Mexico with work on HIV/AIDS is USAID.

now believe it is their responsibility to take stands on significant social, economic, and political issues, a belief that has produced implicit and explicit criticism of government actions" (Camp 2003, p. 139).[52]

It is interesting to note that, according to Camp (2003, p. 89), close to two-thirds of Mexicans were interested in redefining the Catholic Church's role in society and in seeing it more involved in social work, health, and education. Yet there are some indications that most Mexicans do not agree with the sex morals dictated by the Vatican; a phenomenon that has been referred to as a quiet revolution (González Ruiz 2001, p. 91). According to a poll conducted by GIRE in 1994,[53] in spite of the Church's strong condemnation of abortion, 72.6 per cent of the polled declared that it should be allowed when the mother has HIV/AIDS, while 54.4 per cent supported it for eugenics-based reasons. A few years later, and according to a poll by 'Alducín y Asociados' (July 1998), 70 per cent of the people living in Mexico City opined that abortion should be allowed in certain cases, and 72 per cent thought it should be debated (Camp 2003, p. 77). Moreover, among Mexicans who rank the Church at the very top of trusted institutions, it is regarded also as the last source for political beliefs. In fact, scholars argue that for most of the population in Mexico, Catholicism is much more Guadalupean (the widespread cult of the Virgin of Guadalupe) and of a "pre-colonial nature;" the religion's appeal is more mystical and less ideological (Gruzinky 1994, p. 199-214; 1999, p. 277-299). As put by Lumsden (1991, p. 92), most religious people might respond violently to an alleged insult to the Virgin of Guadalupe. It is doubtful, however, that they would react in like fashion when it comes to support demands on the part of the Catholic Church for the state to intrude in the private sex lives of the population.

When it comes to the religiosity of congresspersons, there are significant differences according to political party affiliation. Not surprisingly, members of Congress from the right-of-centre PAN are more religious and more Catholic than the Mexican population as a whole; in the LVI Legislature (1994-1997), amongst PAN members 97 per cent defined themselves as practicing Catholics, while only 3 per cent were Protestant. Amongst PRD congresspersons, two-thirds declared no religious affiliation, and one third identified themselves as Catholic. Meanwhile, PRI congresspersons are most representative of the population at large, with 87 per cent of Catholics, 10 per cent with no religious affiliation, and just 3 per cent Protestants (Camp 2003, p. 141). These differences among political parties play themselves out in the effectiveness of the Catholic Church and other religious and socially conservative groups in influencing public officials and affect policymaking.

Without making overgeneralizations or reaching definite conclusions, it is a fact that in Mexico, social conservatism, intolerance, and discrimination of all kinds have been historically associated with the Catholic Church. In contrast, a significantly higher percentage of Mexican Protestants and atheists tend to favour social change and tolerance (Camp 2003, p. 86). In modern Mexican history, tensions between the

---

[52] Salinas also established official diplomatic relations with the Vatican, and appointed a prominent politician as his personal representative to the Holy See (Camp 2003, p. 140).
[53] A Mexican NGO dedicated to the analysis of gender issues and women, see http://www.gire.org.mx

Catholic Church and Protestants go back at least to 1914, when the Church tried to blame the Revolution on the role of teachers who were said to be protestant and homosexuals (See González Ruiz 2002). The 'Guerras Cristeras' (1926-1929) (See chapter three, section 3.1) were also characterized by confrontations between Catholics and Protestants, and it is possible to trace the origins of many conservative and powerful groups back to these conflicts. More recently, in 1966, a far-right student movement with anti-Protestant tendencies was founded at the National University (UNAM): 'University Movement of Renovating Orientation' (MURO[54]). Its long list of members includes Luis Pazos, who was the PAN's Governor candidate in the state of Veracruz in 1998, and a National Congress representative (2000-2003). Today, there are several other powerful and influential conservative anti-Protestant organizations that remain active, such as the 'Catholic Association of Mexican Youth' (ACJM[55]) and the 'Knights of Columbus' (See González Ruiz 2003).

The Catholic Church has openly manifested its conservative and to some extent intolerant position on issues related to sexuality. The recently retired archbishop and Cardinal Norberto Rivera as much as his predecessor, Ernesto Corripio Ahumada, were very much against the use of condoms and sex education, and supported various conservative groups and PAN officials in their political campaigns for public office. Back in 1989, Genaro Alamilla, who was then the spokesperson for the archbishop, said publicly that it was a "stupidity" on the part of the then secretary of health, Guillermo Soberón, to say that HIV/AIDS was a problem of public health and not of public morals (*Proceso*, July 17, 1989). In 1997, the archbishop Norbeto Rivera asked to add a warning on all condoms stating that the product itself was a health hazard (*Excélsior*, August 25, 1997).[56] The Church's hierarchy has worked closely with PAN and other conservative groups in order to influence public officials and the state's position on issues regarded as of their immediate concern. One of these Catholic organizations is the National Committee of PROVIDA, which was founded in 1978 by Jaime Aviña Zepeda to actively fight against abortion. Aviña Zepeda later joined PAN and was elected a Congress member in the LIV legislature (1988-1991), eventually becoming the Secretary of the Commission on Population and Development. Between 1987 and 2001, Jorge Serrano Limón was a very active and vocal president of this group, and was successful in strengthening the links with PAN and with some of the most powerful Mexican entrepreneurs (González Ruiz 2002, p. 133-138)). In Mexico City, for example, PAN's Secretary for Women's Issues, Camila Zavala Valencia, publicly stated that "PROVIDA coincides with the party's principles and doctrine, therefore we can speak the same language" (González Ruiz 2001, p. 136). One of the main targets of PROVIDA has been the group 'Catholics

---

[54] Movimiento Universitario de Renovadora Orientación.

[55] Asociación Católica de la Juventud Mexicana.

[56] Additionally, there have been various incidents of open discrimination against sexual minorities across the country. In the city of Veracruz, for example, the local bishop, Luis Gabriel Cuara Méndez, declared that "the government has the responsibility to fight perversities and moral wrongs that affect society." (*La Jornada*, January 19, 2001). This declaration was made in support of the decision by the city government – PAN member and Mayor Ramón Gutiérrez de Velasco – to violently "remove" sex workers and homosexuals from the downtown and touristic areas.

[Women] for the Right to Decide[57],' which belongs to an international group called 'We are Church,' whose main goal is the legalization of abortion. In 2003, its Mexican leader, Pilar Sánchez, openly referred to the need to combat the double moral standards of the Church, particularly in its way of dealing with nuns and priests who are HIV carriers (See *Notiese* 2003). At the end of 1993, PROVIDA and a group of PAN members, together with another conservative group 'Feminine Civic Association' (Ancifem[58]), unsuccessfully tried to block the appointment of Luis de la Barreda as the first Ombudsman of Mexico City, arguing that his stand on abortion was unacceptable to them (González Ruiz 2002, p. 137). Other targets of PROVIDA have been Mexfam,[59] the National Population Council (CONAPO), CENSIDA, and all parties or candidates who in any way or under whatever circumstances support the women's right to abort and the use of condoms. In reference to the moral and political battles of the Vatican, John Paul II compared the activists of PROVIDA in Mexico with martyrs (González Ruiz 2002, p. 199).

Amongst other groups, religious organizations with enormous economic and political power such as 'Los Legionarios de Cristo' and the 'Opus Dei' strongly support the Vatican and the Church's authorities in Mexico on these issues (González Ruiz 2002, p. 204).[60] The 'Legionarios de Cristo' was founded in 1941 by the late Marcial Maciel Degollado, who was very close to John Paul II and was found to sexually abuse underage boys. This organization has a variety of affiliated groups in Latin America, the United States, and Spain (González Ruiz 2002, p. 199). In 2000, one of its members, Ana Teresa Aranda, was appointed by Fox as the head of the public federal institution for 'Integral Family Development' (DIF[61]), and repeatedly and publicly defended the traditional definition of the family and opposed "alternative" sexual conducts (See *Notiese* 2003). There are other conservative groups and organizations that, due to their influence and support, deserve special attention (See Appendix 4.4, for a review of some other powerful conservative organizations in Mexico). Among the most prominent ones, there is the 'Mexican Civic Action' (ACM[62]) group, which was founded in 1929, and which is one of those organizations that were formed by disbanded Catholic groups that emerged from the 'Guerras Cristeras.' ACM is an umbrella organization, and in the 1960s it was headed by the late Carlos Castillo Peraza (prominent PAN member and former head of the national committee) (González Ruiz 2002, p. 176). Another one is the 'Sinarquist National Union,'[63] founded in León, Guanajuato, in 1937, which was also a product of the

---

[57] Católicas por el Derecho a Decidir.

[58] 'Asociación Cívica Femenina,' which was founded in 1975 with support from the National Parent's Union UNPF.

[59] 'Fundación Mexicana para la Planeación Familiar, A.C' (Mexfam) is and NGO specialized in sex and education, founded in 1965. See website: http://www.mexfam.org.mx.

[60] The 'Opus Dei' runs the private university 'Universidad Panamericana', and the graduate centre for business education 'Instituto Panamericano de Alta Dirección de Empresas'. While 'Los Legionarios de Cristo' founded another important private university: 'Universidad Anáhuac de México.'

[61] Desarrollo Integral de la Familia.

[62] Acción Cívica Mexicana.

[63] Unión Nacional Sinarquista.

'Guerras Cristeras,' whose political arm became the now disbanded 'Mexican Democratic Party' (PDM[64]). Its most important leader was Salvador Abascal Infante (father of Vicente Fox's Secretary of Labour, José Carlos María Abascal Carranza), from 1940 to 1941 (González Ruiz 2002, p. 180).

The links between the Catholic Church, religious groups, and PAN go back to the origins of the party. The very same founder of PAN, Manuel Gómez Morín, recruited many of the initial members from the 'Knights of Columbus' and other Catholic groups. As a consequence, the level of agreement on policies between the Church and PAN has no parallel to that with other political parties in Mexico. In August of 2000, for example, the Catholic Church publicly welcomed the decision by the State Congress of Guanajuato (dominated by PAN) to approve a reform to the state's *Criminal Code* that ordered the incarceration of all women who aborted, regardless of the circumstances - even if the pregnancy had been a consequence of rape (See *Notiese* 2003). A similar but unsuccessful initiative was put forward in the state of Chihuahua under the government of Francisco Barrio Terrazas,[65] who was a close collaborator of Vicente Fox and a member of his cabinet.[66] In most cases, PRI and PRD representatives in state legislatures have redressed these types of reforms.

The opposition from conservative groups and the Catholic Church has repeatedly manifested itself with regards to policies for the prevention and control of HIV/AIDS. In 2000, for example, there was a project funded by UNAIDS to implement prevention campaigns in 'dark rooms' at gay bars, but conservative groups put pressure on the government so that instead of taking place in gay bars the program would consist of itinerant interactive 'virtual' rooms in private universities (Interviews with members of 'Colectivo Sol', who were in charge of this project, Mexico City, 2001). Although public authorities knew that the real problem of HIV transmission among MSM would not be addressed that way, they gave in to these pressures, fearing the reaction of other powerful conservative groups to the investment of any money on programs for the homosexual population. Additionally, around that same time, pressure from conservative groups was successful in forbidding gay bars from offering condoms, alleging that it was against public morality and that it would in fact promote sexual misconduct (Confidential interviews with gay and HIV/AIDS activists and with owners of some gay bars in Mexico City, 2001/2006). In those cases, when an inspector arrived at a bar and found out that condoms were publicly displayed, the bar would be immediately closed down. Not surprisingly, there was a strong reaction from gay activists, arguing that actions like those would prevent homosexual men from making informed decisions according to their concrete and undeniable sexual needs and the reality of the epidemic.

---

[64] Partido Demócrata Mexicano.

[65] Francisco Barrio Terrazas had a close relationship with Salinas de Gortari during his presidency, from whom he had full support during his term as Governor of Chihuahua (1992-1998). He also got immediate recognition from the Catholic Church, given his close links to conservative groups and the 'good' record he had as Mayor of Ciudad Juárez showing a strong hand fighting "morally reprehensible behaviours" (prostitution and homosexuality) (*El Heraldo de Chihuahua* (local Mexican Newspaper), October 4, 1992).

[66] 'Secretario de la Contraloría y Desarrollo Administrativo' (Secretariat in charge of the Inspection of Public Spending), up to 2003.

After the 2000 elections, with PAN as the winner of the presidential race, and as a response to the long history of association of PAN with the most socially conservative groups, gay and HIV/AIDS activists feared the worst. However, the appointment of Julio Frenk as Secretary of Health, and his clear position regarding the high priority given to prevention campaigns for MSM and access to ARV drugs, allowed some HIV/AIDS and gay activists to consolidate their positions as integral and influential members of the policy network. This does not mean that, as argued by the late Mexican intellectual and writer Carlos Monsiváis, the Catholic Church and conservative groups stopped intimidating Frenk and other public officials (Interview with Carlos Monsiváis, Mexico City, August 13, 2002). On the contrary, and as seen in many of the above cases, it is clear that as put by Camp (2003, p. 142), the Church's and religious groups' openly critical posture on and efforts to influence policy issues related to health and sexuality are very likely to continue into the future. Moreover, in the case of Mexico, the power and influence of the Church and socially conservative groups are also supported by the existence of links between them and the private sector (See Appendix 4.5, for a further overview of these links). In fact, Manuel J. Clouthier, who was a socially conservative impresario, became the PAN candidate in the presidential race of 1988. His candidacy was of no minor significance for the analysis of the links between the business sector and the government, especially if one considers its subsequent impact. During his campaign, Clouthier recruited other businessmen, one of which was none other than Vicente Fox Quezada (Camp 2003, p. 144). As it is well known, some years later, Fox decided to run as a PAN candidate and won the state election for the governorship of Guanajuato in 1994, to then succeed in the presidential race of 2000. As president of Mexico, not only did he strengthen the links between the government, socially conservative groups, and the private sector, but he also brought along a good number of conservative businessmen to collaborate with him in government. Yet the successful formation of the HIV/AIDS policy network and their renewed efforts to continue with their work on HIV/AIDS policies prevented a conservative backlash and secured the ongoing public efforts, under Fox, against the pandemic.

Admittedly, the links between the private sector and socially conservative groups is very strong. Yet the significance of looking at the role of the private sector goes beyond this association and includes their economic interests and capacity to influence public policy to undermine the gains made by the HIV/AIDS policy network. As stated before, changes in social security have triggered the emergence of new and the strengthening of old actors with vested interests in the reform and privatization of the system. Traditionally, although the business sector was excluded from the party structure (PRI), it has been quite influential in the decision-making process (Camp 2003, p. 158; Teichman 1988, p. 143), and as we have seen, it gained access to formal political power in Fox's and Calderón's administrations (See D'Artigues 2002; Ortega Ortíz and Somuano Ventura 2015). Another characteristic of the private sector in Mexico is the strong influence of individual capitalists on corporate decision-making, which is greater than what is found in most post-industrial societies (See Camp 2003; Roett 1998; Thacker 1986; Shadlen 2000). More concretely, and with regards to the health sector, the reforms to IMSS introduced under president Zedillo raised the expectations of private investors (domestic and foreign) for new profit-making opportunities, particularly in the health insurance market (See Leal 2001a; 2001b). Additionally, in the context of the globalist-inspired NAFTA and other international trade agreements (See discussion in chapter three), increasing foreign investment - originated mostly in the United States - has resulted in the proliferation of privately run Health Maintenance Organizations (HMOs) (See Leal F. 2001a),[67] and the growing share of foreign-based Pharmaceuticals in the national drug market (See Leal and Martínez 2001a).[68]

With respect to private insurance, NAFTA opened the market to foreign companies, raising the allowed share of foreign ownership from 30 per cent before 1998 to 100 per cent by 2001 (Leal 2001b, p. 103). Additionally, reforms to IMSS allowing the reimbursing of fees have been a great incentive for the sector, given that there is a reimbursement of 70 per cent for the companies that provide the needed services or private insurance (Leal 2001b, p. 108).[69] After the 1994 financial crisis, according to Manuel Aguilera Verduzco (president of the National Commission of Insurance and Bails[70]), the sector would not have survived if it was not for the reforms to IMSS, which allowed private insurance companies to be incorporated into the social security system (*El Financiero*, May 17, 2000). In 1995, out of 48 insurance companies only 4 dominated 66 per cent of the market ('Comercial-América-Semex,' 'Grupo Nacional Provincial,' 'Monterrey-Aetna' and 'Inbursa'). The sector has been

---

[67] HMOs in conjunction with insurance companies offer tourist-like packages, extending their reach throughout the socio-medical sector and sharing in many cases the same doctors between private and public hospitals.

[68] In the early 1990s, there was a boom in U.S. investment in private hospitals in Mexico, but after realizing that most people could not afford their prices most of them left (*Reforma*, April 10, 2000). Yet after a decade of retrenchment, there has been an increasing interest in the hospital sector from foreign and national investors. For instance, the 'American British Cowdray Medical Centre' (Hospital 'ABC'), became one of the largest medical centres in Latin America, with the construction of a new facility in Santa Fé, Mexico City. This was possible due to a loan of US$44 million from the IFC of the World Bank, the Inter-American Investment Corporation of the IDB and the California Commerce Bank (Leal 2001a, p. 96). Mexican investors are also increasingly interested in this area and, as expressed in 2000 by Ernesto Perusquía (President of the National Association of Private Hospitals), they are "very much looking forward to the opening [reversion of fees] of IMSS … that would allow us to provide service to 4 to 5 per cent of its affiliates" (*Reforma*, December 26, 2000). These expectations were encouraged by Fox's and Frenk's declarations regarding the right of each individual to choose his/her family doctor (*Reforma*, December 27, 2000; See also Secretaría de Salud 2001). According to some critics, however, this is impractical, in terms of the geographically uneven availability of facilities and the restrictions imposed by insurance companies in the selection of doctors and service providers (Leal 2001a, p. 91). Furthermore, although there are almost two thousand private hospitals in Mexico, of these only 69 have more than 50 beds and are found in just 13 states, while the rest are considered clinics that do not have all the necessary equipment (Leal 2001a, p. 92). Additionally, only 139 of all private hospitals have been certified – a program of quality certification initiated during Zedillo's administration (La *Jornada*, December 19, 2000).

[69] One of major arguments in favour of allowing companies and individuals with private insurance to claim the IMSS fees, paid according to the law, has been the fact that even before the reforms of the total of people with private medical insurance, 65 per cent were also affiliates of IMSS, which means that some individuals were paying twice for a similar service.

[70] Comisión Nacional de Seguros y Fianzas.

expanding, and growing in real terms, with the major increases in health insurance, pensions, life and medical expenses.[71] The U.S.-based 'Blue Cross' and 'Blue Shield' entered the market (*Reforma*, October 26, 2000), with special investments in health and in 'Insurance Institutions Specialized in Health.'[72] Before 2001, foreign companies' share of the national market was between 25 and 28 per cent, but after the selling of 'Comercial-América-Semex' to 'ING', it went up to close to 50 per cent (Leal 2001b, p. 106). For its part, 'Aseguradora Hidalgo', the fifth major domestic insurance company sold close to 51 per cent of its shares to foreign investors (Leal 2001b, p. 106). As critics have pointed out, as a consequence of the increasing predominance of private insurance and the reversion of IMSS fees, there has been a series of problems related to the low quality of services, the lack of choice regarding doctors and clinics/hospitals, as well as the de-capitalization of IMSS.

For its part, the foreign pharmaceutical industry's share in the economy has grown. In 2000 alone, the growth in sales for this sector reached 25 per cent or US$4,692 million (*El Financiero*, December 4, 2000). According to the 'National Chamber of the Pharmaceutical Industry' (Canifarma[73]), the government represents 50 per cent of total volume of sales - with sales to IMSS alone representing close to $US1,500 million (*Vértigo*, October 11, 2003) - while the private sector accounts for 44.8 per cent of the volume and 87.3 per cent of the total sales in pesos (*Reforma*, June 12, 2012). The industry's growth has been accompanied by increased efforts to lobby public authorities to protect their interests from being negatively affected by public policies regarding HIV/AIDS treatment and access to drugs. Under pressure from the HIV/AIDS policy network, however, and in order to protect their public image, some Pharmaceuticals have reduced their prices (See *Notiese* 2003-2015). Ironically, when Merck, Sharp and Dhome first reduced the prices of some of its ARVs, some public health authorities refused to buy the drugs at the new prices on the basis that they had already authorized a budget under which they would be purchased at the original price (Confidential interviews with high-level directives of some of the largest pharmaceutical companies, Mexico City, 2001/2002). In the case of ARVs, most domestically owned Pharmaceuticals do not have the capacity for their production, and in the cases of those with the capacity, they would have to wait for the expiration of the patents to be able to produce their generic versions (See Appendix 4.6, for an overview of industry's situation in Mexico).

The industry has had strong supporters within the government. Under president Zedillo, for example, during the discussion in Congress of an initiative regarding drugs' patents and the authorization of generic drugs (1998), a high-level Secretariat of Health official was in permanent contact with some members of the pharmaceutical industry, in order to inform them of the developments of the discussions (Confidential

---

[71] The market continued to be divided as follows: almost 10% health insurance; life insurance 33%; auto-insurance 25% (Based on data by the 'Asociación Mexicana de Instituciones de Seguros' (AMIS) (In Leal 2001b, p. 103).

[72] 'Instituciones de Seguros Especializadas en Salud,' which contrary to Frenk's expectations are not interested in covering the informal sector (*La Jornada*, February 17 2001).

[73] Cámara Nacional de la Industria Farmacéutica.

interview with a high-level directive of a pharmaceutical company, Mexico City, August 13, 2002). The initiative being debated came from the Congressional representatives of the Green Party (PVEM),[74] and consisted of the introduction of 'generic medicines.' Not surprisingly, one of the major beneficiaries of this initiative would turn out to be no other than Víctor González Torres (the brother of the Green Party's founder, Jorge González Torres). Yet the direct representation of the brand pharmaceutical industry's interests within the government, and the pressure put on Zedillo's administration to prevent the initiative from being passed were not enough. In the end, the HIV/AIDS policy community was successful in exercising pressure for the authorization and introduction of generic drugs, which was approved by Congress and confirmed by Zedillo's Secretary of Health.[75] The reduction of the patent rights from 20 to 10 years, however, which was part of the original proposal, was dismissed.

In sum, the private sector interests regarding investment in health insurance and marketing and sales of patented drugs are often at odds with the interests of the HIV/AIDS policy network. So far, the latter has been successful in positioning itself at the centre of the public policymaking process and in guaranteeing access to treatment for all. Yet their future successes will depend on the continuing process of political transformation in Mexico, and the capacity of the policy network to keep corporate interests in check.

CONCLUDING REMARKS

The formation and relative consolidation of a domestic HIV/AIDS policy network has been an integral part of the political, economic, and social changes experienced in Mexico in the last few decades. This phenomenon has strengthened the role and influence of various members of the policy community, and has facilitated the inclusion of formerly marginalized groups in the process of decision-making and implementation of HIV/AIDS-related policies. As such, the HIV/AIDS policy network is integrated by a subset of actors within the policy community who are directly or indirectly participating in the policymaking process. These actors engage in exchanges involving the sharing of information, expertise, and political support. This policy network represents a set of structures that assign roles, resources and capacities, which affect how groups behave as well as policy outcomes. One very important element of this policy network is the presence of state actors - such as the

---

[74] See minutes of the debate on http:camaradediputados.gob.mx.

[75] As a result of the 1998's decision on the commercialization of generic drugs, Victor González Torres has established a national chain of drugstores called 'Farmacias Similares', offering prices that are in average 57 per cent cheaper than the brand ones, with a share of the market of almost 10 per cent. Victor González Torres has become a controversial figure in Mexico, who declared himself a candidate for the presidency in 2006. He is the owner of more than 1,500 drugstores nation-wide, and has created a private social insurance program through his drugstores chain. See http://www.esto. com.mx/040203/atletismo/7atletismo.asp. Through its chain of drugstores, González Torres has also promoted the sales of condoms, especially the 'SIMIcondón', which has been the source of a strong confrontation with the conservative group PROVIDA.
(http://www.imagenmedica.com.mx/datos/modules.ph.?name=News&file=article&sid=360).

head of CENSIDA and the Secretary of Health - who to a significant extent determine the way in which access to power and resources are distributed among members of the policy community at large. This, in turn, creates different patterns of public-private relationships that provide the context for policy deliberations and the delimitation of the policy network.

Several groups have actively participated in the formation and functioning of the network. On the one hand, HIV/AIDS NGOs with the necessary expertise and financial resources have created the conditions for the open discussion of some taboo topics related to sexuality and health, with very concrete results in terms of access to treatment and prevention campaigns. Or as put by a Mexican gay activist, "the existence of important funds dedicated to the prevention and control of the pandemic together with the visibility of prominent gay men in key public positions have forced all domestic actors to look at 'los putos' (faggots) and sex workers" (Confidential interview with gay activist, Mexico City, October 20, 2001). On the other hand, socially conservative groups and the Catholic Church have also been strengthened in the broader process of transition to democracy and the weakening of the PRI regime. Although these forces have not been able to position themselves within the HIV/AIDS policy network, their efforts and power have put public health officials under increasing pressure to respond to the conservative agenda. For his part, the Secretariat of Health, being at the core of the policy network, has to protect the gains made and at the same time negotiate with other members of the policy community, such as socially conservative groups and some powerful members of the private sector. In this context, and in the eyes of most members of the HIV/AIDS policy community at large, CENSIDA (whose functions were carried out by CONASIDA prior to 2003) has been an accomplishment at the federal level, due to the incorporation of civil society groups within its structure. This has resulted in the creation of an inclusive HIV/AIDS policy network that allows for resistance against socially conservative and sexually repressive agendas.

In spite of the accomplishments at the federal level, most critics agree that there is a great deal to be done at the state and local levels. With the exception of the cases of Jalisco and Mexico City, deficiencies are found not only in the way state governments have confronted the disease, but also in the absence of a strong NGO activism. It must also be emphasized that despite the fact that the federal HIV/AIDS policies show a strong stand in some issue areas, such as the right to access to treatment and prevention campaigns among MSM, critics point to some shortcomings. Access to cheaper drugs, for example, has faced important challenges, and as we saw in chapter two, in contrast to the case of Brazil where the government took decisive measures regarding the domestic production of ARVs, Mexico faces severe limitations due to pharmaceuticals' pressure and international trade regimes rules.

CHAPTER 5

General Conclusions

It was with the goal of better understanding the significance and implications of the overall response to the pandemic that we inserted our analysis within a conceptual framework that considers it as part of an ongoing quest for human rights and development. At the outset, it was emphasized that today's world reality is very much shaped by the phenomenon of globalization and the neo-liberal globalist agenda, both of which have had a major impact on Mexico's quest at many different levels. Thus, in looking at the responses to the HIV/AIDS pandemic by the Mexican government and some civil society groups, it became evident that they have been significantly shaped by globalization and, in turn, have been integral to the processes of economic, social, and political transformations of the last few decades.

In engaging with such a fascinating and complex reality, one can decide to focus on a long list of problems and obstacles for the formulation and implementation of HIV/AIDS public policies. But bad news or pessimistic assessments are in oversupply, given that it is often easier, albeit useful, to expose the shortcomings of any set of public policies. Thus, in addition to pointing to the problems, obstacles, and challenges, the current analysis focused on the inroads made by some civil society actors in partnership with government officials in Mexico. Furthermore, it has been argued that external forces have galvanized certain changes we are witnessing in some of the central features of the Mexican political system. This is particularly true for the case of a more inclusive and democratic process of policymaking regarding HIV/AIDS and some health-related policies. As such, the exercise of setting the framework and providing the evidence to support this argument responds to the personal and strongly felt need to uncover some of the opportunities and obstacles faced by Mexico in its elusive search for human rights and development.

It is necessary to recognize that the findings presented above and the conclusions that follow pertain to a policy area that is of a special nature, given the urgency of the pandemic and the type and variety of actors involved in the fight against it, most of whom have been actively engaged in the formation of the policy networks, both domestically and internationally.

A New Label for an Old Wine? Policy Networks Vis-à-vis Traditional 'Camarillas'

As a country with a political system in transition, Mexico shows signs of a declining presidency, with the legislative and judicial branches, as well as political parties and some civil society groups growing in influence. The new set of rules, as put by Camp (2003), is being built on a contradictory political culture that includes liberal and authoritarian qualities. As pointed out above, defined in classic procedural terms (namely free and fair electoral contestation for governing offices based on universal suffrage, guaranteed freedoms of association and expression, accountability through the rule of law, and civilian control of the military), one cannot deny the significant steps taken towards a more democratic regime in Mexico. The unfolding of the transition to democracy, however, has been determined and shaped by the ways in which more and less authoritarian factions within the state react to growing civic pressure from below. Similarly, domestic and external forces associated with globalism represent real obstacles and challenges for the realization of human rights and sustainable human development for the local people, not just in Mexico but in all countries around the world.

As such, the process of democratization has been the result of the weakening of the PRI regime, after a long period of economic crisis and the accompanying loss of legitimacy, and the actions of an effervescent civil society. As we saw in the revision of the different historical moments of civil mobilization, various groups have been the driving forces for the democratic gains and the inroads made in terms of increasing participation in politics of a wider segment of the population. More concretely, we are witnessing the emergence of new opportunities for civil society participation in some policy domains. In fact, and in contrast to the past, civil society groups do not need to have access to the highest possible level in the Executive in order to influence HIV/AIDS and health-related public policies. In the wake of this new reality and due to the current disenchantment with political parties, civil society organizations have looked for alternative channels for participation. Under these circumstances, and given the increasing trust in the work of NGOs, some civil society groups have participated in the creation of an HIV/AIDS policy network that has come to represent a new and relatively more democratic way of making public policy. Therefore, it is fair to conclude that the HIV/AIDS policy network represents an institutional arrangement of a different nature and is deserving of a new label to distinguish it from the traditional 'camarillas.'

Furthermore, the activism of some civil society groups, such as those engaged in the struggle for the recognition of sexual minorities' rights, has been successful in opening up the debate of formerly taboo issues that are central to public policymaking discussions around sexuality and health. Both their role in the creation of the HIV/AIDS policy network and their positioning within it have allowed them to exercise greater influence, regardless of the political party in office. We find evidence of this in their successful participation in the negotiations of the World Bank loan at the end of Zedillo's administration (PRI); in their continuing work at the federal level with Fox and Calderón (PAN) between 2000 and 2012; or in their engagement with the last four local governments of Mexico City (PRD). Thus, it can be argued that the pressure from below has been an essential component of the continued opening up of the policy process in this specific field. Overall, the analysis of the changes experienced in the formulation and implementation of HIV/AIDS and health-related initiatives in Mexico helps to underscore the significance of direct citizen participation in contributing to developmental policies.

Domestic health-care policies have traditionally derived from governmental initiatives and largesse, rather than as a response to organized trade unions or civil society mobilization. More recently, however, some HIV/AIDS policies concerning treatment and prevention campaigns have reflected the presence of a more inclusive and responsive process. From the establishment of CONASIDA in 1986, as a timid program with few resources and a non-existent civil society participation, to the creation of the Department of Civil Society Organizations as part of CENSIDA in 2003, we have witnessed an extraordinary opening of the policymaking process. This example of civil society-state synergy, in the fight against the pandemic, appears to be based on what has been defined as embeddedness, that is, on the institutional ties that connect citizens and public officials across the public-private divide. But not only civil society actors deserve the credit for the changes in the national HIV/AIDS program. In fact, in the Mexican case, state actors interested in changing the status quo and who arguably needed allies in civil society in order to counterbalance the power of entrenched elites contributed as well. As a result, civil society groups gained new leverage in the battles for participation and influence on public policymaking.

As stated in the introduction, beyond electoral participation and a competitive political party system, the politics of economic and social policymaking can tell us much more about the non-electoral dimensions of democratization. Indeed, and in contrast to the HIV/AIDS policymaking process, perhaps the most obvious shortcoming and challenge is found in the economic policy arena. As we have seen before, in recent years, presidents narrowed the range of acceptable policy alternatives in the economic realm - with a globalist agenda dominating the debate. In this sense, it is of major significance the fact that it was former president Carlos Salinas de Gortari, whose questionable victory in the 1988 elections led to protests and a lack of legitimacy in the eyes of many, who as a convinced globalist led the country to the negotiation, signing, and implementation of NAFTA. So that in spite of some positive developments, the policymaking process faces greater obstacles than what might be apparent. Important issues around decision-making and accountability arise, and remain critical in the context of globalization and democratization. In fact, we are witnessing the inertial resistance of a highly entrenched political system, even more so after the 2012 PRI victory and the election of Enrique Peña Nieto as president. Very concrete actors and vested interests that represent the old forces act against the process of democratization, and against a more transparent and participatory process of policymaking. Political cliques, technocratic enclaves, economic interests, political parties afraid of losing control and the trust of their constituencies, corporate interests, conservative groups, and some policy networks themselves try to exclude some voices and certain ideas from entering the debate.

Yet it is also true that we are witnessing significant changes in the role of camarillas. But due to the highly entrenched nature of the PRI regime, even after the defeat of the PRI in the presidential election of 2000, some of them remained very much alive and in some cases well-positioned in the new PAN governments. In some cases, camarillas retained a significantly higher degree of control over their policy areas, such as with the appointment of Francisco Gíl Díaz as Secretary of Finance under Fox. Thus, in spite of the Vicente Fox's electoral platform for change, there was a great deal of continuity in the way the economic policymaking process was defined. This continuity was also evidenced by the decision to keep globalist Santiago Levy as director of IMSS. So that more than indifference to popular demands on the part of the state, such decisions can be seen as the expected actions of a government - supported by an economic elite - that is fully committed to the neo-liberal/globalist agenda. Thus, it is argued here that in the run-up to the election of 2000, it became clear that although the entrenched bureaucracy and PRI camarillas naturally opposed the loss of office to the right-of-centre PAN, Mexico's private sector and foreign economic interests could live with it, given Fox's globalist allegiances.

The continuing presence of some members of the PRI-era camarillas in the economic cabinet and social security bureaucracy represented a further obstacle for an open debate on a wider variety of alternatives for the future of health-care. Thus, the importance of looking at the impact of some of the globalist reforms for the analysis of HIV/AIDS policies in Mexico. These reforms have limited the options for social policies and shaped the reforms introduced to the health sector in the last three federal governments of PRI before 2000, in both PAN administrations (2000-2012), and once again under PRI since 2012. As such, the long-term implications of these reforms are not very encouraging for sustainable human development, given the lack of both a strong health-care infrastructure and a clear commitment to create it.

In contrast, the formation of a new and institutionalized HIV/AIDS policy network provides a hopeful picture; a more participatory process of policymaking in health and a more optimistic view of democratization in Mexico. In fact, the response to the pandemic has had significant positive effects on the growing visibility, both domestically and internationally, of marginalized groups, whose voices are increasingly part of the policy dialogue regarding the need to address the concerns of sexual minorities and HIV/AIDS patients. Therefore, it can be argued that the responses to the pandemic and the interaction between domestic and external actors represent catalyzing forces for democratization in Mexico. Furthermore, the links between domestic and international policy networks are not only seen in the collaboration between civil society individuals and groups, but also in the way that public officials have strengthened their relations with members of the international community. And in the course of the last few years, some members of traditional health camarillas have become part of the more inclusive HIV/AIDS policy network. In the case of the Health Secretariat, for example, although it is true that some of its recent heads belonged to one of the strongest health camarillas (that of Soberón's), they have also strengthened their links with the international health policy community. Julio Frenk, for example, as an expert on health policies and as a long-term collaborator of international organizations such as the WHO, came to office with the legitimacy and credentials that resulted in a clear commitment to health for all. Once there, Frenk fostered the relations between the Secretariat and the NGO community. This gave rise to a stronger HIV/AIDS policy network conducive to an agenda that, otherwise, would have been rejected by socially conservative governments. Furthermore, the HIV/AIDS policy network has been able to resist the pressure from some powerful groups with socially conservative and sexually repressive agendas. What we have witnessed in the case of HIV/AIDS, represents an example of Camp's (2003) statement regarding the ways in which "groups or individuals desirous of influencing the decision-making process have an increasing number of avenues to use or affect institutions that determine actual policy outcomes" (p. 183). In fact, through the formation and operation of a policy network, NGOs seem to have found new ways to enhance their impact on the policy-making process.

In its original usage, the policy network analysis was mainly employed in the study of domestic public policies. Yet it has been expanded in order to incorporate external actors and the links established between them and domestic ones. Thus, the concept of policy networks represents an appropriate tool to analyze the way in which different levels of government, national and global civil society groups, and international institutions interact and define the creation of policy communities that give rise to the formation of networks in different sectors. Additionally, the fruitful use of the policy network analysis, as a conceptual tool to understand more about the impact of external variables on the policymaking process, suggests new lines of research and allows us to better understand certain aspects of globalization. Fashioning explanations about why policy networks take particular forms remains at an elementary stage though. Therefore, empirical research on policy community linkages must be further developed. The impact of core variables – the degree of integration of a policy community and the type of policy network in place – on patterns of mediation is virtually unknown thus far. Do these patterns vary significantly as policy sectors shift back and forth between "normal" politics and unsettled times? What is the impact of particular mediation efforts on the legitimacy of certain political and economic ideas or of particular groups, and on the distribution of power within, and across, policy communities?

Obviously, the concept of policy networks cannot be seen as the panacea for the analysis of public policymaking in Mexico, but it should be regarded as a useful conceptual tool that allows for the incorporation of some of the recent changes. In particular, the use of the policy network analysis allows us to point to the relatively greater inclusiveness that characterizes the process of HIV/AIDS policy formulation and implementation. Furthermore, by focusing on the health sector, it contributes to the understanding of the transformation of traditional camarillas and their incorporation into these more broadly defined networks: thus, *a new label for a new wine*. Additionally, this approach allows us to look beyond the public-private divide or to simply focus on the role of political parties. It facilitates the incorporation into the analysis of policymaking of formal and informal linkages between members of the policy community and the network. This has clearly been the case in our investigation and analysis of HIV/AIDS, through which we were able to determine the network's permeable nature, its more inclusive decision making process, and the higher levels of information/expertise sharing and of political support. Yet as we have seen before, there are still some differences between members based on resources and influential power (i.e., the core vs. the periphery). Therefore, there is a need to investigate more about the institutionalization of power relations both within the network and in the broader economic, political, and social context.

Significantly, the adoption and use of the policy networks approach facilitated the incorporation of globalization into our analysis. The presence of civil society organizations and their positioning, simultaneously, at the core of domestic and international policy networks, such as ICASO, MSF, and the International HIV/AIDS Alliance, together with the role of key individuals such as Peter Piot, Julio Frenk, Arturo Díaz, Jorge Saavedra, to name just a few, represent a catalyzing force for the increasing participation of a diverse set of actors. These actors have engaged in exchanges involving the sharing of information, expertise, and political support. As a result, the domestic and international HIV/AIDS policy networks comprise a set of individual and group actors whose various roles, resources, and capacities determine their behaviour as well as their influence on policy outcomes. One very important element of these policy networks is the presence of state or governmental actors - such as the head of CENSIDA and the Secretary of Health, or the heads of UNAIDS and the WHO - who to a significant extent determine access to influential power and resources among members of the policy community at large. This, in turn, creates different patterns of public-private relationships that provide the context for policy deliberations and the delimitation of the policy network.

However, as some members of the HIV/AIDS policy network often point out, the ultimate goal of some key members of the federal government is to radically change the role of the state in the health-care system. Admittedly, although the social security institutions are in need of restructuring, globalists want to go beyond some reforms to IMSS and ISSSTE, and privatize the entire health-care system. For the moment, and aware of these intentions, members of the NGO community see themselves as taking advantage of the opportunity created by the fight against the HIV/AIDS pandemic to position themselves within the policy network. More concretely, in the short term, the network has been successful in pressing for increased public funding for prevention and treatment. It has also succeeded in convincing Mexican public authorities that in order to stop the spread of the epidemic they need to target those groups that are particularly vulnerable and guarantee their access to public health-care. As part of a long-term strategy, however, civil society groups are looking for ways in which they can link the more narrowly defined HIV/AIDS battle with the broader one; namely the protection and strengthening of the role of the state in the provision of health-care for all. In collaborating with the government, NGOs seem to be aware that they might be indirectly supporting the same globalist trend of devolving the responsibility to civil society groups and away from the state. Yet they also know that they need to take advantage of the resources available to strengthen their position, and to secure their participation in the policy network as well as in ongoing and future policy debates.

Additionally, some shortcomings in the public efforts against the pandemic are related to the process of decentralization and the intolerance of local authorities. On the one hand, with regards to decentralization, as discussed above (chapter three), not even in Mexico City or Jalisco the necessary infrastructure exists to provide the kind of holistic or integral attention that the national program establishes. On the other, at the local level, intolerance persists, resulting in a lack of enforcement of human rights legislation that has been passed to protect citizens, from the sharing of private information and against discrimination, to the protection of social and civic rights.[76] In this regard, it is important to point out that although some socially conservative groups and globalism-committed actors do exercise significant influence, they are not inside the network, which is in itself a very important finding. One of the possible explanations for this is the fact that common sources of funding for HIV/AIDS (both external and governmental) represent a uniting force both for the HIV/AIDS NGO community and CENSIDA, which triggers further collaboration between them. Also, private Mexican foundations, with a weaker tradition of funding, do provide fewer resources for socially conservative organizations that have not been traditionally favoured by international governmental institutions. It is true though that in Mexico, and contrary to the case in other countries with a more liberal private sector, there is a significant association between powerful members of the corporate elite and socially conservative groups. And even if they do not belong to the policy network, they do exercise a different type of influence, which is more difficult to quantify and report on, such as the setting of a policy environment that determines the options and boundaries for public policy maneuvering.

Although we have focused on gay men and MSM, the emergence of HIV/AIDS and the need to fight the stigma attached to it triggered a more active public and political engagement of marginalized groups, which has benefited sexual minorities in general. Moreover, the fight against HIV/AIDS naturally led to some unusual convergences, since it entailed new forms of co-operation between heterogeneous actors, such as public officials, politicians, epidemiologists, physicians, gay and HIV/AIDS activists, sexual workers, and people living with the virus. So that in Mexico, as in most other countries affected by the pandemic, HIV/AIDS has contributed to the visibility of issues not previously discussed publicly, such as homosexuality – or indeed, sexuality – and to make them an inevitable issue for the public agenda, regardless of the ideology of the party in power. It is in this sense that the fight against HIV/AIDS acted as a catalyst for the inclusion of members of the homosexual community into the policy network, further strengthening the movement in terms of the ability to publicly debate their demands for certain rights. This has also been possible due to the significance of epidemiological strategies that emphasize

---

[76] Among other discriminatory practices, there is a continuing mandatory screening for employment, violation of confidentiality, layoffs due to HIV positive status, as well as a lack of access to medical attention and other services.

individual responsibility over social surveillance, as well as to the global hegemonic influence of liberal values of respect for individual and minorities' rights.

By denouncing discriminatory attitudes and demanding anti-discriminatory campaigns, the HIV/AIDS policy network has publicly and strongly criticized other government's actions (and inactions). Important moments and very symbolic ones attest to the relative success in advancing sexual minorities' concerns. For instance, the first march or protest against stigma and discrimination based on homophobia, which took place in Mexico City during the XVII International AIDS Conference on August 2, 2008, was led by UNAIDS director Peter Piot, and it surprisingly included the then Secretary of Health José Ángel Córdova Villalobos and the director of IMSS Juan Molinar Horcasitas; two PAN members and collaborators of conservative president Calderón. Similarly, Mexico's Supreme Court (Suprema Corte de Justicia de la Nación, SCJN) declared the constitutionality of same-sex marriage in 2010, and as a response to a petition put forward before the judiciary by president Felipe Calderón himself against the recently passed law in Mexico City. Later on, in March 2012, the SCJN also revoked a sentence denying the registration of a same-sex partner with IMSS, and in 2015 ruled in favour of the celebration of same-sex marriages nationwide, when declaring as unconstitutional the denial of their celebration by some states' authorities.

In a country like Mexico, with a long history of a deeply-entrenched centralized and authoritarian political system, it is expected to see a difficult transition to a more open and democratic one, with strong resistances and some setbacks. Major obstacles are associated with the ongoing challenges of extreme poverty, inequality, or income polarization. Therefore, a good way of assessing the overall success in the process of democratization is to look at the quality of citizenship engagement, defined as a meaningful participation in the process of political transformation. The question would then be; what is the right proportion of fully engaged citizens for a democracy to be called as such? As a minimum, we should look at the recognition of minorities' rights. One should also look for opportunities available for civil society embeddedness in the form of institutional channels conducive to the negotiation and re-negotiation of goals and policies. As such, it is of major significance to witness the formation of the HIV/AIDS policy network, in which civil society groups play a key role both as part of the consultative arena and in making the government accountable.[77] This policy network represents a new phenomenon in Mexican politics, perhaps too new to be able to accurately portray its composition and ways of operation, as well as to tell the extent to which it will grow and become a permanent feature of the Mexican political system. Based on the previous analysis, however, it can be argued that in order to be effective the HIV/AIDS policy network has directed its efforts as much to the democratization of public health and education about the pandemic, as to addressing the human, social, and political rights of those who have

---

[77] See the previous discussion on the notion of a 'consultative arena,' defined as a network of decision-making bodies linked to specific areas of policy which bring together state officials and representatives of key groups in civil society (Chapter one).

been most immediately affected by it. In sum, the analysis of HIV/AIDS and health-related policies in the last thirty years or so uncovers some democratic openings in the process of policymaking in this policy area, and in doing so it contributes to a better understanding of the broader process of democratization in Mexico.

SUCCESSES AND CHALLENGES

As argued at the very outset, democracy and human rights ought to be regarded as integral to any quest for sustainable human development, especially in a country like Mexico, which has been undergoing a difficult and profound process of economic, social, and political transformations in the last few decades. Democracy is essential for the implementation of social policies that can effectively address the most urgent needs of the population, including an effective response to HIV/AIDS and access to health-care. Moreover, the democratic exercise of political and civil rights, particularly those related to the guaranteeing of open discussion, debate, criticism, and dissent, is central to the process of generating informed choices and essential for inducing effective policy responses to economic and social rights and needs. Thus, the discussion of development has allowed us to emphasize the fact that as a middle-income country, Mexico presents significant levels of extreme poverty, inequality, income polarization, and the lack of a strong welfare state. As such, these factors limit the state's capacity to respond to some of the new global health challenges such as the HIV/AIDS pandemic.

It has also been argued that any attempt to understand the complexities of the changing Mexican reality must go beyond the national level of analysis. This is essential for us to address the gap between the theory behind development and the reality of an overwhelming number of people living under dire conditions in Mexico and other LMICs. Increasingly, it has become essential to look at the international environment and the ways in which it influences domestic policies today. And although the international side of the analysis requires further research, we can see the significance of discussing the interaction between several domestic and international factors and their impact on HIV/AIDS and health-related policy options in the context of globalization. Thus, and notwithstanding its limitations, based on the current analysis, we can see how the fight against HIV/AIDS shows innovative partnerships that effectively cross the public-private divide, both locally and globally. In fact, and contrary to the arguments around the notion of globaliphobia, some civil society actors have embraced globalization, as it facilitated the rise of new and the strengthening of old social networks as active political actors at the national and international levels. This is particularly true for social groups that have been highly marginalized, whose basic human rights have been traditionally violated, and who suffer from a notorious vulnerability due to their living conditions and identity. In that sense, the response to the HIV/AIDS pandemic helps to diffuse the idea that civil society-state synergy is a real possibility for a country like Mexico and other LMICs trying to enhance the welfare of their citizens. Furthermore, both locally and globally, the fight against HIV/AIDS has the attraction of having developed substantial international and trans-national networks and contacts, among political activists, medical researchers, and policy makers. It is an area where considerable efforts have been made by international and national health organizations to model and project the future spread of HIV, in an effort to strategically design prevention and treatment programs.

Although there is still an ongoing contrast between de jure and de facto citizenship, as shown by persistent homophobic crimes, the gains made so far must be recognized for their concrete and symbolic importance, the consolidation of which will depend on the capacity and will of the state to make those reforms effective. Also, further scrutiny of the increasing role of civil society organizations and their close engagement with state agencies represents an analytical challenge for those of us interested in better understanding the long-term effects of NGOization. In developing a prospective analysis, contemporary sociological considerations of politicized identities and their function in public life might help us in understanding HIV/AIDS and sexual minorities' activism. As argued by Bhambra and Margree (2010), among others, the politicized identities of some individuals or groups are social constructions that respond to the need to mobilize in order to overcome structural sociopolitical and economic barriers for full participation in the public sphere. One of the central goals of the assertion of those identities in the public sphere is the construction of more inclusive and democratic futures in conversation with other actors. Bhambra and Margree further argue that such identities tend to weaken when the conditions that originated their politicization disappear, which forces us to identify the ongoing circumstances that continue to justify the mobilization of HIV/AIDS and sexual minorities' organizations and their active engagement with the state. In this case, some individuals and groups were already politicized before, yet they went through a process of professionalization or NGOization, with a change of orientations or a broadening of their agendas once the epidemic hit. Others were created as a direct response to it. Furthermore, in analyzing and understanding their engagement with the state, it is useful to consider Judith Butler's (2002) contention that public institutions make us desire the state's desire, in the sense that for activists, as for most other citizens, it is often hard to resist the narrative of the state; and we would add, with the risk of being fooled and suddenly finding themselves caught up in the same game of neoliberal discourses and structures.

Despite the cautionary considerations mentioned above, in the case of Mexico, there seem to be some NGOs and individuals who work on HIV/AIDS that have been able to keep some distance from the state's narratives and agendas, with a focus on their own strategic and long-term goals. The challenge though, as Jessop (1990, p. 10) reminds us, for individuals and NGOs alike, lies in finding ways to negotiate the terms of entry into public life, since a given type of state and regime will be more accessible to some according to the strategies they adopt. Thus, NGOization can be seen as a process equivalent to an attempt by social movements to participate as "free citizens" in the elaboration of alternative discourses. In the case of Mexico and HIV/AIDS-related policies, the fact that certain offices within government have been created and penetrated by some civil society organizations and activists might serve as evidence of how the state itself is being reshaped or reconstituted (metamorphosed), by the ways in which governmental actors and activists interact in the process of government. This case can also help us recognize the fact that it is actual individuals, who belong to some of these different organizations and who join and position themselves within certain key departments or public bodies, which makes it impossible for them not to bring other dimensions of their identities to their functions as officials. In the process, they help transform or reshape, even if only partially, the same state they end up being part of. Seriously considering activists' protagonist role in the promotion of a new approach and a set of policies, together with the ongoing challenges, might allow us to draw more nuanced conclusions about the current state of, and prospects for, the struggles confronted by the HIV/AIDS community at large.

In fact, and contrary to early warnings regarding their lack of autonomy, we have seen a kind of hybrid character of some of those HIV/AIDS and sexual minorities' NGOs, whereby they engage as both experts and critics of the status quo. Or, as paraphrasing Colombian feminist and sociologist Magdalena León (cited in Álvarez, 2009, p. 178), they have been mainstreamed and "sidestreamed," spreading horizontally, becoming a veritable tangle of networks ("un enredo de redes"), both formal and informal, which in the case of HIV/AIDS allows them to keep what we would like to refer to as two different fronts or two pathways. Along these lines and in an honest revision of her own critical formulations on the NGOization of the feminist movement in Latin America, Sonia Álvarez (2009) has more recently acknowledged that the effects of civil society groups' professionalization are not so clear-cut. Thus, Álvarez acknowledges the hybrid character of many NGOs, arguing that although they have established a formal structure on paper, this does not always correspond with the continuing informal and flexible structures shown by many of them in reality. So that often, what we have is a formal or a more bureaucratic structure side by side with another more "real" and flexible one of the social movement. Moreover, she asserts that the data and analyses generated by NGOs have provided vital foundations for more effective advocacy in a variety of settings, mobilizing ideas and not just people (Álvarez, 2009, p. 178), effectively promoting rights at the local level through the use of global resources. Similarly, for the case of HIV/AIDS in Mexico, what we have is a tangle of international and domestic networks, with doctors and activists in key positions within CENSIDA, PAHO, the International Aids Society (IAS), and UNAIDS, some of which also work hand in hand with NGOs and social movements. They do engage with governments or the state in order to influence public policy, while at the same time some among them continue their support for social action and mobilization. Thus the image of two pathways or two fronts: one along expertise on sexual health and HIV/AIDS and the other along sexual minorities' rights. Although it could be argued that the engaged front is more "well-behaved" than the other one, which tends to be more confrontational or combative, both are joined by the human rights discourse. Also, these two pathways or fronts have simultaneously developed at both the national and the global levels. More concretely, we have witnessed the positioning of some gay activists within national and international bodies engaged in the fight against the epidemic, which resulted in the empowerment of the LGBT community at large. This is similar to what Keck and Sikkink (1998) have called the "boomerang effect," which is used to show how domestic and transnational social movements unite to bring pressure from above and from below on national governments to accomplish human rights change. This resulted in a set of HIV/AIDS policies that was more responsive to the demands of the most affected, which has been defined by increased budgets for prevention and universal coverage. These inroads in the public sphere then led to antidiscrimination legislation against homophobia and mistreatment of HIV/AIDS patients, even under two consecutive socially conservative PAN administrations in Mexico. Furthermore, they resulted in the passing of legislation in favor of same-sex marriage and adoption in Mexico City and other states. Thus, it can be argued that the professionalization of some civil society groups has had some very concrete and positive effects, giving continuity to HIV/AIDS policies.

Obviously, some challenges remain. First of all, it is necessary to consider whether it will be possible to maintain those two fronts or pathways. In other words, the challenge consists in consolidating the position, visibility, access, and influence achieved so far, without neglecting other groups within the larger sexual minorities' community. After all, some of them developed and adopted the politicized identities that allowed their mobilization in the first place. In this regard, the nature of the LGBTT community as a minority makes it hard to think of a radical change in circumstances, so that it would be unnecessary to keep a united front, despite class issues and other differences. Thus, an emphasis on monitoring and contestation will also continue to be indispensable, together with the additional challenge of criticizing the government and other institutions without risking their funding and support. Those activities are indispensable in order to secure the actual implementation of hard-won policy gains, which requires further public pressure, not only through policy monitoring but also aiming at deeper or broader changes in public opinion and attitudes toward sexual minorities. This might also require a stronger engagement within counter-hegemonic spaces, which may prompt some NGOs to move away from the project-centered logic fueled by NGOization and back towards a process-oriented logic. The latter tends to be more fluid, open-ended, and continuous, though not linear, with the aim to reform legal and cultural codes.

So far, it might be argued that through being contentiously entangled with national and global struggles in favor of human rights associated with sexual and social justice, HIV/AIDS and sexual minorities' activists have in fact contributed to the knowledge production and discourse around the epidemic. As such, we might also be able to argue that their NGOization is not so scandalous after all (See Torres-Ruiz 2013). However, it is also clear that we must continue to investigate and problematize the genealogy and development of NGOs in order to offer sounder prospective analyses of the effects of their engagement with the state on the construction of a vibrant and more democratic public sphere.

Another major challenge, in the context of globalization, is the consideration of international actors (governmental and non-governmental alike), which could be regarded as being increasingly domestic or 'Mexican' participants in terms of their functions and influence. Yet some of those same organizations, such as the WTO or TNCs, seem to be even further removed from domestic democratic accountability than the local political parties, civil society groups, or the government. In fact, we have witnessed the increasing prominence of pharmaceuticals—with improved access to decision-making within the UN system and the WTO—which is not always balanced by special access to aid or loan-recipient countries, HIV/AIDS activists and marginalized groups. In contrast, for some international organizations, namely UNAIDS and the World Bank, experiences of participation (albeit sometimes loosely defined) have also come to be integral to welfare policy. It is important to remember, however, that the notion of participation has sometimes been romantically loaded and often failed to fulfill the raised expectations. Thus in practice, the meaning of participation, its importance, and effects vary depending on policy area. For the case of HIV/AIDS, it has been shown that the participation of many actors in the formation of policy networks has represented a real force for change. Yet as we saw in contrasting the case of health-care financing with that of HIV/AIDS, at first, it is not always easy to discern who will benefit from the formation of policy networks in the present context of globalization. But once again, in the specific case of HIV/AIDS, it has become clear that the international/trans-national policy network in place has allowed socially progressive groups to create significant openings for influence at the global and domestic levels. This is particularly true for those affected by the pandemic, and especially so for sexual minorities, who have made significant gains due to the strengthening of the links between members of the domestic and international HIV/AIDS policy networks. In this case, activists must be given recognition for their efforts, since they have demanded more than what actual liberal representative democracies would offer, and have been advocates for direct participation in all decision making, locally and globally. Or as put by a Mexican gay activist, the existence of important funds dedicated to the prevention and control of the pandemic, together with the visibility of prominent gay men in key public positions, have "forced all domestic actors to look at 'los putos' (faggots) and sex workers" (Confidential interview with gay activist, Mexico City, October 20, 2001).

On the other hand, socially conservative groups and the Catholic Church have also been strengthened in the broader process of transition to democracy and the weakening of the PRI regime. Their efforts and power have put public health officials in a situation where they find themselves under increasing pressure to respond to their conservative agenda. As a consequence, being at the core of the policy network, the Secretariat of Health has to protect the gains made, and at the same time negotiate with other members of the policy community, including socially conservative groups and some powerful members of the private sector. In this context, and in the eyes of most members of the HIV/AIDS policy community at large, CENSIDA has been a great accomplishment at the federal level, due to the incorporation of civil society groups within its structure. This has resulted in the creation of an inclusive HIV/AIDS policy network that allows for resistance against socially conservative and sexually repressive agendas.

It must also be emphasized that despite the fact that the HIV/AIDS policies of the federal government show a strong stand in some issue areas – such as the right to access to treatment and prevention campaigns among MSM - critics also point to some shortcomings. Access to cheaper drugs, for example, has faced important challenges. And as we have seen in our analysis of the international context, in contrast to the case of Brazil, where the government has taken decisive measures regarding the domestic production of ARVs by the generic industry, Mexico faces severe limitations due to Pharmaceuticals' pressure and international trade regimes rules. Most critics agree also that there is a great deal to be done at the level of the states and other lower level jurisdictions. For instance, deficiencies are found not only in the way local governments have confronted the disease, but also in the absence of a strong NGO activism.

Overall, and as a result of the increased plurality of the Mexican political system, domestic and international policy networks are facing new opportunities and challenges. In the case of HIV/AIDS, this relatively significant plurality has resulted in the increasing effectiveness of pressure from a greater variety of social and political actors. In fact, the major political changes of the recent past have represented important tests to the permeability, or lack thereof, of all policy networks, including the market-reform ones. However, the fact that the activities of international organizations, such as the World Bank and even some NGOs are not subject to thorough public scrutiny and that the content of their policy priorities and recommendations have not been widely debated in public, still raises important questions around the democratic character of these changes. Thus, the jury is still out concerning the democratizing effect of international or trans-national policy networks, with examples supporting both sides of the argument (i.e., health care financing vs. HIV/AIDS). But in looking at the impact of policy networks the focus goes beyond the presence of formal democratic institutions, and it is placed on specific public policies as the more telling indicators of the profound changes now fully under way in Mexico.

Admittedly, it would be inappropriate to generalize about the effect of all policy networks on democracy, human rights, development, and health. Some of them have been exclusionary and as such have been all but democratic. In fact, in cases such as market reform policy networks, it can be argued that they have not been particularly inclined to open debate. Obviously, the assessment of the impact of policy networks (e.g., market reform and health-care financing) on the structuring and reform of the health-care system is quite complex, given that there are many different forces and interests struggling and pulling in different directions. For instance, the globalist agenda's influence on health leads to budgeting practices that focus on direct costs, underestimating the importance of social costs and relegating HIV/AIDS in the prioritizing of resource allocations. More often than not, this forces policymakers to be confronted with the difficult decision of investing in prevention programs, the effectiveness of which is not easily determined, or the allocation of resources for the treatment of patients with AIDS and other diseases. It is clear that the discussion regarding the allocation of resources for the health-care system and the decision about who will pay for the costs of treatment is a matter of political struggles, and not just a technical/budgeting decision. Yet this fact does not seem to be recognized by globalists, and the cost-effectiveness analysis that takes place for the definition of basic health services is limited to economic rationales and the allocated budgets for health. This is a perverse condition, in the sense that it forces health programs to compete among themselves for an already very restricted budget (i.e., Cancer vs. AIDS). Alternatively, it could be argued that the budgeting exercise should be extended to broader areas of public revenues and spending (i.e., military budgets and tax cuts for the rich) in order to protect programs of social development, health, and education, which are more conducive to sustainable human development. Thus, even the success of the HIV/AIDS policy network must be qualified.

Unfortunately, although civil society groups have had the support of a globalist institution like the World Bank in their fight against the pandemic, their efforts might not be as successful in changing or influencing the broader and more central globalist agenda of health-care privatization. As previously discussed, privatization is at the core of the global commerce of ideas, with networks of consultants consistently pushing for the globalist agenda and its dominant U.S. ethics in health-care, which view it as a predominantly private commodity. Confronted with this reality, and in contrast to openly anti-globalist groups, like those protesting in Seattle in 1999 and other international meetings after that, some NGO members of the HIV/AIDS network have decided to work within the system. As a result, some of them have a foot in the door, while others have been invited to sit at the table, with varying degrees of influence on policy outcomes. Here, it is also important to refer to the case of some of the IDB officials mentioned before (gay men with personal and informal links with members of the HIV/AIDS policy network). The fact that they actually sit at the negotiating table also represents a major supporting force for the network from within the system.

Interestingly, as seen in the case of Latin America, little by little, some of the groups linked to the HIV/AIDS policy network have begun to attach the agenda of access to 'Health for All' to their fight against the pandemic. If they are successful in this endeavor, it might further reinforce the argument that it is through trans-national alliances that norms and rules at the national and global level can be shifted, linking reforms from within to those from without. In other words, the increasing density and influence of more inclusive international policy networks might generate growing pressures for global reform.

One must also recognize the evident inequalities in power, whereby ideas, values, and beliefs of the more powerful are spread either coercively (i.e., policy conditionality) or consensually (i.e., intellectual leadership or ideological hegemony). Due to the force of the globalist agenda, the convergence of policy content is occurring within a circumscribed ideological universe, yielding a narrow set of policies inextricably linked to asymmetrical power relations. The WTO's TRIPS agreement, for example, may make sense according to international economic theory, but it is sometimes contrary to the health interests of LMICs' populations and basic human rights for all. Moreover, the fact that trade and economics have become dominant over other concerns explains why certain actors, such as international trade lawyers and economists, have become the handmaidens of the globalist agenda.

As argued at the outset, globalism represents a hegemonic discourse that has permeated to the national and local levels. In Mexico, the policy networks in charge of market reform have been some of its firmest believers. In this regard, it must be underlined that the concept of hegemony does not necessarily imply conspiracy intent or collusion by the powerful over the less powerful. Yet it is necessary to point to the definition of hegemonic consensus, which lies in the nature of the process of exchange of ideas and its openness to critically assess the appropriateness of policies to specific contexts. This was hardly the case with structural adjustment programs, since they were the result of a closed and exclusionary process of policy formulation based on a very specific economics-based interpretation of reality. Moreover, the problem with globalism is that the information and knowledge in the hands of the so-called experts is so "sophisticated" (or some would argue, purposefully convoluted) and often obscured, that what are needed are counter-experts, capable of translating their discourse. In contrast, the emergence of more inclusive policy networks, such the HIV/AIDS one, represents an example of the kind of effort that can mitigate the undemocratic character of international agencies and lead to a shift in the hegemonic discourse behind globalization.

The previous analysis has also allowed us to address some of the dangers of the overwhelming corporate sector's power associated with globalization and the globalist agenda. Interestingly, although they have had some significant successes in the economic front, these have not been matched with regards to their moral/religious agenda (especially at the domestic level in the case of Mexico). However, particularistic economic interests, which are highly related to the signing of trade agreements, represent persisting challenges for the global fight against HIV/AIDS. This is especially true for the case of Pharmaceuticals and insurance companies, and their interest in the privatization of the health sector. Mexico is not alone in this respect, and as many other countries it faces significant challenges that require the strengthening of its response capacities. Otherwise, the effects of some of these trade agreements on inequality might contribute to perpetuating the already highly unequal character of the Mexican society and its health-care system, making the idea of "Health for All" to remain a remote dream.

In discussing Mexico's participation in the world economy and trade, and the challenges this poses for the protection of health for all and access to health-care for HIV/AIDS patients, the question is not so much whether to engage in strong international linkages or not. The central concern is the need to explore what steps have been or can be taken to ensure that the increasing economic interdependence does not compromise the ability to make autonomous decisions, regarding economic and social policies that are more inclusive and responsive to the needs of the national population. After all, as a signatory to an array of international agreements to promote access to health-care as a fundamental human right, Mexico has acquired other responsibilities as well. Amongst them, it has a responsibility to work together with the international community in order to strengthen and renew international health regulations on monitoring and containing communicable diseases, and to attain higher levels of health for all of its population. Within these circumstances, it is interesting to see the ways in which strong HIV/AIDS policy networks – capable of responding to the increasing challenges of global health – have been formed and act to protect vulnerable groups from the impact of international trade agreements, and from TNCs looking for new profit-making opportunities. In this challenging global context, attention must also be directed to other policy areas such as the environment, education, agricultural practices, and fair trade in general, where the inclusion of civil society actors might lead to greater influence and a real impact on actual policy outcomes.

In recognizing the limitations of the present analysis, it has also become clear that further research is needed, particularly regarding an in-depth investigation of the day-to-day activities of NGOs, their work relations, the way power is handled and distributed, their stated and actual goals, their ideological consistency, and their life cycles. It is necessary also to learn more about the level of preparation and commitment of their members and leaders, the paths through which they go up the ladder and the survival of these groups. Similarly, more work needs to be done to find out what other variables, beyond expertise and personal links, are key in determining which groups are included and which ones are excluded at the national and international levels. In other words, a very important question is the diversity and inclusiveness of the selection or self-selection process of members of the policy network. In sum, and having in mind the aforementioned reservations, it is argued here that we are witnessing the establishment and potential consolidation of domestic and international policy networks. In some instances, these networks incorporate civil society groups, with the necessary expertise to exercise an increasing influence on the decision-making process of international bodies and organizations that are having a greater impact on domestic politics. And if we consider health as part of the global commons, these networks might be the means through which local alternatives can be articulated at the national and international levels, allowing people to reclaim those commons.

BEYOND HIV/AIDS AND HEALTH

Beyond the specifics of the fight against the pandemic, the current analysis has allowed us to uncover much about the effects of globalization on Mexico's elusive quest for development and the overall transformation of its social reality. Fortunately, the Mexican state and society did not wait until the epidemic could have reached the catastrophic dimensions as those seen in Sub-Saharan Africa, and have fully perceived it as a major social and health problem, with some important steps taken in the right direction.

It is also important to emphasize that the current analysis purposefully sees all generations of human rights, democracy, and development as inextricably intertwined. Furthermore, it has been argued that in studying and analyzing democratization and development, we need to look closer at specific policies and issues, and the effects that they are having on real people's lives, in an effort to reject labels and classifications of political regimes and developmental models that tend to generalize, some of which respond to discussions that show a bias against any non-liberal/non-globalist democratic regimes and policies. And as has been mentioned above, although this is part of a broader discussion that falls beyond the scope of the current analysis, it is one that we aim to develop and that entails an epistemological critique of the current and most dominant comparative development and democratic theory literatures. In fact, the importance and emergency of the HIV/AIDS pandemic have forced people in different fields and areas of activity to rethink many of the preconceived notions and believes that are often associated with human rights, development, and democratization. For instance, the fight against it has been increasingly associated with the struggle for universal access to publicly funded health services, and it has provided a great opportunity for minorities to be heard and represented. In most cases, minority groups and activists involved in the fight against HIV/AIDS are not limiting their efforts to the health sector, but their strategies include sexual and minorities' rights more broadly defined, with some of their actions having already helped redefine the social status of homosexuality in different contexts. Yet discrimination and social recognition operate at different societal levels and, therefore, no congruence between them will necessarily exist. Thus the struggle for full acceptance of sexual minorities will continue as part of the ongoing process to guarantee human rights protection, sustainable human development, and democratization.

Additionally, one of the central aims of the current analysis has been to determine where the pressure for change in the health sector originates, the direction this is taking, and the role that national and international policy networks are playing. As such, we have been able to unveil the ways in which the actions of domestic and international networks have been translated into an increasing politicization of sectoral and sub-sectoral policymaking processes. As a consequence, the implications of the current analysis, even if limited to one policy area, speak to more general issues related to the process of democratization experienced in Mexico. It is too early to tell, however, whether this politicization represents a long-lasting change in the nature of policy networks and the process of policymaking. Yet what we can assert is that the existing HIV/AIDS policy networks show signs of greater permeability, allowing for new actors and ideas to enter the policy process, and to have an effect on policy outcomes. Regarding the transformation of camarillas and their incorporation into policy networks in the health sector, the analysis should be extended to other policy areas too.

And regarding the nature of globalization and the world-wide impact of globalism, it would be interesting and useful to extend the policy network approach to the analysis of HIV/AIDS and health policymaking in other LMICs in the Latin American region and beyond. In fact, it should be extended not only for the case of HIV/AIDS, but for other emerging issues in which trans-national co-operation is growing and becoming central to the finding of solutions (i.e., environmental and other human rights concerns). The intention would not be to make generalizations or to engage in the search of a "new model" for development. On the contrary, such an exercise must be guided by the specifics of local realities and political transformations, all of which are being affected by the process of globalization and the globalist agenda. As suggested by the current analysis, the types of networks being created include members from various nations and international bodies, whose support is indispensable for the attainment of suited solutions for those locals facing daily struggles. Thus, it is likely that constraints on the market and on the globalist agenda as a whole will continue to arise spontaneously, in response to specific social problems and needs, and not as elements of any alternative grand vision or universal model. After all, some social needs seem to be universally human, such as security from starvation and the protection from disease, so that the universality of these needs will eventually and necessarily force governments and communities to push against imposing visions such as globalism, and to find their own suited solutions. As part of this push, the campaigning of civil society groups such as MSF, ICASO, or the HIV/AIDS Alliance in favour of access to essential drugs and against unbalanced liberalized trade has been and will continue to be critical.

To end with a cautionary note, one must acknowledge that civil society can also be 'uncivil' (i.e., undermine social justice as in the case of trans-border criminal networks), offering flawed policy prescriptions, poor internal democratic criteria, or provide inadequate representations of relevant interests. In fact, the perceived lack of transparency and accountability among the many international actors and organizations continues to raise concerns, with the risk of the overall accountability falling between the cracks. Another risk, of course, is that international health co-operation might focus on much narrower programs of disease control, which lend themselves to monitoring, and neglect issues such as developing good quality and accessible health-care systems. However, and in spite of the shortcomings and risks, one would expect that the opening up of political spaces for potential democratization of policymaking might result at worst in unclear mandates, and at best in innovative and successful partnerships. In some cases, through networks and partnerships, the influence of non-state actors goes beyond efforts directed at influencing the formal processes of government decision making, to becoming part of the decision-making structure formerly reserved for a few. Our hope is that in spite of the specifics associated with HIV/AIDS politics, this analysis might speak to larger changes in public policymaking in health and the political system in Mexico as a whole. After all, for Mexico, as for other LMICs, the emergence of relatively new health problems such as HIV/AIDS and the prevalence of the so-called diseases of poverty pose new challenges in the pursuit of sustainable human development, such as the need to optimize scarce resources and to allow for greater inclusiveness and participation of marginalized groups in the definition of public policies. We also hope that the study of Mexico's response to HIV/AIDS will contribute to the analysis of other cases in Latin America and other regions facing similar circumstances of economic, social, and political transformations.

REFERENCES

Books and Academic Journals

Abbasi, K. 1999, "The World Bank on World Health: Under fire," *British Medical Journal*, No. 318, pp. 1003-1006.

Adams, Bill 1993, "Sustainable Development and the Greening of Development Theory," in Frans J. Schuurman (ed.), *Beyond the Impasse: New directions in development theory*, London and New Jersey: Zed Books.

Aguayo Quezada, Sergio 1998, *El Panteón de los Mitos: Estados Unidos y el nacionalismo mexicano*, Mexico: Grijalbo, El Colegio de México.

Aguilar M., Alonso 1970, "Problemas y perspectivas de un cambio radical," in Fernando Carmona et al., *El Milagro Mexicano*, Mexico: Editorial Nuestro Tiempo.

Alba Vega, Carlos 1996, "Los Empresarios y el Estado durante el Salinismo," *Foro Internacional*, No. 36, January, pp. 31-79.

Altman, Dennis 2001, *Global Sex*, Chicago: University of Chicago Press.

Alvarez Béjar, Alejandro 2003, "Notas Sobre la Crisis Política Nacional y la Crisis del PRI, sobre la Coyuntura Económica y la Impunidad Neoliberal," Unpublished Manuscript, Mexico: UNAM.

Álvarez, S. E. 2009, "Beyond NGO-ization? Reflections from Latin America," *Development*, 52 (2), 175–184.

Ames, Barry 1987, *Political Survival: Politicians and Public Policy in Latin America*, Berkeley: University of California Press.

Amin, S. 1974, Accumulation on a World Scale, New York: Monthly Review Press.

Amin, S. 2000, "Democratising Globalisation," *Al-Ahram Weekly*, April, Issue 478, pp. 20-26.

Anderson, Benedict 1991, *Imagined Communities*, London & New York: Verso.

Andrain, Charles F. 1998, *Public Health Policies and Social Inequality*, Washington: Macmillan Press Ltd.

Aninat, Eduardo 2000, "Making Globalization Work for All," Remarks by the Deputy Managing Director of the IMF at the German Foundation for International Development, Berlin, March 4: http://www.imf.org/external/np/speeches/2000/031400.htm

Apter, David 1965, *The Politics of Modernization*, University of Chicago Press.

Ávila-Burgos, Leticia, Edson Servan-Mori, Verónica Wirtz, Sandra Sosa-Rubí and Aarón Salinas-Rodríguez, 2013, "Efectos del seguro Popular sobre el gasto en salud en hogares mexicanos a diez años de su implementación," *Salud Publica de México*, vol. 55, supl. 2, pp. S91-s99.

Ávila Figueroa, Carlos 1999, "La Epidemia de VIH/SIDA en el contexto de las Reformas del Sector Salud en América Latina," in *El SIDA en América Latina y el Caribe, una visión multidisciplinaria*, Mexico: FUNSALUD.

Aziz Nassif, Alberto (coord.) 2003, *México al Inicio del Siglo XXI: Democracia, ciudadanía y desarrollo*, Mexico: CIESAS, Miguel Angel Porrúa.

Bachrach, P. and M. Baratz 1970, *Power and Poverty: Theory and Practice*, New York: Oxford University Press.

Baer, M. Delal 1999, "Mexico's coming backlash," *Foreign Affairs*, July-August, Vol. 78, issue 4, pp. 90-99.

Bailey, John 1988, *Governing Mexico: The statecraft of crisis management*, New York: St. Martin's Press.

Bailey, John 1994, "Centralism and Political Change in Mexico: The Case of National Solidarity," in Wayne Cornelius, Ann Craig and Jonathan Fox (eds.), *Transforming State-Society Relations in Mexico: The National Solidarity Strategy*, Centre for U.S.-Mexican Studies, San Diego.

Barber, Benjamin 1995, *Jihad vs. McWorld*, Times Books.

Barros, Rodrigo 2008, "Wealthier but Not Much Healthier: Effects of Health Insurance Program for the Poor in Mexico," *Discussion Document of the Stanford Institute for Economic Policy Research*," at http://economics.stanford.edu/files/JMP_RBarros.pdf

Barro, Robert J. 1996, *Getting It Right: Markets and Choices in a Free Society*, MIT Press.

Barry, Tom, Harry Brown and Beth Sims 1994, *The Great Divide: The Challenge of U.S. – Mexico Relations in the 1990s,* Grove Press.

Bates, Robert 2001, *Prosperity and Violence: The political economy of development*, London: W.W. Norton & Company.

Bauman, Zygmunt 1998, *Globalization: The Human Consequences*, Cambridge: Polity Press.

Baumgartner, Frank R. and Brian D. Jones (eds.) 2002, *Policy Dynamics,* The University of Chicago Press.

Bayon, Maria Cristina, Bryan Roberts and Georgina Rojas 2002, "New Social Labour Market Challenges to Social Policies in Mexico," in Louise Haagh and Camilla T. Helg¢, *Social Policy Reform and Market Governance in Latin*

America, Palgrave Macmillan in association with St. Antony's College, Oxford, pp. 101-120.

Benedek, Wolfang, et al. (eds.) 2007, *Economic Globalisation and Human Rights,* Cambridge: Cambridge University Press.

Benson, J.K. 1982, "A Framework for Policy Analysis," in D. Rodgers, D. Whiton et al. (eds.), *Intergovernmental Coordination,* Ames, Iowa State University Press.

Berlinguer, G. 1999, "Health and equity as a primary global goal," *Development*, Vol. 42, No. 4, pp. 17-21.

Berman, Peter (ed.) 1995, *Health sector reform in developing countries: Making health development sustainable*, Harvard School of Public Health.

Berry, Albert 2003, "Who Gains and Who Loses? An Economic Perspective," in Richard Sandbrook (ed.), *Civilizing Globalization: A survival guide*, State University of New York Press.

Bertranou, Julián F. 1998, "Mexico: The Politics of the System for Retirement Pensions," in María Amparo Cruz-Saco and Carmelo Mesa-Lago (eds.), *Do Options Exist? The reform of pension and health care systems in Latin America*, University of Pittsburgh Press.

Beuchot, Mauricio 2005, *Interculturalidad y Derechos Humanos*, Mexico: Siglo XXI and UNAM, Facultad de Filosofía y Letras.

Bhambra, Gurminder K., and Victoria Margree, 2010, "Identity Politics and the Need for a 'Tomorrow'" *Economic and Political Weekly* 45.15: 59-66.

Bhargava, A., Jamison, D.T., L. J. Lau and C.J.L. Murray 2000, "Modelling the Effects of Health on Economic Growth," Geneva: WHO, Global Programme on Evidence Discussion Paper.

Birdsall, Nancy 1993, *Social Development is Economic Development*, Washington, D.C. World Bank.

Bizberg, Ilán 1990, *Estado y Sindicalismo en México*, Mexico City: El Colegio de México.

Bizberg, Ilán 2015, "Los nuevos movimientos sociales en México: el Movimiento por la Paz con Justicia y Dignidad y el #YoSoy132," *Foro Internacional*, January-March, Vol. LV, Num. 1.

Block, F. 1986, "Political choice and the multiple 'logics' of capital," *Theory and Society*, 15, pp. 175-92.

Bobadilla, José Luis 1996, In Janowsky, Katja (Ed.) *Health policy and systems development*, WHO, Geneva.

Boltvinik, Julio 2000, "Las Obsesiones que Empobrecen," *Proceso*, No. 1244, September 3, pp. 26-27.

Boltvinik, Julio 2001, "La Economía Moral," *La Jornada*, April 19.

Bonfil Batalla, Guillermo 1987, *México Profundo: Una Civilización Negada*, Mexico City: Grijalbo.

Bossert, Thomas 1997a, "Decentralization of health systems: Decision space, innovation and performance," DDM Working Paper Num. 36.

Bossert, Thomas 1997b, "Decentralization: A governance option for health care policy," Harvard School of Public Health, Conference on social policy, poverty alleviation and governance, sponsored by the UNDP and Harvard Institute for International Development, November 14.

Brachet-Márquez, Viviane and Margaret Sherraden 1994, "Political Change and the Welfare State: the case of health and food policies in Mexico (1970-93)," *World Development Journal*, Vol. 22, September, pp. 1295-1312.

Branco, Manuel Couret 2009, *Economics Versus Human Rights,* New York: Routledge.

Bronfman, Mario, Ana Langer and James Trostle 2000, *De la Investigación en Salud a la Política: La Difícil Traducción*, Mexico: Instituto Nacional de Salud Pública, Manual Moderno.

Bronfman, Mario, Leyva Flores, R., & Negroni, M. J. (2002a). "HIV prevention among truck drivers on Mexico's southern border," Culture, Health & *Sexuality*, Vol. 4, Issue 4, pp. 475–488.

Bronfman, Mario, Leyva Flores, R., Negroni, M. J., & Rueda, C. M. (2002b). "Mobile populations and HIV/AIDS in Central America and Mexico: Research for action," *AIDS*, Issue 16, pp. 29–42.

Brooks, David and Jonathan Fox (eds.) 2002, *Cross-Border Dialogues: U.S.-Mexico Social Movement Networking*, La Jolla, California: Center for U.S.-Mexican Studies, University of California, San Diego.

Bruhn, Kathleen 1997, *Taking on Goliat: The Emergence of a new Cardenista party and the Struggle for Democracy in Mexico*, Pennsylvania: Pennsylvania State University.

Bruntland, H. 1987, *Our Common Future* (for the World Commission on Environment and Development), Oxford: Oxford University Press.

Brysk, Alison 2000, "Democratizing Civil Society in Latin America," Journal of Democracy, Vol. 11, Issue 3, pp. 151-165.

Burki, Sahid Javed and Guillermo E. Perry 1996, "The Long March: A Reform Agenda for Latin America and the Caribbean," Washington, D.C.: World Bank.

Burki, Sahid Javed and William Perry 1998, "Beyond the Washington Consensus: Institutions Matter," Washington, D.C.: World Bank.

Burt, Jo-Marie 1996, "Local NGOs in Peru Devise an Alternative Anti-Poverty Program," *NACLA Report on the Americas*, No. 6, May-June.

Buse, K., S. Fustukian and K. Lee (eds.) 2002, *Health Policy in a Globalising World*, Cambridge University Press.

Butler, J. 2002, "Is kinship always heterosexual?" *Differences: A Journal of Feminist Cultural Studies*, 13(1), 14–44.

Cabrero Mendoza, Enrique 1999, "La Experiencia Descentralizadora Reciente en México: Problemas y Dilemas," Documento de Trabajo No. 28, Mexico: Centro de Investigación y Docencia Económicas.

Cabrero Mendoza, Enrique 2000, "Usos y costumbres en la hechura de las políticas públicas en México. Límites de las policy sciences en contextos cultural y políticamente diferentes," in *Gestión y Política Pública*, Vol. IX, N. 2, Second semester, Mexico: Centro de Investigación y Docencia Económicas.

Cáceres, Carlos 1999, "Dimensiones Sociales Relevantes para la Prevención del VIH/SIDA en América Latina y el Caribe," in *El SIDA en América Latina y el Caribe, una visión multidisciplinaria*, Mexico: FUNSALUD.

Camp, Roderic 1996, *Democracy in Latin America: patterns and cycles*, Scholarly Resources.

Camp, Roderic Ai 1980, *Mexico's Leaders*, University of Arizona Press.

Camp, Roderic Ai 1990, "Camarillas in Mexican politics: The case of the Salinas Cabinet," Mexican Studies/ Estudios Mexicanos, 6, No. 1.

Camp, Roderic A. 1994, "The Cross in the Polling Booth: Religion, politics and the laity in Mexico," *Latin American Research Review*, No. 29, pp. 37-68.

Camp, Roderic Ai 1999a, *Politics in Mexico: The Decline of Authoritarianism*, Oxford University Press.

Camp, Roderic Ai 1999b, "Democracy through Mexican lenses," *The Washington Quarterly*, Summer, Vol. 22, issue 3, pp. 229-236.

Camp, Roderic Ai 2001, *Citizen Views of Democracy in Latin America*, University of Pittsburgh Press.

Camp, Roderic Ai 2002, *Mexico's Mandarins: Crafting a Power Elite for the Twenty-First Century*, University of California Press.

Camp, Roderic Ai 2003, *Politics in Mexico: The Democratic Transformation*, Oxford University Press.

Cardoso, F.H. 1972, *Dependecy and Development in Latin America*, Berkeley, CA: University of California Press.

Carrillo Flores, Antonio 1977, "Introduction," in Eduardo Suárez, *Comentarios y Recuerdos*, 1926-1946, Mexico City: Porrúa.

Cárdenas, Sergio, Edgar Ramírez, and David Sánchez 2012, *Levantamiento del panel de la Encuesta Nacional de Afiliados al Seguro Popular. Informe final*, Mexico: Centro de Investigación y Docencia Económicas, at http://seguropopular.cide.edu/documentos/130486/130726/201201_panel.pdf

Casaburi, Gabriel and Diana Tussie 2000, "From Global to Local Governance: Civil Society and the Multilateral Development Banks," in *Global Governance: A Review of Multilateralism and International Organizations*, Volume 6, N. 4, Oct-Dec.

Castells, M. 1996 and 2010, *The Rise of the Network Society*, London: Blackwell.

Castells, M. 1998, *End of Millenium*, Oxford: Blackwell.

Castro, José Alberto 2000, "El Reto para Fox, una Economía con Responsabilidad Social," *Proceso*, No. 1237, July 16, pp. 20-21.

Centro de Estudios de Finanzas Públicas (CEFP), *Evolución del Gasto Social 2003-2010*, Mexico: CEFP, at http://www.cefp.gob.mx/intr/edocumentos/pdf/cefp/2009/cefp0782009.pdf

Cerny, P. 1995, "Globalization and the changing logic of collective action," *International Organization*, 48, pp. 595-625.

Chalmers, Douglas A. and Kerianne Piester, "Non-governmental Organizations and the Changing Structure of Mexican Politics," in *Changing Structure of Mexico: Political, social, and economic prospects*, ed. Laura Randall, M.E. Sharpe.

Chen, L., D. Bell and L. Bates 1996, "World health and institutional change", in *Pocantico retreat: enhancing the performance of international health institutions*. Cambridge, Massachusetts: Rockefeller Foundation, Social Science Research Council, Harvard School of Public Health, pp. 9-21.

Chen, L., Evans, T.G., and R.A Cash 1999, "Health as a global public good", in I. Kaul, I. Grunber, and M.A. Stern (eds.), *Global public goods: International co-operation in the 21st century* (pp. 284-304), New York: Oxford University Press.

Chen, L., Leaning, J., and Vasant Narasimhan (eds.) 2003, *Global Health Challenges for Human Security*, Cambridge and London: Harvard University Press.

Chen, T.T.L. and A.E. Winder 1990, "The Opium Wars Revisited as U.S. forces Tobacco Exports in Asia," *American Journal of Public Health*, No. 80, pp. 659-662.

Child, Raquel 1999, "VIH/SIDA y la organización de las respuestas", in *El SIDA en América Latina y el Caribe, una visión multidisciplinaria,* FUNSALUD.

Chomsky, Noam 2002, 9-11, Seven Stories Press.

Clapham, Christopher 2002, "The Challenge to the State in a Globalized World," *Development and Change*, Vol. 33, pp. 775-795, Oxford, UK: Blackwell Publishers.

Clark, Dana, Jonathan Fox and Kay Treakle (eds.) 2003, *Demanding Accountability: Civil-Society claims and the World Bank Inspection Panel*, Maryland, USA: Rowman & Littlefield Publishers, Inc.

Clarkson, Stephen 2002, *Uncle Sam and Us: Globalization, Neoconservatism, and the Canadian State,* University of Toronto Press, Woodrow Wilson Center Press.

Clarkson, Stephen 2003, "An Illusive Problem: Governance in North America," Manuscript, September 16.

Clarkson, Stephen 2004, "Global Governance and the Semi-Peripheral State: The WTO and NAFTA as Canada's External Constitution," in Clarkson, Stephen, and Marjorie Griffin Cohen (eds.), *Governing under Stress: Middle Powers and the Challenge of Globalization.* Fernwood Publishing.

Cleary, Edward L. 1995, "Human Rights Organizations in Mexico: Growth in turbulence," *Journal of Church and State*, Vol. 37, No. 4, Autum.

Cohen, Edward S. 2001, "Globalization and the Boundaries of the State: A Framework for Analyzing the Changing Practice of Sovereignty," *Governance*, Vol. 14 Issue 1, pp. 75-97.

Coleman, W.D. and A. Perl 1999, "Internationalized Policy Environments and Policy Network Analysis," *Political Studies*, XLVII, pp. 691-709.

Colombani, Jean-Marie 2002, *Tous Américains ? Le monde après le 11 septembre 2001*, Fayard.

Collins, Charles and Abdrew Green 1994, "Decentralization and primary health care: Some negative implications in developing countries," *International Journal of Health Services*, Vol. 24, No. 3, pp. 459-475.

Commission on Macroeconomics and Health 2001, "Macroeconomics and Health: Investing in health for economic development," *Report*, Geneva: World Health Organization.

Conyers, D. et al. 1995, "Decentralization and health systems change: A framework for analysis", WHO Document WHO/SHS/NHP/93.2, Revised Working Paper.

Cook, Maria Lorena, Kevin J. Middlebrook and Juan Molinar (eds.) 1994, *The Politics of Economic Restructuring, State-Society Relations and Regime Change in Mexico*, Center for US-Mexican Studies, UCSD.

Cordera, Rolando 1997, *La Economía Mexicana en Peligro*, Mexico City: Cal y Arena.

Cordera, Rolando 2000, *Las Políticas Sociales de México: descentralización, diseño y gestión*, Mexico: Coordinación de Humanidades, Facultad de Economía, Instituto de Investigaciones Sociales de la Universidad Nacional Autónoma de México.

Cordera, Rolando and Julio Boltvinik 1984, *La Desigualdad en México,* Mexico City: Siglo XXI Editores.

Córdova Villalobos, José Ángel, Samuel Ponce de León, and José Luis Valdespino (eds.) 2008, *25 años de sida en México: Logros, desaciertos y retos*, Mexico: Secretaría de Salud.

Cornelius, Wayne 1996, *Mexican Politics in Transition: The breakdown of a one-party-dominant regime*, San Diego: University of California.

Cosío Villegas, Daniel 1997, *Problemas de América*, Mexico City: Editorial Clío/El Colegio Nacional.

Cox, Robert 1996, *Approaches to World Order*, Cambridge University Press.

Crespo, José Antonio 2008, *2006: hablan las actas / Las debilidades de la autoridad electoral mexicana*, México, D.F.: Random House Mondadori.

Cronin, Bruce 2002, "The Two Faces of the United Nations: The Tension between Intergovernmentalism and Transnationalism," *Global Governance*, Jan-Mar, Vol. 8 Issue 1, pp. 53-71, Boulder.

Cruz-Saco, María Amparo and Carmelo Mesa-Lago (eds.) 1998, *The Reform of Pension and Health Care Systems in Latin America: Do Options Exist?* University of Pittsburgh Press.

Cutler, David M 1998, "The third wave in health care reform," Harvard University and National Bureau of Economic Research (U.S.A.) Preliminary manuscript, April Seminar, Centro de Investigación y Docencia Económicas (CIDE), Mexico.

Cutler, D.M. and E. Richardson 1998, "The Value of Health: 1970-1990," *American Economic Review*, No. 88, pp. 97-100.

Cutright, Philips 1965, "Political Structure, Economic Development, and National Social Security Programs," *American Journal of Sociology*, 70, March.

D'Artigues, Katia 2002, *El Gabinetazo*, Mexico City: Grijalbo.

Daalder, Ivo H. 2003, *America Unbound: The Bush revolution in foreign policy*, Brookings Institution.

Dahl, Robert 1957, "The concept of power," *Behavioural Science*, Vol. 2, pp. 201-215.

Dahl, Robert 1971, *Polyarchy: Participation and Opposition*, New Haven, Yale University Press.

Dahl, Robert 1989, *Democracy and Its Critics*, Yale University Press.

Dahl, Robert and Charles Lindblom 1953, *Politics, Economics and Welfare*, New York: Harper.

Dahrendorf, Ralf 1981, *Class and Class Conflict in Industrial Society*, Stanford University Press.

Dahrendorf, Ralf 1988, *The Modern Social Conflict: An essay on the politics of liberty*, Weidenfeld & Nicolson.

Dahrendorf, Ralf 1994, "The Changing Quality of Citizenship," in Bart van Steenbergen (ed.) *The Condition of Citizenship*, Sage.

Dahrendorf, Ralf 1996, "Citizenship and Social Class," in Martin Blumer and Anthony M. Rees, *Citizenship Today*, UCL Press.

Daniels, N., B.P. Kennedy and I. Kawachi 1999, "Why justice is good for our health: The social determinants of health inequalities," *Daedalus*, Vol. 128, No. 4, pp. 99-134.

Davis, Diane E. 1994, "Failed democratic reform in contemporary Mexico: from social movements to the state and back again," *Journal of Latin American Studies*, Vol. 26, May, part 2, pp. 375-405.

De Feyter, Koen 2005, *Human Rights: Social Justice in the Age of the Market,* London and New York: Zed Books Ltd.

De Gaay Fortman, Bas 2011, *Political Economy of Human Rights: Rights, realities and realization,* New York, N.Y.: Routledge.

De Keijzer, Benno 1992, "Participación popular en salud, logros, retos y perspectivas," in Menéndez y García de León (eds), *Prácticas populares, ideología médica y participación social*, U. de G. y CIESAS.

De la Dehesa, Rafael 2010, *Queering the Public Space in Mexico and Brazil: Sexual Movements in Emerging Democracies,* Duke University Press.

De Mora, Juan Miguel 1973, *Tlatelolco 68: !Por fin toda la verdad¡* Editores Asociados.

De Sousa Santos, Boaventura 2014, *Epistemologies of the South: Justice against epistemicide*, Boulder and London: Paradigm Publishers.

Diamond, L. and Juan Linz. 1989, *Democracy in Developing Countries,* Volume 4: Latin America, Lynne Rienner.

Diamond, Larry Jay and Leonardo Morlino, eds. 2005, *Assessing the quality of democracy,* Baltimore, Maryland: The Johns Hopkins University Press.

Diamond, Larry Jay, Jonathan Hartlyn, Juan J. Linz, and Seymour Lipset 1999, *Democracy in developing countries: Latin America.* Boulder, CO: Lynne Rienner Publishers.

Díez, Jordi 2015, *The politics of same-sex marriage in Latin America: Argentina, Chile and Mexico*, Cambridge University Press.

Dolowitz, David P. and David Marsh 2000, "Learning from Abroad: The Role of Policy Transfer in Contemporary Policy-Making," *Governance*, Vol. 13, Issue 1, pp. 5-23.

Domínguez, Jorge I. and James A. McCann 1996, *Democratizing Mexico: Public Opinion and Electoral Choices*, Baltimore: Johns Hopkins University Press.

Domínguez, Jorge I. and Rafael Fernández de Castro 2001, *The United States and Mexico: Between Partnership and Conflict*, Routledge.

Dowding, K. 1994, "Policy Networks: Don't stretch a Good Idea too Far," in P. Dunleavy and J. Stanyer (eds.), *Contemporary Political Studies*, vol. 1, Belfast, Political Studies Association.

Dowding, K. 1995, "Model or Metaphor? A Critical Review of the Policy Network Approach," *Political Studies*, vol. 43, num. 1, pp. 136-158.

Duquette, Michel 1999, *Building New Democracies: Economic and social reform in Brazil, Chile, and Mexico*, University of Toronto Press.

Eckstein, Harry 1960, *Pressure Group Politics*, Stanford.

Eckstein, Susan (ed.) 1989, *Power and Popular Protest: Latin American social movements*, University of California Press.

Eckstein, Susan Eva and Tymothy P. Wickham-Crowley 2003, *Struggle for Social Rights in Latin America*, Routledge Press.

Escobar Latapí, Agustín 2002, "The PROGRESA Programme and Social Change in Rural Mexico," in Louise Haagh and Camilla T. Helg¢ (eds.), *Social Policy Reform and Market Governance in Latin America*, Palgrave Macmillan in association with St. Antony's College, Oxford.

Evans, M. and J. Davies 1997, "Evolving Networks in Local Governance: The New York Case," University of York, Department of Politics, Working Paper, Num. 14.

Evans, P. 1992, "The state as problem and solution", in S. Haggard and R. Kaufman, eds. *The politics of economic adjustment*, Princeton University Press, pp. 139-81.

Evans, P. 1995, *Embedded Autonomy: States and Industrial Transformation*, Princeton University Press.

Evans, P. (ed.) 1996, *State-Society Synergy: Government and social capital in development*, Elsevier Science Ltd. and University of California at Berkeley.

Evans, P. et al. (eds.) 1985, *Bringing the state back in*, Cambridge University Press.

Evans, P., Harold K. Jacobson and Robert D. Putnam (eds.) 1993, *Double-Edged Diplomacy*, University of California Press.

Farber, Samuel 2011, *Cuba Since the Revolution of 1959: A critical assessment*, Chicago, Ill.: Haymarket Books.

Farmer, Paul 2001, *Infectious Diseases and Inequalities: The modern plagues*, University of California Press.

Farmer Paul 2003, "Pestilence and restraint: Guantánamo, AIDS, and the logic of quarantine," in *Pathologies of Power: Health, Human Rights, and the New War on the Poor,* Farmer Paul and Amartya Sen, Berkeley, Calif: University of California Press.

Farmer, Paul and Amartya Sen 2003, *Pathologies of Power: Health, human rights, and the new war on the poor*, University of California Press.

Fernández de Villegas, Manuel and Naomi Adelson 2000, "Civil Society Participation in World Bank and Inter-American Development Bank Programs: The Case of Mexico," in *Global Governance: A Review of Multilateralism and International Organizations*, Volume 6, N. 4, Oct-Dec.

Fidler, David 2000, *International Law and Public Health: Materials on and analysis of global health jurisprudence*, New York: Transnational Publishers.

Fidler, David P. 2003, "Disease and Globalized Anarchy: theoretical perspectives on the pursuit of global health," *Social Theory & Health*, 1, pp. 21-41.

Fidler, Stephen 1996, "Mexico: what kind of transition?" *International Affairs*, Vol. 72, No. 4, pp. 713-725.

Fink, Sheri 2003, "Cuba's Energetic AIDS Doctor," *American Journal of Public Health*, May; 93(5): 712–716.

Fishlow, Albert 1995, "Inequality, Poverty, and Growth: Where do we stand?" Paper presented at the World Bank Conference on Development Economics, Washington, D.C.

Flamand, Laura and Carlos Moreno-Jaimes 2015, "La protección social en salud durante el gobierno de Calderón. Avances y rezagos en el diseño y la implementación del Seguro Popular (2006-2012)," *Foro Internacional*, January-March, Vol. LV, Num. 1.

Flamand, Laura and Carlos Moreno-Jaimes 2014, *Seguro popular y federalismo. Un análisis de política pública*, Mexico: Centro de Investigación y Docencia Económicas.

Foweraker, Joe and Ann L. Craig (eds.) 1990, *Popular Movements and Political Change in Mexico*, Boulder, Colo.: Lynne Ryenner.

Fox, Jonathan 1994, "The difficult transition from clientelism to citizenship: lessons from Mexico," *World Politics*, V. 46, Jan 1994, p. 151-184.

Fox, Jonathan 1997, "The World Bank and Social Capital: Contesting the Concept in Practice," *Journal of International Development,* Vol. 9, No. 7.

Fox, Jonathan, and L. David Brown (eds.) 1998, *The Struggle for Accountability: The World Bank, NGOs, and grassroots movements*, The MIT Press.

Frank, G. 1967, *Capitalism and Underdevelopment in Latin America: Historical Studies of Chile and Brazil*, New York: Monthly Review Press.

Frenk, Julio (ed.) 1995, *Economía y Salud: Propuestas para avance del sistema de salud en México*, Mexico: FUNSALUD.

Frenk, Julio (ed.) 1997, *Observatorio de la Salud: Necesidades, Servicios, Políticas*, Mexico: FUNSALUD.

Friedman, Edward 1999, "The Painful Gradualness of Democratization: Proceduralism as a Necessarily Discontinuous Revolution," in Howard Handleman and Mark Tessler (eds.), *Democracy and Its Limits*, Notre Dame, Indiana: University of Notre Dame Press.

Friedman, Elisabeth Jay, Kathryn Hochstetler and Ann Marie Clark 2001, "Sovereign limits and regional opportunities for global civil society in Latin America,"

Latin American Research Review, 36.3: 7-35.

Friedman, Thomas L. 2002, *Longitudes and Attitudes: Exploring the world after September 11*, Farrar, Strauss and Giroux.

Fukuyama, Francis 1992, *The End of History and the Last Man*, New York: HarperCollins.

Fukuyama, Francis 1995, *Trust: The social virtues and the creation of prosperity*, The Free Press.

FUNSALUD 1995, *Salud: La sociedad civil frente a los desafíos nacionales, X aniversario de FUNSALUD*, Mexico: FUNSALUD.

Gallup, J.L. and J. Sachs 1998, *The Economic Burden of Malaria, Centre for International Development*, Cambridge, M.A.: Harvard University Press.

Galván Díaz, Francisco, Roberto González-Villarreal and Rodolfo Morales 1991, "AIDS, Government and Society in Mexico," in Ian Lumsden, *Homosexuality, Society and the State in Mexico*, Canadian gay Archives and Solediciones, pp. 101-122.

García-Junco Machado, David 1997, "Confronting Poverty in Mexico: An Overview of Social Policy," Documento de Trabajo No. 48, Centro de Investigación y Docencia Económicas, Mexico.

García Murcia, Miguel, Magdalena Andrade Briseño, Ricardo Maldonado Arroyo and Claudia Morales Escobar (eds.) 2010, *Memorias de la Lucha contra el VIH en México. Los primeros años,* Mexico: Historiadores de las Ciencias y las Humanidades A.C., Consejo Nacional para Prevenir la Discriminación: colección estudios.

Garrett, G. and P.Lange 1996, "Internationalization, Institutions and Political Change", in R. Keohane and H. Milner (eds), *Internationalization and Domestic Politics,* Cambridge.

Garret, Laurie 1996, "The Return of Infectious Disease," *Foreign Affairs*, January/February, pp. 66-79.

Gibney, Matthew J. (ed.) 2003, *Globalizing Rights,* New York: Oxford University Press.

Gibson, Edward L. 1997, "The Populist Road to Market Reform: Policy and Electoral Coalitions in Argentina and Mexico," *World Politics* 49, April, pp. 337-370.

Giddens, Anthony 1990, *The Consequences of Modernity*, Cambridge: Polity Press.

Giugale, M., Olivier Lafourcade and Vinh H. Ngugen 2001, *Mexico: A Comprehensive Development Agenda for the New Era*, Washington, D.C.: World Bank.

González-Block, M.A., René Leyva et al., 1989, "Health services decentralization in Mexico: Formulation, implementation and results of policy," *Health and Planning*; Vol. 4, No. 4, pp. 301-315, Oxford University Press.

González-Block, Miguel Angel 1994, "Access Policies and Utilization patterns in Prenatal and Child Delivery Care in Mexico," *Health Policy and Planning*, Vol. 9, No. 2, Oxford University Press.

González-Block, Miguel Angel and Enrique Gutiérrez 1998, 'State Government and Federal Health Expenditures for the Uninsured in Mexico. Their Contribution to Equity and Efficiency," Mexico City: FUNSALUD.

González-Block, Miguel Angel and Ana Luisa Liguori 1992, *El SIDA en los Estratos Socioeconómicos de México*, Perspectivas en Salud Pública, No. 16, Cuernavaca, Mexico: Instituto Nacional de Salud Pública.

González Bustos, Marcelo 1995, *La rebelión campesina del EZLN en Chiapas*, Mexico: Universidad Autónoma Chapingo.

González Pérez, César Octavio 2001, "La Identidad Gay: Una Identidad en Tensión," *Desacatos*, Spring-Summer, CIESAS, Mexico.

González Ruiz, Edgar 2002, *La Sexualidad Prohibida: Intolerancia, sexismo y represión*, Plaza y Janés.

Gourevitch, P. 1978, "The second image reversed: the international sources of domestic politics", *International Organization*, 32, pp. 881-912.

Gray, Charlotte 1996, "Debate Over NAFTA's Effect on Health Care a Sign Medicare will be Dominant Election Issue", *Canadian Medical Association Journal* 1996; 154: 1549-1551.

Gray, John 1998, *False Dawn: The delusion of global capitalism*, New York: The New Press.

Gray, John 2003, *Al Qaeda and what it means to be modern*, London: Faber and Faber.

Grayson George 1989, *The Mexican Labour Machine: Power Politics and Patronage*, Washington, D.C.: Centre for Strategic International Studies.

Grayson, George 1998, *Mexico: From Corporatism to Pluralism?* Harcourt Brace.

Green, Daniel 1995a, "European Medicines Evaluation Agency: Fast-track Approvals Service, *Financial Times*, April 25.

Green, Daniel 1995b, "EU Body to Speed Up Approval of New Drugs," *Financial Times*, January 26.

Green, Duncan 1995, *Silent Revolution: The rise of market economics in Latin America*, Cassell.

Grinspun, Ricardo and Maxwell Cameron (eds.) 1993, *The Political Economy of North American Free Trade*, St. Martin's Press.

Gruzinski, Serge 1994, *La Guerra de las Imágenes*, Mexico: Fondo de Cultura Económica.

Gruzinski, Serge 1999, *La Pensée Métisse*, France: Librairie Artheme Fayard.

Guest, D. 1980, *The Emergence of Social Security in Canada*, University of British Columbia Press.

Gutiérrez, Juan Pablo and Mauricio Hernández-Ávila 2013, "Cobertura de protección en salud y perfil de la población sin protección en México, 2000-2012," *Salud Pública de México*, vol. 55, supl. 2, pp. S83-s90

Haagh, Louise and Camilla T. Helg¢ 2002, *Social Policy Reform and Market Governance in Latin America*, Palgrave Macmillan in association with St. Antony's College, Oxford.

Haas P. 1992, "Introduction: Epistemic Communities and International Policy Co-ordination", *International Organization*, 49 (1), p. 1-35).

Habermas, Jurgen 1994, "Three Models of Democracy", Constellations 1.

Haggard, Stephen and Robert R. Kaufman 1994, "The Challenges of Consolidation", *Journal of Democracy*, 5, pp. 5-16.

Hagopian, Frances and Scott P. Mainwaring. 2005. *The Third Wave of Democratization in Latin America: Advances and setbacks*. New York, NY: Cambridge University Press.

Halbert, Debora J. 2005, *Resisting Intellectual Property Rights*, London and New York: Routledge.

Hamilton, Nora 1982, *The Limits of State Autonomy: Post-Revolutionary Mexico*, Princeton: Princeton University Press.

Hammer J. 1997, "Economic analysis for health projects", *World Bank Research Observer*, 12 (1), pp. 47-71.

Hassenteufel, Patrick 1995, "Do policy networks matter? Lifting decriptif et analyse de l'État en intercation", in Patrick Le Galés et Mark Thatcher (eds.), *Les Réseaux de Politiques Publiques, débat autour des policy networks*, L'Harmattan.

Hausman, Ricardo 1994, *Sustaining Reform: What role for social policy?* Washington, D.C., Inter-American Development Bank.

Hay, C. 1995, "Structure and Agency", in D. Marsh and G. Stoker (eds.), *Theory and Methods in Political Science*, Basingstoke, Macmillan, pp. 189-208.

Haynes, Jeff 1997, *Democracy and Civil Society in the Third World*, Polity Press.

Heclo, H. and A. Wildavsky 1974, *The Private Government of Public Money*, London, Macmillan.

Held, D. McGrew, A., Goldblatt, D. and Perraton, J. 1997, 'The Globalization of Economic Activity,' *New Political Economy*, Vol. 2, No. 2, July, pp. 2557-2577.

Held, D. McGrew, A., Goldblatt, D. and Perraton, J. 1999, *Global Transformations: Politics, economics and culture*, Cambridge: Polity Press.

Herod, Andrew, Gearoid Tuathail and Susan Roberts 1998, "Negotiating Unruly Problematics" in Herod, Tuathail, and Roberts, *An Unruly World?* Routledge.

Hernández Avila, Mauricio, Susan Vandale Toney and Ana Luisa Liguori (eds.) 1995, *Enfoques de Investigación sobre VIH/SIDA en Salud Reproductiva*, Perspectivas en Salud Pública No. 19, Instituto de Salud Pública, Mexico.

Hernández Cabrera, Porfirio Miguel 2001, "La Construcción de la Identidad Gay de Jóvenes de la Ciudad de México", *Desacatos*, Spring-Summer, CIESAS, Mexico.

Hewitt de Alcántara, Cynthia 1998, "Uses and Abuses of the Concept of Governance", *International Social Science Journal*, No. 155, March, pp. 105-114.

Hirst, Paul and Grahame Thompson 1996, *Globalization in Question*, Polity Press.

Hoffman, Stanley 1981, *Duties beyond borders: On the limits and possibilities of ethical international politics*, Syracuse University Press.

Hongju Koh, Harold and Ronald C. Slye (eds.) 1999, *Deliberative Democracy & Human Rights*, Yale University Press.

Horcasitas, Juan and Jeffrey Weldon 1994, "Electoral Determinants and Consequences of National Solidarity," in Wayne Cornelius, Ann Craig and Jonathan Fox (eds.), *Transforming State-Society Relations in Mexico: The National Solidarity Strategy*, Centre for U.S.-Mexican Studies, San Diego.

Howse, Robert and Kalypso Nicolaidis 2003, "Enhancing WTO Legitimacy: Constitutionalization or Global Subsidiarity?" *Governance*, Vol. 16, Issue 1, pp. 73-94.

Hughes, Sallie 2000, "Culture Clash in the Newsroom: New Media Transformation in a Liberalizing Regime, The Case of the Mexican Press," Paper presented at the Latin American Studies Association Conference, Miami, Florida, March 2000.

Hurst, J. 2000, "Challenges for Health Systems in Member Countries of the OECD," Bulletin of the WHO, No. 78, pp. 751-760.

IDB 1994, "Report on the Eighth General Increase in the Resources of the Inter-American Development Bank", Washington, D.C.

IDB 1997, "Modernization of the State and Strengthening of Civil Society", Washington, D.C., Strategic Planning and Policy Department.

IDB 1997a, "Economic and Social Progress in Latin America: Latin America After a Decade of Reforms," Washington, D.C.: Inter-American Development Bank.

ILO 1998, "World Report: Industrial Relations, Democracy, and Social Stability 1997-98," Geneva: International Labour Office.

IMSS 2004 *Evidencias para el Debate: Resultados y Perspectivas Financieras de la Seguridad Social, Mexico: Dirección de Finanzas y Sistemas*, Coordinación General de Comunicación Social, IMSS.

Inglehart, Ronald, Miguel Basáñez and Neil Nevitte 1994, *Convergencia en Norteamérica: Comercio, política y cultura*, Mexico: Siglo Veintuno Editores, S. A. de C.V.

Irwin, Alexander, Joyce Millen and Dorothy Fallows 2003, *Global AIDS: Myths and facts, tools for fighting the AIDS pandemic*, Cambridge, MA: South End Press.

Izazola Licea, José Antonio and Jorge Huerdo Siqueiros 1999, "A Holistic View", Working Paper, SIDALAC.

Izazola-Licea JA, et al. 1998, "Access to antiretrovirals: the role of political activism in Mexico", paper presented at the 12th International AIDS Conference, Geneva.

Jackman, Robert W. 1975, "Political Democracy and Social Equality: A Comparative Analysis", *American Sociological Review*, 39, February.

Jakarta 1997, "The Jakarta Declaration on Health Promotion into the 21st Century," Geneva: World Health Organization.

Jamison, Dean T., Julio Frenk and Felicia Knaul 1998, "International collective action in health: Objectives, functions, and rationale", *The Lancet*, vol. 351, February 14.

Jessop, B. 1990, *State Theory. Putting the Capitalist State in Its Place*, Cambridge: Polity Press.

Johnson, Chalmers 1982, *MITI and the Japanese Miracle: The Growth of Industrial Policy, 1925-1975*, Stanford University Press.

Johnson, John R. 2002, "How Will International Trade Agreements Affect Canadian Health Care?" Discussion Paper prepared for the Commission on the Future of Health Care in Canada.

Jordan, David 1992, "International Regulatory Harmonization: A New Era in Prescription Drug Approval," *Vanderbilt Journal of Transnational Law*, No. 25, pp. 471-505.

Jordan G. 1990, "Sub-Governments, Policy Communities and Networks: Refilling the Old Bottles?", *Journal of Theoretical Politics*, 2 (3), pp. 319-338.

Jordan, G. et al. 1994, "Characterising agricultural policy", *Public Administration*, 72, 505-526.

Joseph, Gilbert M. and Daniel Nugent (eds.) 1994, *Everyday Forms of State Formation: Revolution and the Negotiation of Rule in Modern Mexico*, Durham: Duke University Press.

Kapstein, E.B. 1999, "Distributive justice as an international public good: A historical perspective," in I. Kaul, I. Grunberg and M.A. Stern (eds.), *Global Public Goods*, (pp. 88-115), New York: Oxford University Press.

Kapur, Devesh, John P. Lewis and Richard Webb (eds.) 1997, *The World Bank: Its First Half-Century*, Brookings Institution Press, Washington, D.C.

Karl, Rohe (ed.) 1990, *Elections, Parties, and Political Traditions: Social Foundations of German Parties and Party Systems*, St. Martin's Press, New York.

Kaufman Purcell, Susan 1973, "Decision-Making in an Authoritarian Regime: Theoretical Implications of a Mexican Case Study", *World Politics* 26, no. 1, October.

Kaul, I., I. Grunber and M.A. Stern (eds.) 1999, *Global public goods: International co-operation in the 21ˢᵗ century*, New York: Oxford University Press.

Kawachi et al. 1997, "Social capital, income inequality, and mortality", *American Journal of Public Health*, September, Vol. 87, No. 9.

Keck, Margaret E. and Kathryn Sikkink 1998, *Activists Beyond Borders: Advocacy networks in international politics*, Ithaca and London: Cornell University Press.

Kellner, Douglas 2003, *From 9/11 to Terror on War: The dangers of the Bush legacy*, Rowman and Littlefield.

Keohane, R. and J. Nye 1977, *Power and Interdependence*, Boston, MA: Little Brown.

Kiely, Ray 2004, "The World Bank and Global Poverty Reduction: good policies or bad data?" *Journal of Contemporary Asia*, Vol. 34, Issue 1, pp. 3-18.

Killick, T. 1998, *Aid and the Political Economy of Policy Change*, London and New York: Routledge.

Knaul, F.M. 1999, "Linking Health, Nutrition and Wages: The evolution of age at menarche and labour earning among Mexican women," Working Paper Series R-355, April, Washington, D.C.: Inter-American Development Bank.

Knaul, Felicia, and Julio Frenk 2005, Health Insurance in Mexico: Achieving Universal Coverage through Structural Reform," *Health Affairs*, vol. 24, num. 6, pp. 1467-1476.

Knight, Alan 1986, *The Mexican Revolution*, Cambridge: Cambridge University Press.

Knoke, David, Urban Pappi, Franz, Jeffrey Broadbent and Yutaka Tsujinaka 1996, *Comparing Policy Networks: Labor Politics in the U.S., Germany, and Japan*, New York, N.Y.: Cambridge University Press.

Koh, Harold Hongju and Ronald C. Slye (eds.) 1999, *Deliberative Democracy and Human Rights*, New Haven and London: Yale University Press.

Korzeniewicz, Roberto Patricio and William C. Smith 2000, "Poverty, inequality, and growth in Latin America: Searching for the high road to globalization," *Latin American Research Review* 35.3: 7-54.

Krasner, Stephen D. (ed.) 1983, *International Regimes*, Cornell University Press.

Kurtz, Marcus 1999, "The Political Economy of Pro-Poor Policies in Chile and Mexico," Paper prepared for the WDR 2001 meetings, August 16-17, Castle Domington, United Kingdom.

Laguarda, Rodrigo 2001, *De lo Rarito al Ambiente: Aproximación a la construcción de la identidad gay en México*, Tesis de licenciatura en historia, Mexico: Universidad Iberoamericana.

Landell-Mills, Pierre 1992, "Governance, Civil Society and Empowerment in Sub-Saharan Africa: Building the institutional basis for sustainable development," June 10, Washington: World Bank, Africa Technical Department.

Laurell, Asa Cristina (coord.) 1994, *Nuevas Tendencias y Alternativas en el Sector Salud*, UAM Xochimilco, Friedrich Ebert Stiftung.

Laurell, Asa Cristina 1997, *La Reforma Contra la Salud y la Seguridad Social*, Ediciones Era, Fundación Friederich Ebert, Mexico.

Laurell, Asa Cristina 2002, "Official Report of Activities," presented by Asa Cristina Laurell at UAM-Xochimilco, Mexico City, August 2.

Laws M. 1996, "International funding of global AIDS strategy: official development assistance", in J. Mann and D. Tarantola, eds., *AIDS in the World II: The Global Policy Coalition*, Oxford University Press.

Lawson, Chappell. 2006. "Preliminary Findings from the Mexico's 2006 Panel Study: Blue States and Yellow States". Available online at: http://web.mit.edu/polisci/research/mexico06/Region_and_demographics8.doc

Laxer, Gordon and Dennis Soron 2003, "Decommodifying Public Life: Resisting the Enclosure of the Commons", Manuscript on "The Globalism Project's" website: http://www.ualberta.ca/GLOBALISM/book%20III.htm.

Leal F., Gustavo 2000, *Agenda y Diseño de la Reforma Mexicana de la Salud y la Seguridad Social*, Universidad Autónoma Metropolitana (UAM), Mexico.

Leal F., Gustavo 2001, "Enigmas, Encrucijadas y Paradojas del Foxismo en la Arena de la Salud," *El Cotidiano: Revista de la realidad mexicana actual*, Universidad Autónoma Metropolitana (UAM), No. 105, January/February, pp. 56-69.

Leal F., Gustavo 2001a, "Conglomerados Hospitalarios Privados, Tendencias Recientes del Sistema Nacional de Salud," *El Cotidiano: Revista de la realidad mexicana actual*, Universidad Autónoma Metropolitana (UAM), No. 109, pp. 88-96.

Leal F., Gustavo 2001b, "¿Aseguradoras frente a Hospitales Privados por el Intermedio de Empresas de Comercio Electrónico? Tendencias Recientes del Sistema Nacional de Salud" *El Cotidiano: Revista de la realidad mexicana actual*, Universidad Autónoma Metropolitana (UAM), No. 110, pp. 103-114.

Leal F., Gustavo and Carolina Martínez S. 2001 "¿En la Ruta del Seattle Sanitario? La Organización Mundial de la Salud y su Informe Sobre la Salud en el Mundo", *El Cotidiano: Revista de la realidad mexicana actual*, Universidad Autónoma Metropolitana (UAM), No. 107, pp. 21-34.

Leal F., Gustavo and Carolina Martínez S. 2001a "Puntos de Vista sobre la Industria Químico-Farmacéutica: Un parpadeo sobre un actor de arena de la política pública de salud y seguridad social", *El Cotidiano: Revista de la realidad mexicana actual*, Universidad Autónoma Metropolitana (UAM), No. 106, pp. 89-104.

Leal F., Gustavo 2002, "Pasaporte al Fracaso. El Foxismo como Tardopriísmo Social, 16 Apuntes Sumarios sobre un Gobierno del 'Cambio que se Traicionó en sólo Cuatro Meses," *El Cotidiano: Revista de la realidad mexicana actual*,

Universidad Autónoma Metropolitana (UAM), No. 111, January/February, pp. 92-98.

Le Gales, Patrick and Mark Thatcher (eds.)1995, *Les Réseaux de Politique Publique: Débat autour des policy networks*, L'Harmattan.

Lee, Kelley and Richard Dodgson 2000, "Globalization and Cholera: Implications for Global Governance," *Global Governance*, Vol. 6, Issue 2, pp. 213-236.

Levy, Daniel C. and Kathleen Bruhn 2001, Mexico, *The Struggle for Democratic Development*, University of California Press.

Liguori, Ana Luisa and Miguel Angel González-Block 1992, "El SIDA en los Estratos Socioeconómicos de México," *Perspectivas en Salud Pública*, No. 16, Instituto de Salud Pública.

Lindermann, Eric 1994, "Importing AIDS Drugs: Food and Drug Administration Policy and its Limitations," *George Washington Journal of International Law and Economics*, No. 28, pp. 133-169.

Linz, Juan 1973, "the Future of an Authoritarian Situation or the Institutionalization of an authoritarian Regime: The Case of Brazil," in A. Stepan, *Authoritarian Brazil: Origins, Policies, and Future*, Princeton University Press.

Loewenberg, Sam 1999, "Businesses Find Ways to Influence World Bank Projects," *Legal Times*, 22 February, p. 1.

Lofchie, Michael F. 1989, "Perestroika Without Glassnost: Reflections on Structural Adjustment," in Beyond Autocracy in Africa, Working Papers from the Inaugural Seminar of the Governance in Africa Programme, The Carter Center of Emory University, Atlanta, Georgia, February 17-18.

Lujambio, Alonso 1995, *Federalismo y Congreso en el Cambio Político de México,* Mexico City: UNAM.

Lujambio, Alonso 2000, *El Poder Compartido*, Mexico: Océano.

Lomas, Jonathan 1996, "Social capital and health: Implications for public health and epidemiology," *Working Papers Series*, McMaster University.

Lumsden, Ian 1991, *Homosexuality, Society and the State in Mexico*, Canadian Gay Archives and Solediciones.

Lustig, Nora 1992, *The remaking of an economy*, The Brookings Institution, Washington D.C.

Malloy, James M. 1979, *The Politics of Social Security in Brazil*, Pittsburgh.

Manokha, Ivan 2008, *The Political Economy of Human Rights Enforcement,* New York: Palgrave Macmillan.

Marsh, D. and M. Smith 2000, "Understanding Policy Networks: towards a Dialectical Approach," *Political Studies*, Vol. 48, 4-21.

Marsh, D. and R.A.W. Rhodes 1992, "New Directions in the Study of Policy Networks," *European Journal of Political Research*, Vol. 21, pp. 181-205.

Marsh, David 1995, "Théorie de l'État et Modele de Réseaux d'Action Publique," in Le Gales, Patrick and Mark Thatcher (eds.), Les Reseaux de Politique Publique: Debat autour des policy networks, L'Harmattan

Marsh, David and R.A.W. Rhodes (ed.) 1992, *Policy Networks in British Government*, Clarendon Press.

Marshall, Catherine and Gretchen B. Rossman 1999, *Designing Qualitative Research*, Sage Publications.

Marshall, Thomas H. 1963, *Sociology at the Crossroads and other Essays*, Heinemann.

Marshall, Thomas and Tom B. Boltomore 1992, *Citizenship and Social Class*, Pluto Press.

Marsiaj, Juan P. 2006, "Social Movements and Political Parties: Gays, Lesbians, and *Travestis* and the Struggle for Inclusion in Brazil," Canadian Journal of Latin American and Caribbean Studies / Revue canadienne des études latino-américaines et caraïbes, Vol. 31, Issue 62, pp. 167-196.

Marsiaj, Juan P. 2010, "NGOization of Civil Society and Social Movement Impact: The case of the Lesbians, Gay, Bisexual and Travesti Movement in Brazil," paper prepared for delivery at the XXIX Meeting of the Latin American Studies Association, Toronto, Canada, October 6-9.

Martinussen, John 1997, Society, State & Market: *A Guide to Competing Theories of Development*, Zed Books Ltd, Fernwood Publishing.

Merry, Sally Engle 2001, "Changing Rights, Changing Cultures," In *Culture and Rights: Anthropological Perspectives*, by Jane K. Cowan, Marie-Benedicte Dembour, and Richard A. Wilson (eds.), Cambridge University Press. PAGES.

Merson, Michael H., Robert E. Black and Anne J. Mills 2001, *International Public Health: Diseases, programs, systems and policies*, An Aspen Publication, U.S.A.

Mesa-Lago, Carmelo 1978, *Social Security in Latin America: Pressure Groups, Stratification and Inequality*, University of Pittsburgh Press.

Mesa-Lago, Carmelo 1992, *Health Care for the Poor in Latin America and the Caribbean*, Inter-American Foundation, PAHO Scientific Publication No. 539.

Miller, Karen Lowry 2001, "How Much Money Should Big Drug Firms Have to Lose to Treat the World's Poorest Patients?" *Newsweek*, November 19, pp. 40-41.

Mills A. et al. 1990, "Health systems decentralization: Concepts, issues and country experience," World Health Organization.

Mills A. et al. 1993, "The costs of HIV/AIDS prevention strategies in developing countries," WHO, GPA/DIR/93.1, Geneva.

Mills, Wright 1959, *The Power Elite*, New York: Oxford University Press.

Moore, G. 1979, "The Structure of National Elite Networks," *American Sociological Review*, Vol. 44, No. 3, pp. 673-692.

Moreno Jaimes, Carlos 2002, "La Descentralización del Gasto de Salud en México: Una Revisión de sus Criterios de Asignación," Gestión y Política Pública, Vol. XI, No. 2, pp. 373-405.

Moyn, Samuel 2010, *The Last Utopia: human rights in history,* Cambridge, Massachusetts and London, England: The Belknap Press of Harvard University Press.

Muller, Pierre and Y. Surel 1998, *L'analyse des politiques publiques*, Paris, Montchrestien.

Nacif, Benito 1997, "La No-Reelección Legislativa: Disciplina de Partido y Subordinación al Ejecutivo en la Cámara de Diputados de México," *Diálogo Debate*, No. 1, July/September, pp. 149-167.

Naím, Moisés 1994, "Latin America: the second stage of reform," *Journal of Democracy*, Vol. 5, No. 4, pp. 32-48.

Naím, Moisés 1999, "Fads and Fashion in Economic Reform: Washington Consensus or Washington Confusion?" *Foreign Policy Magazine*, October 26, Working draft of a paper prepared for the IMF Conference on Second Generation Reforms, Washington,D.C.: http://www.imf.org/external/pubs/ft/seminar/1999/reforms/Naim.HTM

Natale, Denise and Sérgio Pinto de Almeida (eds.) 2002, *AIDS, The Epidemic in Megacities: Networking the response*, Editora Papagaio.

Navarro, V. 1998, Comment: "Whose globalization?" *American Journal of Public Health*, No. 88, Vol. 5, pp. 742-743.

Nelson, Paul 2000, "Whose Civil Society? Whose Governance? Decisionmaking and Practice in the New Agenda at the Inter-American Development Bank and the World Bank," in *Global Governance: A Review of Multilateralism and International Organizations*, Volume 6, N. 4, Oct-Dec.

Nelson, Paul, 1996, "Internationalising Economic and Environmental Policy: Transnational NGO Networks and the World Bank's Expanding Influence," *Millenium* 25, No. 3 pp. 605-633.

Nordlinger, Eric 1988, "The return to the state: Critiques," *American Political Science Review*, Vol. 82, No. 3.

North, Douglas C. 1990, *Institutions, institutional change and economic performance*, Cambridge University Press.

Nun, José 2000, *Democracia: ¿Gobierno del pueblo o gobierno de los políticos?* Siglo Veintiuno de España Editores.

Núñez Noriega, Guillermo 2001, "Reconociendo los placeres, deconstruyendo las identidaes: Antropología patriarcado y homoerotismo en México," *Desacatos*, Spring-Summer, CIESAS, Mexico.

O'Brien, Robert 2003, "Paths to Reforming Global Governace," in Richard Sandbrook, (ed.), Civilizing Globalization: A Survival Guide, State University of New York Press.

O'Donnell, Guillermo A. 1991, "Democracia Delegativa," *Novos Estudos,* CEBRAP, 31: 25 – 40.

O'Donnell, Guillermo 1992, "Transitions, Continuities, and Paradoxes," in Scott Mainwaring, Guillermo O'Donnell, and J. Samuel Valenzuela, eds. *Issues in Democratic consolidation: The new South American democracies in comparative perspective*, University of Notre Dame Press.

O'Donnell, Guillermo 1994, "Delegative Democracy," *Journal of Democracy* 5(1): 55-69.

O'Donnell, Guillermo 2010, *Democracy, Agency, and the State: Theory with Comparative Intent*, Oxford University Press.

O'Donnell, G., L. Whitehead and P. Schmitter 1986, *Transitions from Authoritarian Rule*, 5 volumes, Baltimore and London: Johns Hopkins University Press.

Ortega Ortíz, Reynaldo and Ma. Fernanda Somuano Ventura 2015, "El periodo presidencial de Felipe Calderón," *Foro Internacional*, January-March, Vol. LV, Num. 1.

Ortíz, Mauricio 2006, *El Seguro Popular. Una crónica de la democracia Mexicana*, Mexico: Secretaría de Salud, Funsalud, INSP,FCE.

Ostergard, Robert L. Jr. (ed.) 2007, *HIV/AIDS and the Threat to National and International Security,* New York: Palgrave Macmillan.

Over M. 1996, "HIV infection and other STDs in developing countries: public health importance and priorities for resource allocation," *Journal of Infectious Diseases*, 174, supplement 2, pp. 162-175.

PAHO-WHO 1993, Pan-American Health Organisation XXXVII Meeting, World Health Organisation's XLV Meeting, Washington DC, September-October, Health Promotion in the Americas.

Panebianco, Silvia 2000, "Salud y Justicia. Hecha la Ley, hecha la Trampa: Respetos formales y violaciones reales de los derechos humanos en VIH/SIDA, en América Latina," in Fórum 2000, p. 814.

Parekh, Serena 2008, *Hannah Arendt and the Challenge of Modernity: A Phenomenology of Human Rights,* Routledge.

Parker, Richard, Regina Maria Barbosa and Peter Aggleton (eds.) 2000, *Framing the Sexual Subject: The politics of gender, sexuality, and power,* University of California Press.

Pastor, Manuel Jr. and Carol Wise 1999, "The politics of second-generation reform," *Journal of Democracy*, V. 10, No. 3, July.

Pastor, Manuel and Carol Wise 2003, "A Long View of Mexico's Political Economy: What's Changed? What Are the Challenges?" in Joseph S. Tulchin and Andrew D. Selee (eds.), *Mexico's Politics and Society in Transition*, Boulder & London: Lynne Rienner Publishers, pp. 179-213.

Paul, B.D. (ed.) 1995, *Health, Culture and Community*, New York: Russell Sage Foundation.

Pecheny, Mario 2003, "Sexual Orientation, AIDS, and Human Rights in Argentina: The Paradox of Social Advance amid Health Crisis," in Eckstein, Susan Eva and Tymothy P. Wickham-Crowley 2003, *Struggle for Social Rights in Latin America*, Routledge Press.

Perrot, Marie-Dominique, Gilbert Rist and Fabrizio Sabelli 1992, *La Mythologie programmée: L'économie des croyances dans la societé moderne*, Paris: PUF.

Perroux, François 1961, *L'Économie au XXe siècle*, Paris: PUF.

Peschard, Karine 2003, "Rethinking the Semi-Periphery: some conceptual issues," Manuscript posted in "The Globalism Project's" website: http://www.ualberta.ca/GLOBALISM/book%20III.htm

Peterson, J. 1994, "Policy Networks and Governance in the European Union," in P. Dunleavy and J. Stanyer (eds.), *Contemporary Political Studies*, Vol. 1, Belfast, Political Studies Association.

Peterson, J. 1995, "Decision-making in the European Union: Towards a Framework for Analysis," *European Journal of Public Policy*, Vol. 2, pp. 69-93.

Pierceson, J., Piatta-Crocker, A., Schulenberg, S. (eds.) 2013, *Same-sex marriage in Latin America: Promise and resistance,* Plymouth, UK: Lexington Books.

Poitras, Guy E. 1973, "Welfare bureaucracy and clientele politics in Mexico," *Administrative Science Quarterly*, 18, pp. 18-27.

Polany, Karl 1957, *The Great Transformation*, Beacon Press.

Przeworski, Adam 1991, *Democracy and the Market: Political and Economic Reforms in Eastern Europe and Latin America*, Cambridge University Press.

Przeworski, Adam (ed.) 1995, *Sustainable Democracy*, Cambridge University Press.

Przeworski, Adam (ed.) 2000, *Democracy and Development: Political Institutions and the Well-Being of the World, 1950-90*, Cambridge University Press.

Prud'homme, Jean-François 2015, "La insatisfacción con la democracia en el México actual," *Foro Internacional*, January-March, Vol. LV, Num. 1.

Psacharopoulos, George (ed.) 1993, *Poverty and Income Distribution in Latin America: The story of the 1980s*, Washington, D.C.: World Bank, Technical Department of the Latin American Commission.

Putnam, R.D. 1988, "Diplomacy and domestic politics: the logic of two-level games," *International Organization*, 42, pp. 427-460.

Putnam, Robert 1995, "Bowling alone: America's declining social capital", *Journal of Democracy*, Vol. 6, pp. 65-78.

Pye, L.W. 1966, *Aspects of Political Development*, Boston, MA: Little, Brown & Co.

Rabotnikof, Nora, M. Pía Riggirozzi and Diana Tussie 1999, "Los organismos internacionales frente a la sociedad civil: Las agendas en juego", Program on International Economic Institutions, Working Paper No. 5, Buenos Aires, FLACSO/Argentina.

Rajaee, Farhang 2000, *Globalization on Trial: The human condition and the information civilization*, IDRC-Kumarian Press.

Ralston Saul, John 2004, "The Collapse of Globalism," *Harper's Magazine*, Vol. 308, Iss. 1846, pp. 33-43, March 2004.

Ramírez Sáiz, Juan Manuel 2003, "Organizaciones Cívicas, Democracia y Sistema Político", in Alberto Aziz Nassif, (coord.) *México al Inicio del Siglo XXI: Democracia, ciudadanía y desarrollo*, CIESAS, Miguel Angel Porrúa.

Rawls, John 1989, *A Theory of Justice*, Oxford University Press.

Rayside, David 1998, *On the fringe: Gays & lesbians in politics*, Cornell University Press.

Reding, Andrew 1995, *Democracy and Human Rights in Mexico*, World Policy Institute.

Reinhardt, U. 1999, "Social ethics and the globalization of health reform," in D.E Holmes (ed.), *Reflections on Globalization and Health: Consequences of the 3rd Trilateral Conference*, Washington, D.C.: Association of Academic Health Centres.

Remmer, Karen L. 1990, "Democracy and Economic Crisis: The Latin American experience," *World Politics*, Vol. 42, No. 3, pp. 315-335.

Reno, William 1998, *Warlord Politics and African States*, Lynne Rienner Publishers.

Rhodes, R. 1985, "Power Dependence, Policy Communities and Inter-governmental Networks", *Public Administration Bulletin*, vol. 49, April.

Rhodes, R.A.W. 1986, "Power Dependence, Policy Communities and Intergovernmental Networks", Essex Papers in Politics and Government, num. 30.

Rhodes, R.A.W. 1988, *Beyond Westminster and Whitehall*, London, Unwin Hyman.

Richardson, J. and G. Jordan 1979, *Governing Under Pressure*, Oxford, Martin Robertson.

Rimlinger, Gaston V. 1971, *Welfare Policy and Industrialization in Europe, America, and Russia*, New York.

Risse-Kappen, Thomas 1995, "Bringing Transnational Relations Back In: Introduction," in *Bringing Transnational Relations Back In: Non-State Actors, Domestic Structures, and International Institutions*, ed. Risse-Kappen, Cambridge University Press.

Rist, Gilbert 1996, *Le dévelopment: Histoire d'une croyance occidentale*, Paris: Presse de Sciences Po.

Roberts, Matthew W. 1995, "Emergence of Gay Identity and Gay Social Movements in Developing Countries: The AIDS Crisis as a Catalyst", *Alternatives*, 20, pp. 243-264.

Robinson, Mark and Gordon White (eds.) 1998, *The Democratic Developmental State: Politics and institutional design*, New York: Oxford University Press.

Robinson, N. 1997, "Empirically Suspect and Methodological Mess? Policy Networks as a Tool to Study Agenda Setting", in J. Stanyer and G. Stoker (eds.), *Contemporary Political Studies*, Ulster, PSA.

Roett, Riordan (ed.) 1998, *Mexico's Private Sector: Recent history, future challenges*, Boulder: Lynne Rienner.

Romanow, Roy 2003, "Final Report: Commission on the Future of Health Care in Canada", Government of Canada.

Romero Keith, José 2002, *Gestión Social y VIH en México: Nuevos escenarios de acción política*, UNDP, COESIDA, Jalisco.

Ronfeldt, Donald 1989, "Prospects for Elite Cohesion", In Wayne Cornelius, Judith Gentleman, and Peter H. Smith (eds.), *Mexico's Alternative Political Futures*, San Diego: Center for U.S.-Mexican Studies, University of California.

Rosenberg, Mark B. 1979, "Social Security Policymaking in Costa Rica: A Research Report", Latin American Research Review, 14, 1, pp. 116-133.

Ross, Fiona 2000, "Beyond Left and Right: The New Partisan Politics of Welfare," *Governance*, Vol. 13, Issue 2, pp. 155-183.

Rostow, Walt. W. 1971, *The Stages of Economic Growth: A Non-Communist Manifesto*, Cambridge University Press.

Rubio Carriquiriborde, Ignacio 1994, "El Sida a los 17", *Mundo: Culturas y Gente 68*.

Saavedra, Jorge 1999, "Economía y SIDA en América Latina", in *El SIDA en América Latina y el Caribe, una visión multidisciplinaria*, FUNSALUD.

Saavedra, Jorge et al. (1999), "Costs and Expenditures for AIDS medical care in Mexico," Working Paper, SIDALAC.

Saavedra, Jorge 2007a, "Mexico: Situation of Witnesses to Crime and Corruption, Women Victims of Violence and Victims of Discrimination Based on Sexual Orientation," Issue Paper, Mexico City: CONASIDA.

Saavedra, Jorge 2007b, "Homofobia: Alcances y limitaciones en los servicios de salud," in *Homofobia y Salud*, Guillermo Soberón and Dafna Feinholz (eds.), pp. 87–94. Mexico City: Comisión Nacional de Bioética, Secretaría de Salud.

Sabatier, P. 1988, "An Advocacy Coalition Framework of Policy Change and the Role of Policy-Oriented Learning Therein", *Policy Sciences*, Vol. 21, pp. 129-168.

Sabatier, P. 1991, "Towards Better Theories of the Policy Process", *Political Science and Politics*, Vol. 24, pp. 147-156.

Sabatier, P. and H. Jenkins Smith (eds.) 1993, *Policy Change and Learning: An Advocacy Coalition Approach*, Bolder, Co., Westview Press.

Sánchez, Marco Aurelio 1999, *PRD: La Elite en Crisis*, México: Plaza y Valdés.

Sandbrook, Richard (ed.) 2003, *Civilizing Globalization: A survival guide*, State University of New York Press.

Schadlen, Kenneth C. 2000, "Neoliberalism, Corporatism, and Small Business Political Activism in Contemporary Mexico", *Latin American Research Review*, No. 35, pp. 73-106.

Schaefer, Claudia 1996, *Danger Zones, Homosexuality, National Identity, and Mexican Culture*, The University of Arizona Press.

Schedler, Andreas 1998, "What is democratic consolidation", *Journal of Democracy*, V. 9, No. 2, pp. 91-107.

Scheper-Hughes N. 1993, "AIDS, public health, and human rights in Cuba*,"* Lancet, 342: 965–967.

Scherer Ibarrra, María 2000, "Julio Frenk o Carlos Tena, el posible Secretario de Salud," *Proceso*, No. 1244, September 3, pp. 32-33.

Scherer García, Julio and Carlos Monsiváis 1999, *Parte de Guerra: Tlatelolco 1968*, Nuevo Siglo Aguilar.

Schmidt, Samuel 1991, *The Deterioration of the Mexican Presidency: The Years of Luis Echeverría*, The University of Arizona Press.

Schmitter, Philippe 1974, "Still the Century of Corporatism?" *Review of Politics*, No. 36.

Schmitter, Philippe 1993. "La consolidación de la democracia y la representación de los grupos sociales," *Revista Mexicana de Sociología*, Mar: 3 – 30.

Schmitter, Philippe and Terry Karl 1993, "What Democracy Is ... and Is Not", in *The Global Resurgence of Democracy*, Larry Diamond and Marc Platter (eds.), 39-52, Johns Hopkins University Press.

Schumpeter, Joseph 1987, *Capital, Society and Democracy*, Unwin paperbacks.

Schuurman, Frans J. (ed.) 1993, *Beyond the impasse: New directions in development theory*, Zed Books.

Secretaría de Salud 2000, Conference by José Antonio Fernández González (Secretary of Health 1999-2000), Meeting organized by the Colegio Nacional and FUNSALUD, "Desempeño de los Sistemas de Salud: la Experiencia de México, "Mexico, July 11, 2000, 17 p. (available at URL: http://www.ssa.gob.mx/prueba/discursos/20000711.hrml).

Secretaría de Salud 2001, *Programa Nacional de Salud 2001-2006: La democratización de la salud en México, hacia un sistema universal de salud, Plan Nacional de Desarrollo*, México, IMSS, ISSSTE.

Secretaría de Salud 2015, *Ley General de Salud*:

file:///C:/Users/antonio/Desktop/Book%20Manuscript%202016/Articulos%2
0para%20Actualización%20de%20Investigación/Ley%20General%20de%2
0Salud%202015.pd

SEDESOL 2000, "Está Dando Buenos Resultados PROGRESA? Informe de los resultados obtenidos de una evaluación realizada por el IFPRI (International Food Policy Research Institute)," Mexico City: Secretaría de Desarrollo Social.

Seers, Dudley 1963, 'The Limitations of the Special Case', *Bulletin of the Oxford Institute of Economics and Statistics*, V. 25, No. 2, May, pp. 77-98; reprinted in Gerald Meier, Leading Issues in Economic Development, New York: Oxford University Press, 1976, pp. 53-58.

Sefchovich, Sara 1987, *México: país de ideas, país de novelas: Una sociología de la literatura mexicana*, Mexico City: Grijalbo.

Segall, M. 1983, "Planning and politics resource allocation in primary health care: Promotion of meaningful national policy", *Social Sciences and Medicine*, Vol. 17, pp. 1947-1960.

Semo, Enrique 2000, "Fox y la Cuestión Social," *Proceso*, No. 1240, August 6, pp. 57-58.

Sen, Amartya 1993, "Capability and Well-Being", in *The Quality of Life*, Martha Nussbaum and Amertya Sen (eds.), New York: Oxford University Press, pp. 30-54.

Sen, Amartya 1997, "Development as Freedom," The First Presidential Lecture, Washington, D.C.: The World Bank.

Sen, Amartya 1999, "Democracy as a universal value", Journal of Democracy, Vol. 10, No. 3, July, pp. 3-17.

Sen, Amartya 2009, *The Idea of Justice,* The Belknap Press of Harvard University Press.

Sengupta, Arjun 2000, "Realizing the Right to Development," *Development and Change*, Vol. 31, pp. 553-578, Blackwell Publishers, Oxford, UK.

Sepúlveda Amor, Jaime et al. 1989, *SIDA, Ciencia y Sociedad en México*, Secretaría de Salud, Instituto Nacional de Salud Pública, Fondo de Cultura Económica.

Sharma, Arvind 2006, *Are Human Rights Western? A contribution to the dialogue of civilizations*, Oxford University Press.

SIDALAC 2004, *Cuentas Nacionales en VHI/SIDA*: http://www.sidalac.org.mx.

Shakow, Aaron and Alec Irwin 2000, "Terms Reconsidered: Decoding Development Discourse," in Jim Yong Kim, Joyce V. Millen, Alec Irwin and John

Gershman (eds.) 2000, *Dying for Growth: Global inequality and the health of the poor*, Common Courage Press.

Sierra Magazine Corporation Nation 1999, "Can Corporations be Good Citizens?" *Sierra Magazine*, May/June 1999.

Sklar, Richard 1987, "Developmental Democracy," *Comparative Studies in Society and History*, Vol. 29, No. 4, October, pp. 686-714.

Smallman, Shawn 2007, *The AIDS Pandemic in Latin America,* University of North Carolina Press.

Smith, Peter H. 1979, *Labyrinths of Power*, Princeton, NJ: Princeton University Press.

Smith, Peter H. 1986, "Leadership and Change, Intellectuals and Technocrats in Mexico," in Roderic Camp, *Mexico's Political Stability: The Next Five Years*, Boulder, Colorado: Westview Press.

Smith, Jackie, Charles Chatfield and Ron Pagnucco (eds.) 1997, *Transnational Social Movements and Global Politics*, Syracuse University Press.

Smith, Raymond. A. (ed.) 2013, *Global HIV/AIDS politics, policy, and activism: Persistent challenges and emerging issues* [3 volumes], Santa Barbara, CA: Praeger.

Soler Claudín, Carmen 2002, "Ciudad de México", in Celia Regina de Souza and Letania Menezes (eds.), *AIDS, The Epidemic in Megacities: Networking the response*, Sao Paulo: Editora Papagaio Ltda.

Spalding, Rose J. 1980, "Welfare policymaking", *Comparative Politics*, July, pp. 419-438.

Spencer, Nick 1996, *Poverty and Child Health*, Oxford: Radcliffe Medical Press.

Secetariat of Health/Pan-American Health Organization 1995, "Health Reform in Latin America", Proceedings, Washington, D.C.: Secretaría de Salud (Mexico)/Pan- American Health Organization.

Stahl, Karen 1996, "Anti-Poverty Programs: Making Structural Adjustment More Palatable," *NACLA Report on the Americas*, No. 6, May-June.

Stahler-Sholk, Richard, Harry E. Vanden and Glen David Kuecker 2002, "Globalizing Resistance: The New Politics of Social Movements in Latin America," *Latin American Perspectives,* 153.34.2: 5-16.

Standing, Guy 2000, "Brave New Words? A Critique of Stiglitz's World Bank Rethink," *Development and Change*, Vol. 31, pp. 737-763, Blackwell Publishers, Oxford, UK.

Stiglitz, Joseph 1999, "Whither Reform? Ten Years of the Transition," Keynote Address, Annual World Bank Conference on Development Economics, Washington, D.C. (28-30 April).

Stiglitz, Joseph 2002, *Globalization and its Discontents*, New York: WW Norton.

Stokes, Susan C. 2001, *Mandates and Democracies: Neoliberalism by Surprise in Latin America*, Cambridge University Press, New York, 221 p.

Stone, Diana 2000, "Non-Governmental Policy Transfer: The Strategies of Independent Policy Institutes," *Governance*, Vol. 13, Issue 1, pp. 45-70.

Story, Dale 1986, *Industry, the State, and Public Policy in Mexico*, Austin: University of Texas Press.

Susuki, David and Holly Dressel 2002, *Good News for a Change: Hope for a troubled planet*, Toronto: Stoddart Publishing Co. Limited.

Swidler, A. 1986, "Culture in action: symbols and strategies", *American Sociological Review*, 51.

Tarabusi, C. and G. Vickery 1993, "Globalization and Pharmaceuticals," *OECD Observer*, Vol. 185, No. 41.

Taylor, Charles 1986, "Human Rights, The Legal Culture," in Philosophical Foundation of Human Rights, UNESCO.

Teichman, Judith A. 1988, *Policymaking in Mexico: from boom to crisis*, Allen & Unwin.

Teichman, Judith A. 1995, *Privatization and Political Change in Mexico*, University of Pittsburgh Press.

Teichman, Judith 2001, *The Politics of Freeing Markets in Latin America: Chile, Argentina, and Mexico*, The University of North Carolina Press.

Teichman, Judith 2002, "The Political Challenges of Equitable Development in Latin America", paper presented for the Conference in Honour of Professor Albert Berry: *Social and Economic Impacts of Liberalization and Globalization*, at the Munk Centre for International Studies, University of Toronto, April 19-20.

Teichman, Judith 2004, "The World Bank and Policy Reform in Mexico and Argentina," *Latin American Politics and Society*, Vol. 46, No. 1, Spring, University of Miami.

Tendler, Judith 1997, *Good Government in the Tropics*, Johns Hopkins University Press.

Thacker, Strom C. 1986, *Big Business and the State*, Austin: University of Texas Press.

Torres-Ruiz, Antonio 1997, "Decentralización en Salud: Algunas Consideraciones para el Caso de México", *Working Paper No. 69*, Centro de Investigación y Docencia Económicas, México.

Torres-Ruiz, Antonio 2006, "Nuevos Retos y Oportunidades en un Mundo Globalizado: Análisis Político de la Respuesta al VIH/SIDA en México," *História, Ciencias, Saude,* 13(3), Manguinhos, Brazil.

Torres-Ruiz, Antonio 2011, "HIV/AIDS and Sexual Minorities in Mexico: A Globalized Struggle for the Protection of Human Rights," *Latin American Research Review,* 46 (1).

Torres-Ruiz, Antonio 2013, "The NGO-ization of HIV/AIDS activism in Mexico: Not so scandalous after all?" In Smith, R. A. (ed.), *Global HIV/AIDS politics, policy, and activism: Persistent challenges and emerging issues: Vol. 3. Activism and community mobilization*, Santa Barbara, CA: Praeger.

Torres-Ruiz, Antonio 2017, "Governance versus Governmentality: The professionalization of Mexican and Brazilian HIV/AIDS and LGBT activists," Unpublished draft of Journal Article, available on Academia.edu: https://yorku.academia.edu/AntonioTorresRuiz

Torres-Ruiz, Antonio 2017, "Populism and Democratization in Latin America: A Geo-Politico-Economic Perspective." Paper Presenter for panel on *The New Populist Right, Canadian Political Science Association (CPSA) Conference*, Ryerson University, Toronto, May 30 to June 1, available on Academia.edu: https://yorku.academia.edu/AntonioTorresRuiz

Torres-Ruiz, Antonio 2018, Toxic Democracies and Human Rights: Rethinking Democratic Theory from an International Political Economy Perspective, Unpublished book manuscript.

Torres-Ruiz, Antonio, and Stephen Clarkson 2009, "The Globalized Complexities of Transborder Governance in North America," In *Contentious Politics in North America: National Protest and Transnational Collaboration under Continental Integration*, by Jeffrey Ayres and Laura Macdonald (eds.), 155–176, New York: Palgrave Macmillan.

Torres-Ruiz, Antonio, and Paulo Ravecca 2014, "The Politics of Political Science and Toxic Democracies: A Hemispheric Perspective," *Crítica Contemporánea; Revista de Teoría Política*, Universidad de la República, Montevideo, Uruguay, No. 4, December.

Townsend, Janet G. 2001, "Whose Ideas Count: How can Mexican NGOs Challenge Global Development Fashions? Department of Geography, University of

Durham, UK, http://www.geography.dur.ac.uk/grassroots/Booklets/mexbooklet.htm.

Truby, Katherine 2014, "Bodies on the Border: The state, civil society and HIV at Mexico's *Fronteras*," *Policy and Society*, Vol. 33, Issue 1, pp. 53-64.

Truman, David 1951, *The Governmental Process: Political Interests and Public Opinion*, Knopf, New York.

Tsebelis, George 2000, "Veto Players and Institutional Analysis," *Governance,* Vol. 13, Issue 4, October, pp. 441-474.

Tulchin, Joseph S. and Amelia Brown (eds.) 2002, *Democratic Governance and Social Inequality*, Boulder & London: Lynne Rienner Publishers and the Woodrow Wilson International Center for Scholars.

Tulchin, Joseph S. and Ralph H. Espach (eds.) 2001, *Latin America in the New International System*, Boulder & London: Lynne Rienner Publishers and the Woodrow Wilson International Center for Scholars.

Tulchin, Joseph S. and Andrew D. Selee (eds.) 2003, *Mexico's Politics and Society in Transition*, Boulder & London: Lynne Rienner Publishers.

Tussie, Diana and Gabriel Casaburi 2000, "From Global to Local Governance: Civil Society and the Multilateral Development Banks", in *Global Governance: A Review of Multilateralism and International Organizations*, Volume 6, N. 4, Oct-Dec.

Ugalde, Luis Carlos 2000, *The Mexican Congress: Old player, new power*, Washington, D.C: CSIS Press.

Ugalde, Luis Carlos 2000, *Vigilando al Ejecutivo: El papel del Congreso en la supervisión del gasto público 1970-1999*, Cámara de Diputados LVII Legislatura.

UNDP 2015, *Human Development Report*, United Nations Development Program, At: http://hdr.undp.org/en/2015-report

UNAIDS/WHO 2002, *AIDS Epidemic Update: Under Embargo*, UNAIDS, WHO.

UNAIDS 2015, At http://www.unaids.org/en

UNCTAD 1994, "World Investment Report: Transnational Corporations, Employment and the Workplace," New York: United Nations Conference on Trade and Development.

Van Waarden, F. 1992, "Dimensions and types of policy networks," *European Journal of Political Research*, 21, pp. 29-52.

Vaughan, J.P. et al. 1996, "WHO and the Effects of Extrabudgetary Funds: Is the Organization donor driven?" *Health Policy and Planning*, No. 11, pp. 253-264.

Verweij, Marco and Timothy E. Josling 2003, "Special Issue: Deliberately Democratizing Multilateral Organizations," *Governance*, Volume 16, Issue 1, January, pp. 1-21.

Vincent, Andrew 2010, *The Politics of Human Rights,* Oxford University Press.

Vogel, David 1990, "When Consumers Oppose Consumer Protection: The Politics of Regulatory Backlash," *Journal of Public Policy, October-December*, No. 10, pp. 449-470.

Vogel, David 1998, "The Globalization of Pharmaceutical Regulation," *Governance*, Vol. 11, No. 1, January (pp. 1-22), Malden, MA, USA: Blackwell Publishers.

Ward, Peter 1986, *Welfare Politics in Mexico: Papering over the cracks*, Allen & Unwin.

Watt, R. 1997, "A Historical Relationship between Agency and Structure: Synthesising Actor Network, Policy Network and Advocacy Coalition Interpretations of Policy-making", in J. Stanyer and G. Stoker (eds.), *Contemporary Political Studies*, Ulster, PSA.

Wallerstein, Immanuel 1974, *The Modern World System, Capitalist Agriculture and the Origins of the European World Economy in the Sixteenth Century*, New York: Academic Press.

Wallerstein, Immanuel 1979, *The Capitalist World Economy*, Cambridge University Press.

Walton, John 1989, "Debt, Protest, and the State in Latin America", in Susan Eckstein (edit.) *Power and Popular Protest: Latin American Social Movements*, University of California Press.

Weber, Max 1948, *From Max Weber* (Eds. H.H. Gerth and C. Wright Mills), London: Routledge and Kegan Paul.

Whitehead, Laurence 1995, "An elusive transition: The slow motion demise of authoritarian dominant party rule in Mexico", *Democratization*, Vol. 2, No. 3, Autumn, pp. 246-269.

Whiteside, Alan and Tony Barnett 2002, *AIDS in the Twenty-first Century: Disease and globalization*, Palgrave.

WHO 1946, *Constitution*, in Basic Documents, 40th edition, Geneva: World Health Organization, pp. 1-18.

WHO 1998, *World Health Report*, Geneva: World Health Organization.

WHO 1999, *World Health Report*, Geneva: World Health Organization.

WHO 2003, *World Health Report*, Geneva: World Health Organization.

Wilks, S. and M. Wright 1995, "Networks of Power: Theorizing the Politics of Urban Change", in J. Stanyer and J. Lovenduski (eds.), *Contemporary Political Studies*, Vol. 2, pp. 725-733.

Womack, John Jr. (ed.) 1999, *Rebellion in Chiapas*, New York: The New Press.

World Bank 1987, "Financing Health Services in Developing Countries: An agenda for reform," Washington.

World Bank 1992, "Effective Implementation: Key to Development Impact," Washington, D.C., World Bank, Portfolio Management Task Force.

World Bank 1993, "World Development Report: Investing in health," Washington.

World Bank 1994, "OED [Operations Evaluation Department] Study of Bank/Mexico Relations, 1948-1992", Report No. 12923, Washington, D.C.

World Bank 1997, *Confronting AIDS: Public priorities in a global epidemic, A World Bank Policy Research Report*, Oxford University Press.

World Bank 2014, World Development Indicators, http://data.worldbank.org./data-catalog/world-development-indicators.

WTO 1998, "World Trade Growth Accelerated in 1997, Despite Turmoil in Some Asian Financial Markets," Available at www.wto.org/intltrad/internat.html

WTO 2001, "Declaration on the TRIPS Agreement and Public Health", Adopted on November 14, Doha WTO Ministerial Conference, Fourth Session, Geneva, World Trade Organization.

Wright, M. 1988, "Policy Community, Policy Networks and Comparative Industrial Policies," *Political Studies*, 36, pp. 513-612.

Yach, D. and D. Bettcher 1998, "The globalization of public health I and II,*"* *American Journal of Public Health*, Vol. 88, No. 5, pp. 735-741.

Yong Kim, Jim, Millen, Joyce V., Irwin, Alec and John Gershman (eds.) 2000, *Dying for Growth: Global inequality and the health of the poor*, Common Courage Press.

Periodicals and Other Sources

Mexican Newspapers: *El Financiero, La Jornada (including its monthly insert, Letra S), Milenio, Novedades, La Prensa, Reforma, El Universal.*

Notiese 2000-2017, News Service, Mexico, last accessed: August 2017: http://www.letraese.org.mx

Foro 2003, *Memorias*, II Foro en VIH/SIDA/ITS de América Latina y el Caribe, 7-12 de Abril, Palacio de Convenciones de la Habana, Cuba, CDROM.

Fórum 2000, *ANAIS*, I Fórum e II Conferência de Cooperaçao Técnica Horizontal da América Latina e do Caribe em HIV/Aids e DST, Volumes I and II, 7-8 Novembro, Rio de Janeiro.

Human Rights Watch Americas reports.

Secretaría de Salud 2004, Mexico, Secretariat of Health's web site: http://www.ssa.gob.mx.

Secretaría de Salud 2016, Mexico, Secretariat of Health's web site: http://www.gob.mx/salud

SEDESOL 2004, Secretaría de Desarrollo Social, Mexico, Secretariat of Social Development's web site: http://www.sedeso.gob.mx.

Appendices by Chapter

CHAPTER ONE

Appendix 1.1: Some Notes on the Interviewing Process

Interviews were conducted with two main purposes. First, the goal was to come up with a clear idea of the number of political cliques in the health sector (namely health camarillas) and to identify their central figures. With that goal in mind, the author proceeded with the identification of a set of potential interviewees, through personal and professional contacts in the Secretariat of Health, having access to some public officials and conducting a series of interviews with various members of the medical community in Mexico. The second main goal was to identify the actors involved in the formation and the operation of the HIV/AIDS policy network. Then again, through personal and professional contacts, and after identifying some key individuals within the HIV/AIDS policy community, contact was established with some of them. This led to the interviewing of various activists and public health officials engaged in the fight against the pandemic.

In preparation for my interviews some basic guiding questions were formulated, which varied according to the interviewee. At the time of the actual interviews, a series of open-ended questions were posed. In some cases questions were asked about the existence and make up of political cliques in the health sector. In others, the focus was on the process of HIV/AIDS public policymaking and the role of the various members of the policy community in it. As stated above, the goal was to identify the various 'camarillas' and its members as well as the actors with access to the process of HIV/AIDS policymaking and able to exercise some influence on policy outcomes.

Although most of the interviews were conducted in Mexico, attendance to three HIV/AIDS conferences for Latin American and the Caribbean (Rio de Janeiro in 2000, Havana in 2003, and Mexico City 2008) was essential for the identification of key individuals and in the process of building trust with contacts and potential interviewees. Furthermore, active participation in them (presentation of one poster and a couple of papers) helped in getting access to many more of the relevant actors.

Appendix 1.2: List of Interviews

Non-Confidential

Bertozzi, Stefano, Mexico City, December 13, 2001. Former UNAIDS official, currently working at the National Institute of Public Health in Mexico.

Brito, Alejandro, Mexico City, December 5, 2001. Mr. Brito is the director of 'Letra S.'

Covarrubias, José María, Mexico City, October 20, 2001. Mr. Covarrubias was the founder of the 'Círculo Cultural Gay,' and a human rights activist. He played a significant role in the actions leading up to the investigation of a series of killings of transvestites in the State of Chiapas in 1993.

Díaz Betancourt, Arturo, Mexico City, September 10, 2002. Rio de Janeiro, November 9, 2000. Mr. Díaz Betancourt is a co-founder of 'Letra S' and the editor of its monthly publication in La Jornada. He is also a gay and HIV/AIDS activist, and founder also of the international groups ASICAL and ICASO.

Egremy, Guillermo, Mexico City, June 14 2002. Mr. Egremy is Director of Education and Information of CENSIDA.

Hernández, Juan Jacobo, Mexico City, November 6, 2001. Mr Hernández is a long-time gay activist, founder and director of the HIV/AIDS NGO 'Colectivo Sol.'

Huerdo Siqueiros, Jorge, Rio de Janeiro, November 7, 2000. Mr. Huerdo Siqueiros was the Technical Secretary of the Committee for Citizen Observance and Vigilance of HIV/AIDS (MEXSIDA) and the Director for Latin America of the Global Network of People living with HIV/AIDS.

Izazola, José Antonio, Mexico City, November 27, 2001. Mr. Izazola is the director of SIDALAC.

Leal F., Gustavo, Mexico City, July 13, 2002. Mr. Leal is a well-known academic, based at the Universidad Autónoma Metropolitana (UAM-Xochimilco), with an extensive work on health politics.

Luna Cadena, Anuar I., Mexico City, December 12, 2001. Mr. Luna cadena is the founder and an active member of FRENPAVIH, and works also for 'Colectivo Sol.'.

Monsiváis, Carlos, Mexico City, August 13, 2002. Mr. Monsiváis is a well-known openly gay Mexican writer and intellectual.

Orbinsky, James, Toronto, April 28, 2004. Mr. Orbinsky is former president of Médecins Sans Frontières (MSF).

Panebianco, Silvia, Rio de Janeiro, November 7, 2000. Ms. Panebianco is a co-founder and active member of MEXSIDA.

Pérez Vásquez, Hilda, Mexico City, December 6, 2001. Ms. Pérez Vásquez is a member of 'Colectivo Sol, and is in charge of the national program 'Alianza México.'

Ramos Vargas, Remedios, Mexico City, October 2002. The director of HIV/AIDS NGO 'La Casa de la Sal, A.C.'

Soler, Carmen, Mexico City, September 13, 2002. Ms. Soler is the head of the Mexico City's HIV/AIDS program and 'Clínica Condesa,' and has been participating in the fight against AIDS for more than twenty years.

Tetelboin, Carolina, Mexico City, July 31, 2002. Ms. Tetelboin is a well-known academic, based at the Universidad Autónoma Metropolitana (UAM-Xochimilco), with an extensive work on health politics and community medicine.

Torres, Mary Ann, Toronto, October 23, 2000. Ms. Torres is a member of the International Council of AIDS Service Organizations (ICASO).

Uribe, Patricia, April 10, Havana, 2003. Ms. Uribe is the former director of CONASIDA, now CENSIDA, with a long-time engagement in the fight against HIV/AIDS.

Confidential

Single Interviews

Gay activist, Mexico City, October 20, 2001.

High-level directive of a pharmaceutical company, Mexico City, August 13, 2002.

HIV/AIDS activist, Mexico City, November 13, 2001.

Human rights and HIV/AIDS activist, Mexico City, October 15, 2001.

IMSS' Senior Official, Mexico City, August 23, 2001.

IMSS's high-level officials, Mexico City, 2001-2006.

Senior Official, Health Secretariat, Mexico City, October 25, 2001

Senior Official, Health Secretariat, Mexico City, August 15, 2000.

Transvestite and gay activist, Mexico City, August 20, 2002.

Two Senior Officials, Health Secretariat, Mexico City, November 14, 2001.

UNAIDS official, Rio de Janeiro, November 9, 2000.

Others

Activists and Representatives of various NGOs in Havana, Mexico City, and Rio de Janeiro, 2000-2003 (Fifteen).

CONASIDA officials, Mexico City, 2001-2002 (Three).

Gay and HIV/AIDS activists, and owners of gay bars in Mexico City, 2001/2002 (Fifteen)

High-level directives of some of the largest pharmaceutical companies, Mexico City, 2001/2002 (Three).

IDB officials, Rio de Janeiro and Havana, 2000 and 2003 (Eight).

Members of 'Colectivo Sol,' Mexico City, 2001 (Three).

Members of SIDALAC and MEXSIDA, Mexico City, 2001-2002 (Four).

People living with HIV/AIDS, Mexico City, 2001-2002 (Twenty).

Interviews Breakdown

Government Officials		20
NGO Representatives:		
	Domestic	21
	International	12
Individual Activists		38
Representatives of International Governmental Organizations		12
Academics		5
Representatives of Pharmaceutical Companies		4
Total		112

CHAPTER TWO

Appendix 2.1

Joint United Nations Programme on HIV/AIDS
Composition of the Programme Coordinating Board (PCB)

26 January to 31 December 2016

Member States

1 Brazil	12 Malawi
2 Burundi	13 Monaco
3 Canada	14 Morocco
4 China	15 Netherlands
5 Ecuador	16 Norway
6 El Salvador	17 Russian Federation
7 Ghana	18 Switzerland
8 India	19 Tanzania (United Republic)
9 Iran (Islamic Republic)	20 Ukraine
10 Japan	21 United Kingdom
11 Kazakhstan	22 United States of America

Co-sponsors

1 UNHCR	7 UN Women
2 UNICEF	8 ILO
3 WFP	9 UNESCO
4 UNDP	10 WHO
5 UNFPA	11 The World Bank
6 UNODC	

Representatives of NGOs/People living with HIV/AIDS

1. Africa: Widows Fountain of Life (WFoL)/Uganda Youth Coalition on Adolescent Sexual Reproductive Health Rights and HIV (CYSRA)
2. Asia/Pacific: Youth Leadership Education Advocacy Development (Youth LEAD), India HIV/AIDS Alliance
3. Europe: East Europe and Central Asia Union of People Living with HIV (ECUO)/AIDS Action Europe
4. Latin America/Caribbean: SOMOSGAY/Collaborative Network of Persons Living with HIV of Belize

5. North America: Global Network of People Living with HIV-North America (GNP+NA)/Canadian Aboriginal AIDS Network

Appendix 2.2

An Overview of the World's Pharmaceutical Industry

Globally, the pharmaceutical industry represents one sector that has been characterized by the domination of corporations based in HICs. The United States, Europe and Japan account for 75 per cent of the world's production of medicines and 90 per cent of global pharmaceutical research and development (Jordan 1992, p. 492). This concentration has increased even more in recent years through various mergers. In the 1980s, for example, there were about eighty international pharmaceutical companies, whereas in the 1990s there were only thirty-five left (Leal and Martínez 2001a, p. 90). Furthermore, there has been an increasing co-ordination between the dominating markets. In 1991, for instance, the United States, the then European Community, and Canada sponsored a conference to harmonize the names of health care products. Japan later joined and their efforts led to the creation of the International Conference on Harmonization of Technical Requirements for the Registration of Pharmaceuticals for Human Use (ICH), which includes officials from the US Food and Drug Administration agency, the EU's Committee for the Proprietary Medical Products (CPMP) and the Japanese Ministry of Health and Welfare (MHW), as well as representatives from the largest multinational pharmaceutical companies (Vogel 1998, p. 11). ICH guidelines are likely to become de facto international standards, given that virtually all nations have pharmaceutical industries dominated by American, European or Japanese firms. In fact, the WHO has begun to encourage developing countries to adopt them.

The profits of this industry continue to be exceptionally good, with successful new drugs earning US$1 million per day in global sales revenues (Green 1995a, p. 13), 40 per cent of which are being first approved in the United States (See Green 1995b). Significantly privileged, the US population has almost immediate access to essentially all clinically important drugs that are available anywhere else in the world (Vogel 1998, p. 15). For its part, the European Union accounts for about 40 per cent of global sales (Green 1995a, p. 13). Critics, such as Jefrey Sachs (a professor of economics at Harvard University and co-ordinator of the Macroeconomic and Health Commission of the WHO under Bruntland) (*The Economist*, August 14, 1999), refer to the fact that the United States and Europe have nearly 99 per cent of the patents as a nothing less than a scandal, since this has led to the neglect of research on Malaria and other "diseases of poverty", given that they do not seem profitable from the viewpoint of investors.

With regards to the Latin American markets, they amount to close to 24 billion dollars, representing 10 per cent of the World market. In terms of sales, the three largest LA countries Brazil, Argentina and Mexico account for 13 billion, far behind Europe (Germany, France and Italy combined represent around 37 billion), Japan (51 billion), and the United States (more than 94 billion alone, and together with Canada close to 100 billion) (Leal and Martínez 2001a, p. 90). The drug trade balance for Mexico has a deficit of close to 300 million dollars (Leal and Martínez 2001a, p. 91), with the opening to foreign markets causing the dead of many domestic companies, which in some cases has resulted in a short supply of drugs (Leal and Martínez 2001a, p. 95).

CHAPTER THREE

Appendix 3.1: Economic Reforms between 1970 and 1982.

Following the 1968 events, the recognition of important social welfare problems and the need to appease the regime's critics and opposition forced President Luis Echeverría's administration (1970-1976) to act. Therefore, upon taking office, two years after the 1968 events, Echeverría's major concern was to shift the direction of the economy away from the stabilizing development model towards one of 'shared development.' State involvement and intervention in economic development increased, not without the opposition and resistance from the private sector (See Roett 1998; Story 1986; Thacker 1986). Echeverría developed a wide range of planning activities through the creation of rural development agencies, as well as the promotion of the decentralization of industry and the stimulation of development poles outside Mexico City (See Ward 1985). Additionally, throughout the 70s, the government engaged itself in an indebting dynamics that would prove to have devastating consequences for the country in the following decades. As pointed out in Teichman (1988, p. 38): "Mexico's public foreign debt ... became the adjustment mechanism through which the Mexican government filled the gap between public income, on the one hand, and public investment and expenditure, on the other". By the end of Echeverría's administration, big businesses had withdrawn their capital to foreign bank accounts, reduced industrial production and issued strong anti-government press releases through the Chambers of Commerce and Industry (See Story 1986; Thacker 1986). Consequently, Echeverría's successor José López Portillo's (1976-1982) had as a primary concern to shift the political balance back into the middle ground as a means of restoring the private sector's confidence. In the short term the simple accession to power of López Portillo did much to restore the lost confidence.

At first, López Portillo contracted financial support from the IMF, and with it his administration was obliged to adopt an austerity program. Due to the implementation of the austerity program unemployment was high, and real wages dropped as did public sector expenditure (See Ward 1985). Eventually, circumstances improved and by 1978 the existence of enormous oil reserves became public knowledge, with the consequent flow of loans to Mexico from the international market. With confidence on the exploitation of oil resources, López Portillo decided to ignore the IMF stringency measures and reflated. From then on, his administration tried to capitalize the exploitation of oil resources for national development (See Teichman 1988), neglecting other areas of the economy and creating an increasing dependence on oil export revenues.

Appendix 3.2: Brief Overview of a Globalist Social Program

In 1997, PROGRESA became the core of Zedillo's social policy. However, it represented only one seventh of social programs of the Secretariat of Social Development in Mexico, less than 1 percent of total social expenditure and 0.2 percent of GDP (Escobar Latapí 2002, p.219). At first, it was perceived by most people and critics as a continuation of Salinas's PRONASOL, with its manipulation for electoral purposes and regional variability in its forms of operation and political use, so that the regions that most benefited were not the most marginalized ones. Yet according to Escobar Latapí, the design and operation of PROGRESA – whose target population was 19 million rural poor - made it into something substantially different and more successful than PRONASOL. In terms of PROGRESA's relative success, more than the program itself, the broader macro-economic recovery seems to have been the driving force behind it (See Escobar Latapí 2002). Even Boltvinik (2000) and Leal (2001) – two of the harshest critics of official social policies - recognize some of the achievements of Zedillo's administration in the areas of health and education.

Under Fox, PROGRESA was renamed as Oportunidades (Opportunities), and as such it has expanded into urban areas. In its new phase, community meetings have a merely informational nature and serve to entertain requests for incorporation, with an individual follow-up process of each beneficiary (SEDESOL 2000; 2003). Each individual in the family must comply with the conditions set in the program, in terms of school attendance, medical check-ups and attendance to health training clinics (Escobar Latapí 2002, p. 220). Oportunidades provides direct subsidies in cash and kind to selected families. Health care experts, mothers and doctors have recognized the relatively rapid effect of the nutritional supplement given to undernourished children. However, the program is plagued with many problems, such as the understaffed and ill-equipped health care facilities and clinics of the Secretariat of Health and IMSS-COPLAMAR (National Plan for Depressed Zones and Marginal Groups), and the fact that transportation to these is expensive and time-consuming (Escobar Latapí 2002, p. 229). Given the saturation of clinics, women have received some training for the health evaluation of children and adults, and those who become health promoters manage a small package of 10 medical items (See SEDESOL 2000). Critics have pointed out other shortcomings of this program and stressed the need to move beyond targeted programs and towards the generation of employment opportunities, as well as the strengthening of the health sector as a whole (See Haagh and Helgø 2002).

Appendix 3.3: The Decentralization Strategy in Health

In 1982, the new government of Miguel de la Madrid introduced a major reform of the public administration in order to – at least officially - deepen the process of devolution, de-concentration, and fiscal reform to strengthen local units of government in different areas, including the health sector. In terms of the decentralization of the health sector, the intention was to place the national Secretariat of Health as the head of the national health system to allow for a stronger co-ordination of the system as a whole. Yet given the opposition from different groups at the state level (See Gonzalez-Block et al. 1989), at the beginning the Health Secretariat focused only on those states with less resistance both from governors and local IMSS members. State actors were justifiably afraid of being given greater responsibilities, without enough funds and the technical support (personnel and infrastructure) to be able to carry the reforms and assume the new tasks (See Cardozo 1995). As a result, the first stage of the decentralization process included only 14 states, in which case the Secretariat of Health de-concentrated its regional offices, giving them greater administrative responsibilities (See Torres-Ruiz 1997). The Secretariat of Health continued the supervision and control in the remaining 17 states, which represented an obstacle in its efforts to focus on the planning, co-ordination, and supervision of the sector as a whole.

In general, the administration of de la Madrid's successor, Carlos Salinas de Gortari (1988-1994), was characterized by a lack of continuity in the health sector reform. In spite of this interruption, the process of decentralization of the 1980s allowed for the creation and consolidation of state entities, such as state secretaries of health, or parastatal entities such as health institutes in those 14 states that were part of the first stage.

In 1994, upon taking office, and as part of the second stage of structural adjustment reforms, President Ernesto Zedillo introduced his 'New Federalism' agenda. As such, the 'New Federalism' agenda officially re-launched the decentralization process, with the intention to devolve power to the local level and to transform intergovernmental relations in a significant way (See Cabrero Mendoza 199; Torres-Ruiz 1997). Additionally, a program called 'Healthy Municipality' was considered central in the promotion of and participation in health.

CHAPTER FOUR

Appendix 4.1: Women and HIV/AIDS in Mexico

The few existing organizations working directly with women/HIV/AIDS complain about the lack of reliable data regarding the increasing HIV infection rates among women as well as on underage prostitution, which results in the absence of public policies effectively addressing these issues (See Elvira Madrid Romerto in Fórum 2000). There have been isolated programs such as the distribution of 2 million condoms among female sex workers in 1999, which came mostly as a response to the fears of widespread infection by the then new governments in the states of Querétaro and Mexico (See presentation by 'Coordinadora Regional de Trabajadoras Sexuales: Sor Juana Inés de la Cruz, in Fórum 2000). There are also a few community-based centres for the attention of this population. In downtown Mexico City, for example, there is a centre for the attention of female sex workers in 'La Merced' market, with a special clinic for terminal patients (See work by María Verónica Ortega Hernández, in Fórum 2000). As in the case of sexual minorities, the factors determining the vulnerability of women are associated with poverty and marginalization, such as lack of economic security and education, illiteracy, and discrimination. Married women are particularly vulnerable, given that they cannot freely negotiate and practice safe sex with their husbands (see http://www.gire.org.mx). Studies have shown that temporary legal and illegal male migrants working in the US find themselves at a higher risk of being infected, further putting their wives at risk upon returning to their communities (Bronfman, Langer and Trostle 2000). According to Mabel Bianco, who is the president of the Argentina-based 'Foundation for Women's Studies and Research' (Fundación para el Estudio y la Investigación de la Mujer, FEIM) and co-ordinator of the group 'Women and AIDS', the attention to women is close to non-existent in Latin America. This, in spite of the fact that in some countries in the region – again, especially in the rural areas- there is a feminization of the pandemic (El Financiero, Mexican Newspaper, July 10, 2002, p. 36). In Mexico, some women's groups argue that the government has come up with limited efforts to reduce the vulnerability of women, such as the distribution of 100 thousand female condoms through the different COESIDAS (Interview with Guillermo Egremy, director of education and information of CENSIDA, Mexico City, June 14 2002).

Appendix 4.2: An Overview of Various HIV/AIDS Organizations

There is a great degree of concentration of HIV/AIDS NGOs in Mexico City, which privileges its population, giving it access to a larger variety of services than their counterparts in other states. 'La Casa de la Sal, A.C.,' for example, was established in 1986 and provides medical attention to orphan children and adults. They also visit hospitalized AIDS patients, provide individual and couple psychological therapies, and administer a drug bank (Interview with Lic. Remedios Ramos Vargas, current director, in Mexico City, October 2002). Other similar programs, such as 'Alianza México,' have expanded across different states, and since 1998 they have new facilities in the states of Oaxaca, Yucatán, Puebla, Guerrero, Campeche and Quintana Roo. The population living in Mexico City and the Metropolitan area has access also to a hot phone line, 'Diversitel,' whose mission is to assist sexual minorities between 12 to 29 years of age. Another significant effort is the web-site Amigos contra el SIDA (Friends against AIDS: http://www.aids-sida.org/indice.html), which is not only a good source for general consultations regarding the efforts to combat the disease, but it also represents a valuable source of scientific information for other NGOs and people living with HIV/AIDS. There are other kinds of civil-society groups too, which through theatre performances raise awareness among the population at large regarding prevention and means of infection (See Tirso Clemades Pérez de Corcho, Brigada Callejera de Apoyo a la Mujer "Elisa Martínez, A.C.", Prevención del VIH/SIDA y de otras IT'S A través de la narración oral escénica en trabajadoras/es sexuales mexicanos/as, in Fórum 2000, p. 7630).

Some organizations have made significant efforts to extend their reach beyond the capital region. 'Colectivo Sol' represents a good example of a nation-wide effort in prevention campaigns. One of their programs involves a Condomóvil (a car called like this after a condom), in which they travel providing information on HIV/AIDS, STDs, and unwanted pregnancy, visiting towns and cities in other states (Fórum 2000, p. 794). For its part, the Mexican Network of People living with HIV/AIDS (MEXSIDA), which was founded in 1995 has a reach and a mission that extend beyond the capital region. Recently, they have put together a national campaign against the value-added tax (IVA) on medicines (The slogan for their campaign was 'IVA a medicinas igual a muerte y SIDA' [IVA to medicines equals death and AIDS]). As part of their work, they organize workshops for smaller NGOs from across the country, in Mexico City and Monterrey, in order to talk about empowerment, nutrition, home care, sexuality, and treatment adherence for those living with HIV/AIDS (Fórum 2000, p. 859). The organization 'Ave de México' has also played a central role, since its creation in 1988 by Francisco Estrada Valle – a prominent activist who was assassinated in 1992. Since 1992, Carlos García de León Moreno replaced Estrada as president of the organization and has actively participated in the fight against the pandemic, with much of their efforts focusing on MSM and the end of discrimination based on sexual orientation. Additionally, there are two major media organizations that collect and disseminate information on HIV/AIDS, health and sexuality; the news agency 'Notiese', and 'Letra S.' 'Letra S' is a monthly supplement of the national newspaper La Jornada, while 'Notiese' represents an important archival source that provides services to journalists and researchers. It reaches 45 local newspapers in 26 states, 20 national circulation media, 18 radio shows and the 4 main TV national stations (Fórum 2000, p. 797). Notiese also sends out its information material to 213 different NGOs in Mexico, Latin America, the US, and Europe (http://www.laneta.apc.org/mailman/ listinfo/agencia_notiese). Alejandro Brito and Arturo Díaz Betancourt are among the founders of Letra S and current leading figures within the HIV/AIDS policy network and community.

Appendix 4.3: CONAPRED and CONASIDA's Radio Campaign Transcripts (In Spanish)

SPOT 1: LA CENA
madre: Te ves muy enamorado m'hijito.
hijo: Ay, sí, Mamá.
madre: ¿Y cuánto llevan?
hijo: Ya cinco meses.
madre: ¿Y le gustó la idea de venir a cenar con la familia?
hijo: Sí, le encantó, es más, preparó un postre que te va a fascinar.
madre: Espero que le guste lo que yo cociné . . . Por cierto, ¿cómo me dijiste que se llama?
hijo: Óscar, Mamá, ya te lo había dicho, se llama Óscar.
voz de locutor: ¿Te parece algo raro? La homofobia es la intolerancia a la homosexualidad,
la igualdad comienza cuando todos reconocemos el derecho a ser diferentes. Por un México incluyente, tolerante y plural.

SPOT 2: PREGUNTAS
voz de locutor: Si ves a un homosexual o lesbiana en la calle, ¿ves para otro lado? ¿Sientes ganas de ofenderlo o que desaparezca? Si una persona cercana a ti es gay, ¿le dejas de hablar? ¿Sientes odio por los diferentes a ti? ¿Sabías que lo que tienes es homofobia? Es decir, un odio irracional." La tolerancia a la diferencia sexual es más sana que el odio. Por un México incluyente, tolerante y plural.

Appendix 4.4: Other Powerful Socially Conservative Organizations

The aforementioned 'Unión Nacional de Padres de Familia' (UNPF) was founded in 1917 as a civic association to oppose laic education, and to openly and strongly decry article 3 of the Constitution. They publish printed materials in which they criticize the use of contraceptives, homosexuality, abortion, and masturbation (see UNPF's website: http://www.familia.com.mx). Another one of these organizations is 'Desarrollo Humano Integral y Acción Ciudadana, DHIAC (Integral Human Development and Citizens Action), which was founded in 1975 and has a long list of prominent members and supporters: Luis H. Alvarez, Francisco Barrio Terrazas and Rodolfo Elizondo Torres (PAN members and close collaborators of Vicente Fox); José Luis Luegge (member of Mexico City's PAN); Luis Felipe Bravo Mena (former member and president of COPARMEX [Confederación Patronal Mexicana/ Mexican Association of Employers], and current president of PAN's national committee); Manuel J. Clouthier (former PAN presidential candidate in 1988); and Claudio X. Gonzalez, Lorenzo Servitje and Juan Sánchez Navarro (prominent entrepreneurs associated with the CCE [Consejo Coordinador Empresarial/ Co-ordinating Entrepreneurial Council]) (González Ruiz 2002, p. 145). Some of these personalities have also supported 'Vida Humana,' a group associated with 'Human Life International' (HLI), which has forcefully criticized prevention campaigns by the Secretariat of Health, CONASIDA and Mexfam, stating that to talk about topics such as homosexuality and anal sex must be considered illegal and immoral. HLI is based in Washington, D.C. and was founded in 1981 by Paul Marx with the support of the Pope to lobby the US Congress to oppose any initiatives promoting abortion (see Front Lines Research, vol. 1, No. 1, June 1994. With the election of George W. Bush in 2000, HLI and other conservative groups have found greater receptiveness and support from the US government. During Zedillo's government, UNPF, DHIAC, and 'Vida Humana' put pressure on him to fire his secretary of health, Juan Ramón de la Fuente, for having expressed the idea of opening a public debate regarding abortion (González Ruiz 2002, p. 153).

Appendix 4.5: Overview of the Links between big Entrepreneurs and Socially Conservative Groups

José Barroso Chávez (a magnate of the textile industry and the majority shareholder of the matches-making company 'La Central') has openly defended conservative views on sexuality and sex education. He has publicly made declarations against the condom, arguing without hard evidence that it fails to protect its users 40 per cent of the times (Notiese 2001). Barroso Chávez is also president for-life of the Red Cross in Mexico, and honorary member of the National Committee of PROVIDA, to which he makes regular donations (González Ruiz 2002, p. 241-242). He has also directly participated and continues to have influence on the 'Junta de Asistencia Privada de la República Mexicana' (The Mexican Council for Private Assistance); a body in charge of deciding what private associations can get tax exemptions. Until November of 1994, he was part of the 'Consultative Council of the National Solidarity' (Salinas' PRONASOL). Barroso Chávez is also very close to the Serrano Limón family (See National Union of Parents [UNPF], in chapter five). Their friendship was strengthened when Gustavo Serrano Limón was the director of COPARMEX (The big Private Employers' Union), while Barroso Chávez was a member of the Council.

Lorenzo Servitje and Juan Sánchez Navarro are also amongst some of the most prominent businessmen who strongly support a socially conservative agenda. Lorenzo Servitje is the majority shareholder of 'Grupo Industrial Bimbo'. In 1957, with the support of the Social Secretariat of the Catholic Church founded the 'Social Union of Mexican Entrepreneurs' (Unión Social de Empresarios Mexicanos, USEM), of which various distinguished PAN members are former presidents – amongst other, Carlos Castillo Peraza, a former national leader of PAN who died in 2002. In 1994, USEM's president, Gustavo Mendoza Avila, worked hand in hand with PROVIDA in a campaign to prevent the collaboration of the National Federation of Chambers of Industries (CONCAMIN) with 'Mexfam', in a program of sex education for workers at various private companies and factories in the State of Mexico. For his part, Juan Sánchez Navarro (former head of the Co-ordinating Entrepreneurial Council, CCE) and vice-president of 'Grupo Modelo' (One of the two largest brewery companies in Mexico) is well respected within the business elite and has long being known for his conservative positions on various issues. Additionally, Sánchez Navarro is a founding member of PAN and is considered by some as 'the ideologue" of the private sector. He actively participated in the 'Guerras Cristeras' as a messenger for some leading 'Cristeros' and, according to some sources, collaborated with Spain's Francisco Franco as a spy (González Ruiz 2002, p. 244).

Appendix 4.6: The Pharmaceutical Industry in Mexico

According to data from INEGI and Banco de México, around 200 different companies (including not only pharmaceuticals but also the manufacturers of basic substances for the production of medicines) integrate the industry, and they employ close to 50 thousand people. For 2000, the industry's exports/imports ratio was about 0.5 *(El Financiero,* April 28, 2000). The concentration of the industry manifests itself both geographically and in terms of sales. Close to 92 per cent of all pharmaceuticals are located in Mexico City, the State of Mexico and Jalisco (Leal and Martínez 2001a, p. 91). While 70 per cent of the total sales belong to 40 companies (with just 4 Mexican firms among them). The market in Mexico is dominated by the big international pharmaceuticals. Today, 80 per cent of the drugs sold in Mexico come from 42 foreign-based pharmaceuticals and 24 nationals. This has significantly been a of result of the decision of the Mexican government to protect the drug's patents. Although generic drugs are sold by half the price of brand ones, their share of the market amounts to only 0.3 per cent (*Vértigo,* October 11 2003). Recently, however, Apotex (one of the largest Canadian producers of generic drugs) has strengthened its presence in Mexico with new investments of more than $US30 million (*Reforma,* July 30, 2003).

In the opinion of Mauro Lara Verde, president of the 'National Association of Producers of Medicines, (ANAFAM), the series of neo-liberal policies implemented by the federal government in the last decades were behind the debacle of the domestic pharmaceutical companies, causing the disappearance of 97 of them, while the remaining ones cover only 20 per cent of the national demand (Leal and Martínez 2001a, p. 93). The participation of the national industry in public biddings has fallen from close to 80 per cent, to less than 50 per cent throughout the 1990s (Leal and Martínez 2001a, p. 94). On the other hand, between 1994 and 2000, prices of medicines in Mexico have increased fivefold, at an average of 38.5 per cent, above the annual inflation of 22.6 per cent (Leal and Martínez 2001a, p. 97). As a result, the burden on people's health expenditures has increased significantly. According to Evaristo Jiménez, leader of the 'Unión de Propietarios de Farmacias' (The Union of Drugstores Owners), it is estimated that each individual spends almost three days of a monthly salary to buy a medicine *(La Jornada,* October 5, 2000).

CPSIA information can be obtained
at www.ICGtesting.com
Printed in the USA
LVHW081628250419
615550LV00003B/52/P